Egg Consumption and Human Health

Special Issue Editor
Maria Luz Fernandez

MDPI • Basel • Beijing • Wuhan • Barcelona • Belgrade

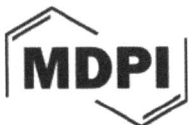

MDPI

Special Issue Editor
Maria Luz Fernandez
University of Connecticut
USA

Editorial Office
MDPI AG
St. Alban-Anlage 66
Basel, Switzerland

This edition is a reprint of the Special Issue published online in the open access journal *Nutrients* (ISSN 2072-6643) in 2015–2016 (available at: http://www.mdpi.com/journal/nutrients/special_issues/egg-consumption-human-health).

For citation purposes, cite each article independently as indicated on the article page online and as indicated below:

Lastname, F.M.; Lastname, F.M. Article title. *Journal Name.* **Year**. *Article number*, page range.

First Edition 2018

ISBN 978-3-03842-666-0 (Pbk)
ISBN 978-3-03842-667-7 (PDF)

Table of Contents

About the Special Issue Editor

Maria Luz Fernandez is a Professor of Nutrition at the University of Connecticut, Storrs, CT, U.S.A. Dr. Fernandez is a leading authority on cholesterol and lipoprotein metabolism. Her pioneer work with the guinea pig model has been instrumental in elucidating the mechanisms by which dietary factors affect lipoprotein atherogenicity, hepatic cholesterol homeostasis, systemic inflammation and atherosclerosis. She has conducted over the years a number of clinical interventions to determine how diet, weight loss and physical activity affect dyslipidemias, oxidative stress and inflammation in patients with diabetes, heart disease and metabolic syndrome. Dr. Fernandez has authored 242 peer-review papers and 14 book chapters. Dr. Fernandez has been invited since 2002 by several organizations and universities all over the world as the spokesperson to clarify the lack of evidence between egg intake and heart disease risk.

Preface to "Egg Consumption and Human Health"

Eggs have been a controversial food for many years due to their cholesterol content. In fact, they have been used as icons for dietary cholesterol. The USDA dietary guidelines of 2015 removed the upper limit for cholesterol intake thus dietary cholesterol is no longer a nutrient of concern. The United States was not a pioneer in these recommendations. Many European and Asian countries had already considered that dietary cholesterol and blood cholesterol were not related and had changed their dietary guidelines accordingly, years before US.

Eggs, a highly nutritious food has received bad press across history. Recently the formation of trimethylamine N-oxide (TMAO), a risk factor for heart disease, from dietary sources including choline has brought eggs yet again to the spotlight as a food of concern. However, although not shown in this book, research from my laboratory and from other investigators has demonstrated that eggs increase plasma choline without changing TMAO concentrations.

It is important to understand the historical perspective on how eggs became a food of concern before the positive attributes of eggs are highlighted. Such history is presented in detail as an information piece, on how dietary guidelines were created in the past without having enough evidence derived from rigorous clinical studies or well-analyzed epidemiological data. These recommendations of no more than 300 mg/day of dietary cholesterol still persist in the minds of the consumers and of course the main target of these recommendations are eggs.

Eggs in fact are not only a nutritious food characterized for its very high quality protein as well as being important contributors to the daily recommendations of Vitamin E, selenium and choline but eggs also have components with properties that go beyond nutrition.

Among the bioactive components of interest that are present in eggs are phospholipids. These phospholipids may play a role in decreasing heart disease risk twofold by decreasing cholesterol absorption and by incorporating into HDL and enhancing the uptake of cholesterol into cells and returning to the liver in the process known as reverse cholesterol transport. The protein in egg has also been shown to have anti-bacterial properties as well as antioxidant and anti-inflammatory properties. Lutein and zeaxanthin, two carotenoids present in egg yolk, are also considered bioactive components of eggs because they protect against oxidative stress and inflammation, as has been demonstrated in clinical studies. Further, these carotenoids are selectively taken up by the eye and exert a protective action against age-related macular degeneration, the leading cause of vision loss in adults over the age of 50. These properties of lutein and zeaxanthin are confirmed by animal studies, which have consistently shown how these carotenoids protect the liver, reduce systemic inflammation, and decrease atherosclerosis.

Eggs can also be a highly nutritious food for at-risk populations as has been demonstrated in studies in children from underdeveloped countries, in individuals who live in poverty and even in subjects with metabolic syndrome or those with documented diabetes.

The goal of this book is to demonstrate that eggs in addition to being a highly nutritious food, they also provide additional health benefits and should be considered as part of a healthy diet for all populations.

Maria Luz Fernandez
Special Issue Editor

nutrients

MDPI

Review

Egg and Egg-Derived Foods: Effects on Human Health and Use as Functional Foods

Jose M. Miranda [1,*], Xaquin Anton [2], Celia Redondo-Valbuena [1], Paula Roca-Saavedra [1], Jose A. Rodriguez [3], Alexandre Lamas [1], Carlos M. Franco [1] and Alberto Cepeda [1]

[1] Laboratorio de Higiene Inspección y Control de Alimentos, Dpto. de Química Analítica, Nutrición y Bromatología, Universidad de Santiago de Compostela, 27002 Lugo, Spain; pekenarv@gmail.com (C.R.-V.); procsaa@hotmail.es (P.R.-S.); alexandre.lamas@gmail.com (A.L.); carlos.franco@usc.es (C.M.F.); alberto.cepeda@usc.es (A.C.)
[2] Clavo congelados, S. A. Caldas de Reis, 36650 Pontevedra, Spain; xaquin@clavo.net
[3] Centro de Investigaciones Químicas, Universidad Autónoma del Estado de Hidalgo, Carr. Pachuca-Tulancingo Km. 4.5, 42076 Pachuca, Hidalgo, Mexico; josear@uaeh.edu.mx
*   Author to whom correspondence should be addressed; josemanuel.miranda@usc.es; Tel.: +34-982252231 (ext. 22410); Fax: +34-982254592.

Received: 11 November 2014; Accepted: 15 January 2015; Published: 20 January 2015

Abstract: Eggs are sources of protein, fats and micronutrients that play an important role in basic nutrition. However, eggs are traditionally associated with adverse factors in human health, mainly due to their cholesterol content. Nowadays, however, it is known that the response of cholesterol in human serum levels to dietary cholesterol consumption depends on several factors, such as ethnicity, genetic makeup, hormonal factors and the nutritional status of the consumer. Additionally, in recent decades, there has been an increasing demand for functional foods, which is expected to continue to increase in the future, owing to their capacity to decrease the risks of some diseases and socio-demographic factors such as the increase in life expectancy. This work offers a brief overview of the advantages and disadvantages of egg consumption and the potential market of functional eggs, and it explores the possibilities of the development of functional eggs by technological methods.

Keywords: egg; egg-derived products; functional foods; cholesterol; technological elaboration; omega-3.

1. Introduction

Nowadays, foods are not intended to only satisfy hunger and to provide necessary nutrients for humans, but also to prevent nutrition-related diseases and improve physical and mental wellbeing of consumers [1]. However, human nutrition in developed countries is characterized by an excessive intake of protein, cholesterol, saturated fatty acids (SFA), *n*-6 polyunsaturated fatty acids (PUFA), calories or sodium, whereas consumption is deficient in *n*-3 PUFA, fiber and antioxidants. These imbalances are partly responsible for the high incidence of both obesity and the onset of chronic or degenerative non-transmissible diseases, from which cardiovascular diseases (CVD) are the leading cause of mortality and morbidity globally [2]. The consumption of a lower fat diet is generally accepted in all clinical guidelines on CVD prevention, and is based on total fat consumption of 25%–35% of total calories, of SFA should be no more than 7%–10%, *trans* fatty acids less than 1%, unsaturated fats, mainly monounsaturated fats (MUFA) and *n*-3 PUFA) should represent the rest of the calories from fat and cholesterol, for a total of less than 300 mg/day [3,4].

In order to improve public health, nutritional experts and related organizations, such as the U.S. Department of Agriculture and U.S. Department of Health and Human Services [5] of the Spanish Society of Community Nutrition (SENC) [6], has persistently recommended a reduction in the intake of foods that are related to the occurrence of chronic diseases, and am increased consumption of fruits and vegetables, grains, legumes, low-fat dairy products, lean meats and fish, especially fatty fish species that are high in *n*-3 PUFA. Owing to the persistence of these recommendations, there is a high degree of awareness of this problem in the populations of developed countries, and, fortunately, nutritional composition is already a major factor in the choice of foods by the consumer. However, although there is a significant demand for healthier food, consumers are reluctant to change their dietary habits [7]. This suggests that there is great potential for foods that are consumed regularly when they are converted to functional foods by changing the composition to include certain ingredients that are beneficial to health. Another way to obtain functional foods is to modify the quantity of certain components in the food to make it more suitable to the recommendations of nutrition experts [7].

In this sense, because eggs are a conventional food containing nutrients that play fundamental roles beyond basic nutrition, their promotion as functional foods should be considered [8]. Eggs are of particular interest from a functionality point of view, because they offer a moderate calorie source (about 150 kcal/100 g), a protein of excellent quality, great culinary versatility and low economic cost [9], which make eggs within reach to most of the population. Eggs are also relatively rich in fat-soluble compounds and can, therefore, be a nutritious inclusion in the diet for people of all ages and at different stages of life. In particular, eggs may play a particularly useful role in the diets of those at risk of low-nutrient intakes such as the elderly, pregnant women and children [10]. Additionally, it must be mentioned that eggs can be consumed throughout the world, having no use restrictions on religious grounds [11].

However, eggs are a controversial food for nutritional experts and health agencies, because of the saturated fat content (about 3 g/100 g) and cholesterol content (about 200–300 mg/100 g) [12]. Owing to these two characteristics, during the past 40 years, the public had been warned against frequent egg consumption due to the high cholesterol content in eggs and the potential association with CVD. This was based on the assumption that high dietary cholesterol consumption is associated with high blood cholesterol levels and CVD. Afterwards, subsequent research suggests that, in contrast to SFA and TFA, dietary cholesterol in general and cholesterol in eggs in particular have limited effects on the blood cholesterol level and on CVD [4].

However, the volume of eggs and egg yolk used by food companies in their formulations is constantly increasing. Nowadays, egg-yolk products are largely used by the food industry as a result of three very important properties: manufacture and stabilization of emulsions, foaming stability and thermal gelation, as it is a fundamental ingredient for the elaboration of several food products [13]. Unfortunately, eggs and egg-derived foods are responsible for a large number of food-borne illnesses each year, mainly caused by *Salmonella* [14]. For this reason, as well as for their lower price and ease of handling and storing compared to shelled eggs, the food service industry and commercial food manufacturers have shown an increasing interest in the use of liquid pasteurized egg products instead of fresh whole eggs [15].

Thus, it would be of major interest to develop egg-derived products, appropriate for food companies, with a modified nutritional composition that helps maintain the health of consumers. Nowadays, retail markets for functional eggs are available, mainly enriched with *n*-3 PUFAs or with low cholesterol content. However, in most cases, these eggs are obtained through modification of layer-hen's diet and management, whereas much less attention has been paid to the development of functional eggs by means of technological methods [16]. In this manuscript, the possible development of functional pasteurized liquid eggs by technological methods and their advantages in the food industry and from the point of view of nutritionists are also discussed.

2. Advantages of Egg Consumption for Human Health

Eggs are an inexpensive and highly nutritious food, providing 18 vitamins and minerals, the composition of which can be affected by several factors such as hen diet, age, strain as well as environmental factors [16,17]. Nevertheless, although different compositions have been reported by several authors [10,17], on average, the macronutrient content of eggs include low carbohydrates and about 12 g per 100 g of protein and lipids, most of which are monounsaturated [8,18,19] and supply the diet with several essential nutrients (Table 1). Some of these nutrients, such as zinc, selenium, retinol and tocopherols, are deficient in people consuming a western diet, and given its antioxidant activity, can protect humans from many degenerative processes, including CVD [10].

There is also scientific evidence that eggs contain other biologically active compounds that may have a role in the therapy and prevention of chronic and infectious diseases. The presence of compounds with antimicrobial, immunomodulator, antioxidant, anti-cancer or anti-hypertensive properties have been reported in eggs [11]. Lysozyme, ovomucoid, ovoinhibitor and cystatin are biologically active proteins in egg albumen, and their activity prolongs the shelf life of table eggs [14]. Some of these protective substances are isolated and produced on an industrial scale as lysozymes and avidin. Additionally, eggs are an important source of lecithin and are one of the few food sources that contain high concentrations of choline [8,20]. Lecithin, as a polyunsaturated phosphatidylcholine, is a functional and structural component of all biological membranes, which acts in the rate-limiting step of the activation of membrane enzymes such as superoxide dismutase. It has been suggested that ineffective activation of these antioxidant enzymes would lead to increased damage of membranes by reactive oxygen species. In addition, lecithin increases the secretion of bile, preventing stagnation in the bladder and, consequently, decreases the lithogenicity [8].

Table 1. Nutritional composition of hen eggs.

Component (Unit)	Amount	Component (Unit)	Amount
Egg shell (%)	10.5	Calcium (mg)	56.0
Egg yolk (%)	31	Magnesium (mg)	12.0
Egg white (%)	58.5	Iron (mg)	2.1
Water (g)	74.5	Phosphorus (µg)	180.0
Energy (Kcal)	162	Zinc (mg)	1.44
Protein (g)	12.1	Thiamine (mg)	0.09
Carbohydrates (g)	0.68	Riboflavin (mg)	0.3
Lipids (g)	12.1	Niacin (mg)	0.1
Saturated fatty acids (g)	3.3	Folic acid (µg)	65.0
Monounsaturated fatty acids (g)	4.9	Cyanocobalamin (µg)	66.0
Polyunsaturated fatty acids (g)	1.8	Pyridoxine (mg)	0.12
Cholesterol (mg)	410	Retinol equivalents (µg)	227.0
Iodine (µg)	12.7	Potassium (mg)	147
Tocopherols (µg)	1.93	Carotenoids (µg)	10
Selenium (µg)	10	Cholecalciferol (µg)	1.8

Quantities represent an edible portion of about 100 g.

However, as a component of egg lecithin, choline has numerous important physiologic functions, which include the synthesis of phospholipids, the metabolism of methyl and cholinergic neurotransmission, and it is a required nutrient that is essential for the normal development of the brain [21].

Another important nutritional component from eggs is phosvitin, a phosphoglycoprotein present in egg yolk and represents about 7% of yolk proteins. It has a specific amino-acid composition, comprised of 50% serine, and 90% of which are phosphorylated. This specific structure makes phosvitin a strong metal chelator and, by this mechanism, it acts as an important melanogenesis inhibitor to control excessive melanin synthesis in the melanocytes of animal and human skin [21]. It was suggested that egg-yolk phosvitin has the potential to be used as a natural bioactive compound as a hyper-pigmentation inhibitor for human skin [21].

Other interesting egg components from the nutritional point of view are the carotenoids. Carotenoids are natural pigments in hen egg yolks that confer its yellow color, which can range from very pale yellow to dark brilliant orange. Egg carotenoids represent less than 1% of yolk lipids, and are mainly composed of carotene and xanthophylls (lutein, cryptoxanthin and zeaxanthin) [19,22,23]. The total concentration of lutein and zeaxanthin is 10 times greater than of cryptoxanthin and carotene, combined [23], and are not endogenously synthesized by the human body and tissue levels therefore depend on dietary intake. These natural compounds found in the bodies of animals, and in dietary animal products, are ultimately derived from plant sources in the diet, mainly from dark green leafy plants [24]. Lutein and zeaxanthin content of eggs depends on different factors, such as the feed given to laying hens, or the husbandry system. Thus, variable contents of these carotenoids in non-enriched eggs were recently reported, varying about 167–216 µg/yolk for lutein and about 85–185 µg/yolk for zeaxanthin [22,24]. Additionally, a greater serum response to lutein was reported following the consumption of eggs compared with the consumption of dietary lutein supplements or vegetables [22,24]. This could be related with the fact that carotenoids depend on a lipophilic environment for optimal gastrointestinal uptake [24]. Consequently, eggs are a very important food source of these carotenoids, especially in the case of people that consume low amounts of vegetables with a high content of these substances (as occurs in western developed countries).

These carotenoids are, perhaps, best known for their function in the neural retina, where they are found in high concentration and, along with their isomer mesozaexanthin, are termed macular pigment [25]. Lutein and zeaxanthin are known to serve light-absorbing and blue-filtering optical functions, as well as antioxidant and anti-inflammatory functions, and thereby, is considered to play a role reducing immune-mediated macular degeneration and age-related cataract formation [23–25].

Taking into account the presence of all these components, eggs can be considered a nutritious inclusion in the diet for people of all ages and at different stages of life, but they may play a particularly useful role in the diets of those at risk of low-nutrient intakes [10]. Owing to their high nutritional value, eggs are also an important food that should be included in the planning of diets for patients, and are especially valuable in feeding people with gout, because it is a source of protein that does not add purines. Additionally, for people in sports training, egg proteins may have a profound effect on the training results, because, by its inclusion in the diet, it could be possible to enhance skeletal muscles synthesis [8]. It is well established that essential amino acids stimulate skeletal muscle protein synthesis in animal and human models, and the protein in egg has the highest biological value [26]. Fifteen grams of egg white protein contain about 1300 mg of leucine (the third most common amino acid in egg, after glutamic and aspartic acids), and is also an abundant source of branched amino acids and aromatic amino acids. Recent data showed that leucine induces a maximal skeletal muscle protein anabolic response in young people, which suggests that egg white protein intake might have an important effect on body mass accretion [27]. Specifically, leucine stimulates skeletal muscle synthesis independently of all other amino acids in animal models and is a potent stimulator of the cell hypertrophy mammalian target of rapamycin complex pathway. Additionally, leucine decreases muscle protein breakdown and breakdown-associated cellular signaling and mRNA expression [26].

3. Undesirable Effects of Egg Consumption

Despite their abovementioned nutritional benefits, egg consumption was traditionally associated with adverse factors for human health and nutrition. In this sense, egg whites contain anti-nutritional factors, among which are proteins such as ovomucoid that can inhibit trypsin or avidin, which can bind biotin. However, these factors are thermo-labile and, therefore, these compounds are usually destroyed when cooking eggs, after which they do not cause further detrimental effects. Additionally, eggs have been the subject of numerous recommendations from nutrition experts in order to moderate egg consumption, owing to its high cholesterol and saturated-fat content. Reducing saturated-fat intake is the primary dietary strategy recommended for reducing serum cholesterol levels, and this strategy has often led to a reduction in the consumption of eggs. Nevertheless, substituting eggs for other animal-protein foods in the diet may result in small changes to low-density lipoprotein cholesterol (LDL) [10] and, consequently, egg consumption should be considered in a similar way to other protein-rich foods. Although metabolic studies have shown that dietary cholesterol is a major determinant of serum cholesterol concentrations, other studies failed to detect changes in the serum total-cholesterol concentration when eggs were added to diets that already contained moderate amounts of cholesterol [28]. In this sense, large research works, and even meta-analyses, have been conducted to investigate the effects of eggs on serum cholesterol levels and cardiovascular health, with very different conclusions (Table 2). Several authors state that dietary cholesterol from eggs could be an important risk factor for cardiometabolic diseases including CVD and diabetes [12,29–31]. Furthermore, lecithin (approximately 250 mg in a large egg yolk) is converted by intestinal bacteria to trimethylamine, which is in turn oxidized by the liver to trimethylamine oxide, which is pro-atherosclerotic [32]. In this sense, a meta-analysis found that an intake increment of four eggs per week could possibly increase the risk of CVD by 6% and diabetes by 29% [12]. Nevertheless, a recent systematic review found no clear relation of egg consumption and CVD among diabetic individuals [33].

However, for a large number of researchers, traditional assumptions that dietary cholesterol consumption translates directly into elevated plasma cholesterol levels and the development of CVD in all individuals were deemed to be mistaken [10,34,35]. First, a conservative estimate suggests that only 30% of the population would hyper-respond to dietary cholesterol [29], whereas approximately 70% of humans are hypo-responsive to excess dietary cholesterol consumption [36]. Therefore, clinical studies have clearly shown that plasma compartment changes, resulting from dietary cholesterol consumption, are influenced by several factors such as ethnicity, genetic makeup, hormonal factors and body mass index [36,37]. All of these characteristics determine who would hyper-respond to dietary cholesterol and those who are hypo-responsive to intake. In addition, those individuals who hyper-respond to dietary cholesterol intake generally show increased LDL and high-density lipoprotein cholesterol (HDL) [8], allowing for the maintenance of the LDL/HDL ratio, an important marker for CVD risk. This suggests that, for healthy individuals, the nutritional benefits clearly outweigh the concern surrounding the dietary cholesterol provided by one large egg.

Table 2. Recent works regarding effect of eggs consumption on of serum cholesterol and cardio circulatory human health.

Reference	Study Design	Number and Type of Subjects	Main Conclusion
Djousse, Graziano, 2008a [30]	Prospective cohort study	21,275 US male physicians aged 40–85 years	Egg consumption of ≥ 1 per day was related to an increased risk of heart failure among male
Djousse, Graziano, 2008b [38]	Prospective cohort study	21,327 US male physicians aged 40–85 years	Infrequent egg consumption does not seem to influence the risk of CVD in male. In addition, egg consumption was positively related to mortality, more strongly so in diabetic subjects
Herron, Fernandez 2004 [8]	Expert Opinion	-	Current recommendation about limiting egg consumption are not benefiting the public as a whole and may have negative nutritional implications
Hu *et al.* 1999 [34]	Prospective study	37,851 men aged 40 to 75 years at study outset and 80,082 women aged 34 to 59 years at study outset, free of cardiovascular disease, diabetes, hypercholesterolemia, or cancer	Consumption of up to 1 egg per day is unlikely to have substantial overall impact on the risk of CHD or stroke among healthy men and women
Katz *et al.* 2005 [39]	Randomized crossover controlled trial	49 patients healthy adults with a mean age of 56 years	Short-term egg consumption does not adversely affect endothelial function in healthy adults
Li *et al.* 2013 [12]	Meta-analysis	320,778 included in 14 different studies	A dose-response association between egg consumption and the risk of CVD and diabetes
McNamara, 2000a [36]	Review	-	For the general population, dietary cholesterol makes no significant contribution to atherosclerosis and risk of cardiovascular disease

Table 2. *Cont.*

Reference	Study Design	Number and Type of Subjects	Main Conclusion
McNamara, 2000b [40]	Review	-	Cholesterol feeding studies demonstrate that dietary cholesterol increases both LDL and HDL cholesterol with little change in the LDL:HDL ratio
Nakamura *et al.* 2006 [28]	Prospective study	90,735 Japanese men and women aged 40–69 years	Eating eggs up to almost diary was not associated with an increase in CVD-incidence for middle-aged Japanese men and women
Nakamura *et al.* 2004 [41]	Prospective study	5186 Japanese women and 4077 Japanese men aged 40–69 years	Limiting egg consumption may have some health benefits, at least in women in geographic areas where egg consumption makes a relatively large contribution to total dietary cholesterol intake
Mutungui *et al.* 2008 [42]	Clinical trial	31 men aged 40–70 and with a Body Mass Index of 26–37	Including egg in a carbohydrate-restricted diet results in increasing HDL-C while decreasing the risk factors associated with metabolic syndrome
Natoli *et al.* 2007 [10]	Review	-	Egg consumption results in only a small increase in serum cholesterol levels in most people. The inclusion of eggs in the context of a diet low in saturated fat and containing cardio-protective foods is not associated with increased CVD risk.
Njike *et al.* 2010 [43]	Randomized placebo-controlled crossover trial	40 hyperlipidemic adults	Egg consumption was found to be non-detrimental to endothelial function and serum lipids in hyperlipidemic adults, while egg substitute consumption was beneficial
Quresci *et al.* 2007 [44]	Prospective study	9734 men and women aged 25 to 74 years	Consumption of greater than 6 eggs per week does not increase the risk of stroke and ischemic stroke
Rong *et al.* 2013 [35]	Meta-analysis	5847 incident cases for coronary heart disease, and 7579 incident cases for stroke	Consumption of up to one egg per day is not associated with increased risk of coronary heart disease or stroke
Scrafford *et al.* 2011 [45]	Prospective study	33,994 men and women free of CVD and completed food frequency questionnaire	It was not found a significant positive association between egg consumption and increased risk of mortality from CVD or stroke in the US population
Shin *et al.* 2013 [46]	Meta-analysis	A total of 16 studies were included, including participants ranging in number from 1600 to 90,735	Egg consumption is not associated with the risk of CVD and cardiac mortality in general population
Spence *et al.* 2012 [31]	Prospective study	1262 patients attending vascular prevention clinics, mean age of 61.5 years	Regular consumption of egg yolk should be avoided by persons at risk of cardiovascular disease
Spence *et al.* 2010 [47]	Review	-	It does exist evidence about people al CVD risk must to restrict egg consumption
Tran *et al.* 2014 [33]	Systematic Review	-	Conflicting results prevent broad interpretation to conclude the effects of egg consumption and cardiovascular disease among diabetic individuals
Voutilainen *et al.* 2013 [48]	Prospective study	2682 middle-aged men	No evidence was found that people with cardiovascular risk should restrict egg consumption

Table 2. *Cont.*

Reference	Study Design	Number and Type of Subjects	Main Conclusion
Weggemans *et al.* 2001 [29]	Meta-analysis	17 studies including 556 subjects, 422 men and 134 women	Dietary cholesterol from eggs raises the ratio of total to HDL cholesterol and, therefore, adversely affects the cholesterol profile
Zampelas 2012 [49]	Invited Commentary	-	Although it becomes increasingly clearer that, eggs consumption is not associated with CVD risk in healthy populations, the evidence cannot be considered as conclusive in high risk populations
Zazpe *et al.* 2011 [50]	Prospective study	14,145 Mediterranean university graduates	No association between egg consumption and the incidence of CVD was found

In addition to the consumer individual response, there are other important factors of egg cholesterol that can play an important role in the effect on human health, such as the food matrix in which it is presented or the total diet consumed. Thus, previous studies have suggested that egg-yolk consumption raises serum cholesterol to a greater extent than crystalline cholesterol dissolved into a solution or incorporated into a diet [51]. On the other hand, another important factor in the individual response to egg cholesterol is the diet consumed. The egg consumption in countries with typical western diets, such as the United States, accounts for 26%–32% of the total dietary cholesterol intake, whereas egg consumption accounts for about 48% of total dietary cholesterol intake in Japan [28]. These differences are of major interest from a nutritional point of view, because an increase in serum cholesterol in response to increased egg consumption is 1.7 times greater when the background diet is high in saturated fat compared with a low-saturated-fat background diet. The effect may be attenuated even further in the case of overweight, insulin-resistant people [10].

In addition to nutrition-related risks, egg consumption can also represent a risk for consumers derived by other factors, such as their microbiological status. *Salmonella*, and serovars Enteritidis and Typhimurium are responsible for most food-borne illnesses associated with the consumption of eggs and egg products. In Europe, S. Enteritidis and S. Typhimurium are the most commonly isolated serotypes in human cases of salmonellosis, and contaminated eggs still remain the most important source of infection with S. Enteritidis for humans [14].

In fact, between 1993 and 2002, 9364 food-borne outbreaks were reported in Spain, 4944 (52%) of which were caused by *Salmonella* and 3546 (37.8%) of which were associated with egg products, constituting an obstacle to the well-being of populations and a source of high economic loss [52].

In order to have safe products, European Commission [53] requires the absence of *Salmonella* in 25 g or 25 mL of eggs and egg-derived foods, and limits the presence of Enterobacteriaceae to a maximum of 100 cfu/g after the pasteurization treatment. Limits are also given for 3OH-butyric acid (10 mg/kg dry matter), an index of the presence of incubator reject eggs, and for lactic acid (1000 mg/kg dry matter), a chemical index of hygienic quality of the raw material, which are to be measured before treatment [54]. Additionally, to ensure their safety, egg shells must be clean, dry, fully developed, and with no cracks; although, cracked eggs can be used if they are processed as soon as possible [55]. Eggs must be broken in a manner that minimizes contamination, from the shells themselves in particular, and egg contents may not be obtained by centrifuging or crushing the eggs [54].

Despite this strict safety normative, in some countries, the use of fresh eggs to elaborate egg-derived products in restoration is not allowed. For this purpose, it is mandatory to use pasteurized egg products. Although food-service industries other than central kitchens, caterers and restaurants are not bound to use pasteurized egg products, they have shown an increasing interest in their use, because of its convenience and ease of handling and storing compared to shelled eggs [15].

Another important human-health risk related to egg consumption is the potential presence of residues of veterinary drugs, because laying hens treated with pharmaceutical products can produce contaminated eggs [56]. Certain habits can also compromise health by being a source of exposure to environmental contaminants. Many of these potentially toxic pollutants are fat soluble, and thus, any fatty foods (including eggs) may often contain high levels of persistent organic pollutants [57] or dioxins, that are usually present even in free-range and organic eggs [58].

Additionally, egg allergies represent one of the most common IgE-mediated food allergies in infants and young children [59]. This allergy can be influenced on several environmental or demographic factors. Thus, a recent study found that factors as female gender, preterm delivery, having older siblings, maternal smoking during pregnancy or exposure in the first year to pets inversely associated with egg allergy. With respect to demographic origin, this work found that child with a family history of allergy and those parents born in East Asia are at increased risk of egg allergy [59]. Among infants and young children, egg allergy is the second most common food allergy after cow's milk allergy [60]. The overall prevalence of egg allergy in children in the Western Countries is about 1%–3% [61], with prevalence in European countries about 2.5% [60,62].

The five major allergens identified in hens eggs are ovomucoid (Gal d1), ovalbumin (Gal d2), ovotransferrin (Gal d3), lysozyme (Gal d4) and albumin (Gal d5). The majority of allergenic proteins are contained in egg white (Gal d1–4) rather than in egg yolk (Gal d5) [63]. Several other allergens have been identified in egg yolk, including vitellenin (apovitellenin I) and apoprotein B (apovitellenin VI), although their role remains jet unclear [64]. However, various studies have demonstrated that a large number of egg allergic people were able to tolerate heated egg whites [65], an advantage for thermally processed eggs. Recent publications indicate that up to 70% of children with egg allergy can tolerate egg baked in a cake or muffin without apparent reaction. Heat treatment destroys the conformational epitopes that some individuals form IgE against, thus allowing ingestion of the egg without any adverse reaction. In addition to altering the epitopes, heating the egg protein also acting to reduce the allergenicity of the protein by affecting the digestibility of the proteins or making the IgE binding sites less accessible [66].

4. Recommendations and Worldwide Consumption of Eggs

Guidelines from agencies as the U.S. Department of Agriculture and U.S. Department of Health and Human Services [5] or the SENC [6] advise healthy adults to limit dietary cholesterol intake to less than 300 mg each day. However, due to the growing body of scientific literature showing a lack of relationship between egg intake and CVD, recent dietary guidelines indicate healthy people can consume one egg a day as part of a healthy diet [33]. Other guidelines have yielded different points, ranging from no restriction to recommending regular intake of eggs [67]. Despite the recommendations to limit egg consumption, the worldwide production of eggs increased in recent decades and exceeded 64 million tons in 2009, with China as the largest world producer, with 36% of the world's production. For consumers, Mexico is the highest consumer per capita, reaching an average consumption of 355 eggs per person and year, followed by China (344) and Japan (325) [68]. The increase in worldwide egg production and consumption is rational, because egg protein is of excellent quality and low economic cost, whereas a big demand for protein sources are needed in developing countries, in which a third of the population are under nourished [69]. Additionally, the fact that eggs are a good food alternative for the elderly plays an important role in their consumption increase, because it is expected that, by the year 2020, the number of people worldwide over the age of 60 could reach one billion [8]. Although elevated total seric cholesterol values have been shown to predict CVD in middle-aged individuals, this parameter does not seem to be relevant for the elderly demographic. Unfortunately, in the elderly, the restriction of fat and cholesterol from the diet often results in the subsequent inclusion of foods that are high in simple sugars. This change in diet composition can be detrimental, causing increases in seric triglycerides (TG), which are generally accompanied by low HDL levels, which has been identified as the best lipoprotein indicator of CVD risk in elderly individuals. Furthermore, it has been suggested that the consumption of a low-fat diet by elderly individuals may promote insulin resistance as a consequence of increased levels of LDL and TG and decreased HDL levels in serum [8].

Furthermore, another important factor that could raise egg consumption in the near future is the fact that typical factors of modern life, such as frequent travel, busy schedules, little time to cook and eat at home and the inability to eat together as a family, play an important role in the increased consumption of pre-cooked and processed foods. As eggs are common ingredients employed by the food industry for their thickening, gelling, emulsifying, foaming, coloring, and flavoring properties, it is also expected that the worldwide consumption of eggs included in food industry formulations will increase in next years [13].

However, in the case of pre-cooked and processed foods, the use of pasteurized liquid eggs and egg powders are more commonly used than fresh eggs [70]. Food industries chiefly make use of the liquid egg products obtained through the shelling and pasteurization of shelled eggs, and whole egg products are employed as ingredients for the manufacture of egg pasta, mayonnaise, pastry or baked foods [13]. The pasteurization process can accelerate reactions between lipids and molecular oxygen, resulting in losses of nutritional and sensory properties of the egg products. Besides the possible impact of processing on lipid oxidation, the initial composition of raw materials can impact the behavior during processing [70].

Thus, there is a large potential market for functional egg products fortified with bioactive compounds by means of technological methods. Fortification is often the more cost effective and practical way to provide micronutrients to communities in need, especially if the technology already exists and if an appropriate and equitable food-distribution system is in place. It is usually possible to add multiple micronutrients without substantially increasing the total cost of the food product at the point of manufacture [69], especially when they manufacture large quantities of foods.

5. Potential Markets for Egg-Derived Functional Foods

The increasing demand for functional foods during recent decades can be explained by the increasing cost of healthcare, the steady increase in life expectancy and the desire for an improved quality of life in later years. Functional foods may improve the general condition of the body, decrease the risk of some diseases and may even be used to cure some illnesses. Taking into account the progressive aging of the population of developed countries, functional foods are a good alternative for controlling health costs, because medical services for the aging population are rather expensive [1].

Although the term "functional food" has already been defined several times, there is no unitarily accepted definition for this group of foods. In most countries, there is no legislative definition for the term and drawing a line between conventional and functional foods is challenging, even for nutritionist or food experts. The European Commission's Concerted Action on Functional-Food Science in Europe (FuFoSE), coordinated by International Life Science Institute (ILSI) Europe stated that "a food product can only be considered functional if, together with the basic nutritional impact, it has beneficial effects on one or more functions of the human organism, thus either improving the general and physical conditions or/and decreasing the risk of the evolution of diseases. The amount of intake and form of the functional food should be as it is normally expected for dietary purposes. Therefore, it could not be in the form of a pill or capsule, just as normal food form" [1].

Experts like Sloan [71] has estimated the global functional-food market to be 47.6 billion US$, with the United States as the largest market segment followed by Europe and Japan. Some estimations report an even higher global market value (nearly 61 billion US$) [72]. The three dominant markets (USA, EU and Japan) contribute to over 90% of total sales, from which the European market was estimated to contribute around 15 billion US$ in 2006 [73]. It should be emphasized, however, that the European market is heterogeneous, and there are large regional differences in both the use and acceptance of functional foods. In general, the interest of consumers in functional foods in the Central and Northern European countries is higher than in Mediterranean countries, where consumers have appreciated natural, fresh foods and consider them better for health [1]. Additionally, women tend to be slightly more health-oriented than men, and middle-aged and elderly consumers tend to be substantially more health-oriented than younger consumers [74]. It has been suggested that the reason behind women's higher awareness of health issues is the heightened responsibility they feel for the wellbeing of other family members (related to the dominant role of women as the main purchasers of foods in households). Therefore, middle-aged and elderly consumers are more aware of health issues, simply because they, or members of their immediate social environment, are much more likely to be diagnosed with a lifestyle-related disease than younger consumers. However, other recent research based on surveys did not find clear differences in the acceptance of functional foods between ages, gender or the country of origin of consumers [75].

It can be assumed that functional foods represent a sustainable category in the food market [76,77], because it cannot be neglected that functional-food products help to ensure an overall good health and/or to prevent/manage specific conditions in a convenient way [71,72]. Moreover, it is beyond doubt that persuading people to make healthier food choices would provide substantial health effects; therefore, it is in common economic and public interest [77]. This increasing consumer awareness, in combination with advances in various scientific domains, provides companies with unique opportunities to develop a large variety of new functional-food concepts [76]. It should also be considered that functional foods are sold at higher prices, thus containing larger profit margins than conventional foods, which obviously make the sector attractive for the players in the supply chain [73]. In general, price premiums of 30%–50% are observed in high-volume functional-food segments; however, for some products, it can be increased up to 500% [72,73].

Taking into account that eggs and egg-derived products are largely accepted by consumers, owing to their great culinary versatility and low economic cost, the development of functional eggs and egg-derived products could be an important way to value the products and to gain profitability for egg producers and the food industry [8]. Nevertheless, as previously reported [75], functional eggs are still rarely consumed in Europe. Recent polls revealed that consumers mentioned the consumption of functional eggs in only two countries. In Sweden, only 3.8% of those asked consumed eggs enriched with *n*-3 PUFAs, whereas in Spain, only 6.7% of the respondents consumed eggs enriched with *n*-3 PUFAs or eggs that were low in cholesterol. Consumers in all other surveyed European countries reported using no eggs or functional egg products [75].

6. Egg-Derived Products with High Omega-3 Fatty Acid Content

Although the possibility of using other bioactive compounds to obtain functional eggs, such as lycopene [78], was investigated, the most common bioactive compounds used for this purpose were *n*-3 PUFAs [16]. These fatty acids, especially eicosapentaenoic acid (EPA) and docosahesaenoic acid (DHA), have received great attention from nutritionists and the medical community, because it is considered that a clear relationship exists between the consumption of EPA and DHA and the maintenance of normal cardiac function. Thus, *n*-3 PUFA-fortified products (such as eggs) provide a means to achieve desired biochemical effects of these nutrients, without the ingestion of dietary supplements, medications or the need for a major change in dietary habits [19].

Most international agencies and sanitary authorities of western countries recommend a daily intake of *n*-3 PUFA between 1000 and 2000 mg daily [19], almost 200 mg/day of which should come from DHA. Owing to differences in the biological effectiveness, about ten times as much alpha-linolenic acid (ALA) is required to achieve a similar benefit to EPA and DHA. For this reason, European Commission [79] states that, in order to advertise and label food as "source of omega-3 fatty acids", a food must contain at least 0.3 g of ALA per 100 g and per 100 kcal, or at least 40 mg of EPA + DHA per 100 g and 100 kcal, whereas in order to advertise and label food as "high omega-3 fatty acids', it must contain at least 0.6 g of ALA per 100 g and 100 kcal, or at least 80 mg of EPA + DHA per 100 g and 100 kcal.

The content of *n*-3 fatty acids in eggs and egg-derived products can be increased, either through feed modifications for hens or through technological methods (in the case of egg-derived products).

Depending on whether or not we want to produce a product that gets the statement "source of omega-3 fatty acids" or "high in omega-3", we may choose to supplement the product with a specific raw material. Thus, if we want to increase the content of ALA, we can use plant oils as a source. Various plants, such as canola, soybean, walnuts and flaxseed, produce ALA, with the latter being the most concentrated source [80]. Consequently, flaxseed is the most employed matter for the supplementation of hens when aiming to obtain *n*-3 PUFA-enriched eggs by means of increasing the ALA content [16]. However, one of the disadvantages of flaxseed supplementation is that, when the hens feed under such production parameters, the egg characteristics are very contradictory in terms of feed consumption, egg production or egg weight [16].

On the contrary, owing to their EPA and DHA content, marine products, such as fish oils, seaweed or microalgae could be used to obtain egg-derived products with "sources of" or "high in" *n*-3 PUFA [16]. When using fish oil as source of *n*-3 PUFA, it is highly recommended to include an antioxidant substance to prevent sensorial hurdles that are mainly caused by oxidized *n*-3 PUFA in eggs [16]. In this sense, recent research has shown that, when seaweed is used as source of *n*-3 PUFA, it can also act as an antioxidant, as seaweed naturally contains antioxidants such as carotenoids, polyphenols, and vitamins E and C [81]. Additionally, inclusion of fish oil in the hens' diets at levels above 1.5% generates eggs that are generally unacceptable to western consumers, with tastes described as "fishy". In this sense, previous works observed that deodorization of fish oil, in order to reduce the amount of volatiles in the hens' diet, did not improve the acceptability of the eggs [82]. Similarly, feed supplementation with microencapsulated fish oil, which is expected to have greater oxidative stability, still had a negative impact on egg sensory attributes [83]. Oxidative damage in egg yolks fat results only from direct deposition of oxidized lipids from the feed, as lipids are not further oxidized during storage [16,80].

With respect to the microalgae supplementation of hens' diets, autotrophic or heterotrophic microalgae can be employed. For autotrophic microalgae, despite being an excellent source of *n*-3 PUFA and other important bioactive compounds such as carotenoids [84], the high price of production restricts its application in relatively low-value products such as eggs [16]. With respect to heterotrophic microalgae, recent technology has been developed to produce marine microalgae with an extremely high DHA content (about 18% of dry mass) through a fermentation process. Oils obtained of two microalgae, sources of *n*-3 PUFA, has yet obtained authorization by the European Commission to be employed as novel food ingredients, (*Schizochytrium* sp. and *Ulkemia* sp.) [85,86]. Eggs from hens fed heterotrophic microalgae typically show similar PUFA profiles to eggs from hens fed fish oil, yielding eggs with DHA contents up to 200 mg per egg, while maintaining consumer acceptability [16].

Given the relatively limited conversion of ALA into EPA and DHA by the human metabolism, feed supplementation with long chain *n*-3 PUFA in the form of fish oil or microalgae is much more interesting compared to supplementation with their precursor ALA through the addition of flaxseed. In any case, the obtained enriched eggs by supplementation of hens diet does not affect the cholesterol content of the eggs [87] and, consequently, consumers could be reluctant to consume eggs as a source of *n*-3 PUFA, owing to their high cholesterol content [29,34].

Therefore, one way to diversify the supply and to possibly enlarge the market of egg products is to produce *n*-3 PUFA-enriched pasteurized liquid eggs and egg powders. Using technological methods, it is possible to fortify these by-products with *n*-3 PUFAs at the same time as reducing cholesterol content. Moreover, their use as ingredients in a wide range of processed foods could contribute to increased consumption of *n*-3 PUFA among the population [70]. Another important potential advantage of egg-derived products enriched with *n*-3 PUFA is that the lipid profile is better preserved at refrigeration temperatures, because storage at room temperature results in a loss of PUFAs [9]. In some countries, such as those in the EU, it is established that fresh eggs must be stored and transported at a constant temperature and should, in general, not be refrigerated before sale to the final consumer (with the exception of French overseas departments) [88]. However, some egg-derived products, such as pasteurized liquid eggs, are required to be conserved by refrigeration. Thus, in the case of bioactive compounds that need refrigeration for better conservation, this could be an advantage for functional egg-derived products obtained by technological methods with respect to functional fresh eggs obtained by hens' diet supplementation.

7. Eggs and Egg-Based Products with Low Cholesterol and Saturated Fats Contents

Eggs represent the major excretory route of the sterol in hens [89], which is almost entirely contained in the yolk. Different strategies were employed in order to obtain eggs with lower amounts in cholesterol. Most of these strategies have focused on genetic selection or alteration of the laying hens' diet, with various nutrients, non-nutritive factors and pharmacological agents [89–91]. Unfortunately, the vast majority of these experimental approaches only elicited minimal changes (<10%), at best, or, as in the cases of some strategies such as dietary azasterols and triparanol, they resulted in the unacceptable replacement of yolk cholesterol by desmosterol [91]. The relatively poor effectiveness of strategies carried out for reducing yolk cholesterol content was probably due to the relative resistance of yolk cholesterol content to manipulation by genetic selection. Additionally, there is a lack of available pharmacological agents that could greatly attenuate hepatic cholesterol biosynthesis and metabolism, and/or lipoprotein assembly and secretion, without causing a cessation of egg production [89]. In this sense, copper supplementation to laying hens at pharmacological concentrations (>250 mg/kg) has been demonstrated to cause a reduction in egg-yolk cholesterol [92], although other researchers did not find differences in egg-yolk cholesterol after feeding pharmacological levels of dietary cooper [93,94]. On the other hand, the use of atorvastatin in laying hens elicited favorable changes in egg nutrient composition in addition to the reduction in egg-yolk cholesterol. Thus, eggs obtained from hens treated with atorvastatin were lower in fat and higher in high-quality proteins that control the eggs [90]. Regarding modification of hens' diets, feeding hens a diet containing high amounts of fats or oils generally elevates the yolk cholesterol content [89], whereas feeding hens a diet containing low amounts of fats or oils slightly reduces the yolk cholesterol content. Other effective approaches to egg cholesterol reduction include feeding hens garlic paste [95].

In addition to strategies based hen genetic selection or on the modification of the feeding conditions of laying hens, it is also possible to produce eggs that are low in cholesterol by technological methods (Table 3). The simplest way is implemented after dehydrating the yolks and whites separately, developing a new "mix" with more content and less clear yolk, which is where the cholesterol fraction is found [96]. Another strategy is the removal of cholesterol from egg yolks using organic acids such as acetone [97]. However, the use of organic acid reduces the emulsifying capacity of the egg yolk, so detracts technological potential as an ingredient, and could potentially leave residues of these acids in the egg. Another option is the use of supercritical CO_2, an extremely potent solvent for removing cholesterol from egg yolk [98]. This methodology has obtained very promising results, but despite its potential, it is not used a lot on the industrial level because of its high price. Other recent methodology described for this purpose includes the selective degradation of cholesterol in egg yolks using the enzyme cholesterol oxidase together with ultrasound [99] or using different species of microorganisms [100–103]. Alternatively, cholesterol can be removed from egg yolks using microbial degradation or by complexation with β-cyclodextrin, alone or inmobilized in chitosan beads [104,105], high metoxyl pectins [106], Streamline Phenyl® resin [107] anionic chelating agent [108] or low-cholesterol liquid food oil [109,110], or by obtaining egg yolk granules [111].

Table 3. Different strategies employed to obtain egg-derived foods with lower amounts in cholesterol by technological methods.

Reference	Method Employed	Results Obtained
Aihara *et al.* 1998 [100]	Degradation of egg yolk cholesterol by *Rodococcus equi* No. 23	Degradation of about 60% of egg yolk cholesterol content

Table 3. *Cont.*

Reference	Method Employed	Results Obtained
Chiu *et al.* 2004 [105]	Cholesterol absorption by β-cyclodextrin inmobilized in chitosan beads	Reduction of 92% of cholesterol content in egg yolk
Christodoulou *et al.* 1994 [101]	Bioconversion of cholesterol by 3 days of incubation with cholesterol oxidase from *Pseudomonas fluorescens* and *Nocardia erythropolis*	93% of egg yolk cholesterol bioconversion
Froning *et al.* 2008 [98]	Extraction of cholesterol from dried egg yolk using supercritical carbon dioxide	Reduction of about 2/3 of total cholesterol content in egg yolk
Garcia-Rojas *et al.* 2007 [106]	Extraction of cholesterol in liquid egg yolk using high methoxyl pectins	The egg yolk contends of cholesterol decreased about 14%
Garcia-Rojas *et al.* 2006 [107]	Removing egg yolk plasma cholesterol using Streamline Phenyl® resin	70% of egg cholesterol content decreased in yolk plasma
Hsieh *et al.* 1994 [108]	Removing cholesterol and fat from egg by an anionic chelating agent (gum arabic)	Obtaining egg yolk essentially free from cholesterol
Jackeschky 2001 [109]	Dehydrating whole eggs or egg yolks and there upon treating it with an extraction based on a low-cholesterol, liquid food oil	Cholesterol proportion in the egg yolk being lowered by at least 95%
Kijowski, Lombardo 2000 [110]	Removing cholesterol from egg yolk by shearing a mixture of oil:egg yolk:water ratio	Reduction in cholesterol content about 50%–82% in egg yolk
Laca *et al.* 2014 [111]	Different methods to obtain egg yolk granules	Reduction in cholesterol content about 80%–90% in egg yolk granules with respect to egg yolk
Lv *et al.* 2002 [102]	Bioconversion of yolk powder cholesterol by extracellular cholesterol oxidase obtained from a mutant *Brevibacterium* sp	More than 85% of the yolk powder cholesterol was bioconverted
Manohar *et al.* 1998 [104]	Extraction of cholesterol from egg materials based on the use of β-cyclodextrin	Reduction of about 94.5% of total egg yolk cholesterol and esters
Martucci *et al.* 1997 [97]	Extraction of cholesterol from dehydrated hen egg yolk using acetone as solvent	Reduction about 91% of cholesterol content in egg
Sotelo, González 2000 [96]	Elaboration o fan egg powder mixture with a 3:1 proportion of white and yolk	Reduction about 40% of cholesterol content in egg
Sun *et al.* 2011 [99]	Ultrasonic-assisted enzymatic degradation	Cholesterol level in egg yolk was reduced to 8.32% of its original concentration without affecting the quality attributes of the yolk
Valcarce *et al.* 2002 [103]	Bioconversion of egg cholesterol to into pro-vitamin D sterols by the non-pathogenic ciliate *Tetrahymena thermophila*	Cholesterol content in egg yolk was reduced in about 55%

8. Conclusions

Eggs represent a very important food source, especially for some populations such as the elderly, pregnant women, children, convalescents and people who are sports training. The volume of both fresh eggs and eggs used by food companies in their formulations increases constantly. Owing to their higher security, lower price and easier handing and storing properties, food manufacturers prefer to use pasteurized egg products rather than fresh eggs. Additionally, the number of functional-food markets has also increased in recent decades and, owing to some factors such as the progressive aging of the population of developing countries, are expected to continue to increase in the coming years. Nevertheless, the presence of functional eggs in the market and knowledge of such products by the consumers are lower than other groups of foods.

Consequently, the development of functional egg-derived foods through technological methods could be an interesting way to gain profitability for egg producers and the food industry, in addition to improving the general conditions of public health. This could be especially interesting for the addition of bioactive compounds that need to be stored at refrigeration temperatures, because egg-derived products such as pasteurized liquid eggs must be stored under refrigeration during the commercialization process. Additionally, these products are safer from the microbiological point of view, cheaper, easier to hand and store, and because of the heat treatment applied, in some cases are less allergenic than fresh eggs. Thus, functional egg-derived products obtained through technological methods are a very interesting option for food manufacturers.

Acknowledgments: The authors wish to thank the Centro para el Desarrollo Técnico Industrial (CDTI) from the Ministerio de Economía y Competitividad for finance support

Author Contributions: A. Cepeda designed the review. C. Redondo-Valbuena, P. Roca-Saavedra and A. Lamas participated in the process of scientific literature search. X. Anton and J.A. Rodriguez made the tables and formatted the manuscript. J.M. Miranda wrote the manuscript, whereas C.M. Franco contributed in the revision process.

Conflicts of Interest: The authors declare no conflict of interest.

References

1. Siró, I.; Kápolna, E.; Kápolna, B.; Lugasi, A. Functional food. Product development, marketing and consumer acceptance-A review. *Appetite* **2008**, *51*, 456–467. [CrossRef] [PubMed]
2. Mokdad, A.H.; Ford, E.S.; Bowman, B.A.; Dietz, W.H.; Vinicor, F.; Bales, V.S.; Marks, J.S. Prevalence of obesity, diabetes, and obesity-related health risk factors. *JAMA J. Am. Med. Assoc.* **2003**, *289*, 76–79. [CrossRef]
3. Perk, J.; de Backer, G.; Gohlke, H.; Graham, I.; Reiner, Z.; Verschuren, M.; Albus, C.; Benlian, P.; Boysen, G.; Cifkova, R.; *et al.* European Guidelines on Cardiovascular Disease Prevention in Clinical Practice (version 2012). The Fifth Joint Task Force of the European Society of Cardiology and Other Societies on Cardiovascular Disease Prevention in Clinical Practice (constituted by representatives of nine societies and by invited experts). *Eur. Heart J.* **2012**, *33*, 1635–1701. [CrossRef] [PubMed]
4. Eilat-Adar, S.; Sinai, T.; Yosefy, C.; Henkin, Y. Nutritional recommendations for cardiovascular disease prevention. *Nutrients* **2013**, *5*, 3646–3683. [CrossRef] [PubMed]
5. U.S. Department of Agriculture and U.S. Department of Health and Human Services. *Dietary Guidelines for Americans*, 7th ed.; U.S. Government Printing Office: Washington, DC, USA, 2010.
6. Sociedad Española de Nutrición Comunitaria (SENC). Objetivos nutricionales para la población española. *Rev. Esp. Nutr. Comunitaria* **2011**, *4*, 178–199.
7. Martinez, B.; Miranda, J.M.; Vazquez, B.I.; Fente, C.A.; Franco, C.M.; Rodriguez, J.L.; Cepeda, A. Development of a hamburger patty with healthier lipid formulation and study of its nutritional, sensory, and stability properties. *Food Bioprocess Technol.* **2012**, *5*, 200–208. [CrossRef]
8. Herron, K.L.; Fernandez, M.L. Are the current dietary guidelines regarding egg consumption appropriate? *J. Nutr.* **2004**, *134*, 187–190. [PubMed]
9. Carrillo, S.; Rios, V.H.; Calvo, C.; Carranco, M.E.; Casas, M.; Perez-Gil, F. *N*-3 fatty acid content in eggs laid by hens fed with marine algae and sardine oil and stored at different times and temperatures. *J. Appl. Phycol.* **2012**, *24*, 593–599. [CrossRef]

10. Natoli, S.; Markovic, T.; Lim, D.; Noakes, M.; Kostner, K. Unscrambling the research: Eggs, serum cholesterol and coronary heart disease. *Nutr. Diet.* **2007**, *64*, 105–111. [CrossRef]
11. Abeyrathne, E.D.N.S.; Lee, H.Y.; Ahn, D.U. Egg white proteins and their potential use in food processing or as nutraceutical and pharmaceutical agents—A review. *Poult. Sci.* **2013**, *92*, 3292–3299. [CrossRef] [PubMed]
12. Li, Y.; Zhou, C.; Zhou, X.; Li, L. Egg consumption and risk cardiovascular diseases and diabetes: A meta-analysis. *Atherosclerosis* **2013**, *229*, 524–530. [CrossRef] [PubMed]
13. Rossi, M.; Casiraghi, E.; Primavesi, L.; Pompei, C.; Hidalgo, A. Functional properties of pasteurized liquid whole egg products as affected by the hygienic quality of the raw eggs. *LWT-Food Sci. Technol.* **2010**, *43*, 436–441. [CrossRef]
14. Rakonjac, S.; Bogosavljevic-Boskovic, S.; Pavlovski, Z.; Skrbic, Z.; Doskovic, V.; Petrovic, M.D.; Petricevic, V. Laying hen rearing systems: A review of major production results and egg quality traits. *World Poult. Sci. J.* **2014**, *70*, 93–104. [CrossRef]
15. Garcia-Gonzalez, L.; Geeraerd, A.H.; Elst, K.; van Ginneken, L.; van Impe, J.F.; Devlieghere, F. Inactivation of naturally occurring microorganisms in liquid whole egg using high pressure carbon dioxide processing as an alternative to heat pasteurization. *J. Supercrit. Fluids* **2009**, *51*, 74–82. [CrossRef]
16. Fraeye, I.; Bruneel, C.; Lemahieu, C.; Buyse, J.; Muylaert, K.; Foubert, I. Dietary enrichment of eggs with omega-3 fatty acids: A review. *Food Res. Int.* **2012**, *48*, 961–969. [CrossRef]
17. Samman, S.; Kung, F.P.; Carter, L.M.; Foster, M.J.; Ahmad, Z.I.; Phuyal, J.L.; Petocz, P. Fatty acid composition of certified organic, conventional and omega-3 eggs. *Food Chem.* **2009**, *116*, 911–914. [CrossRef]
18. United States Department of Agriculture (USDA). Nutrient Data Laboratory. Available online: https://www.ars.usda.gov/main/site_main.htm?modecode=80-40-05-25 (accessed on 19 January 2015).
19. Kassis, N.; Drake, S.R.; Beamer, S.K.; Matak, K.E.; Jaczynski, J. Development of nutraceutical egg products with omega-3-rich oils. *LWT-Food Sci. Techol.* **2010**, *43*, 777–783. [CrossRef]
20. Zeisel, S.H.; Mar, M.H.; Howe, J.C.; Holden, J.M. Concentrations of choline-containing compounds and betaine in common foods. *J. Nutr.* **2003**, *133*, 1302–1307. [PubMed]
21. Jung, S.; Kim, D.H.; Son, J.H.; Nam, K.; Dong, D.U.; Jo, C. The functional property of egg yolk phosvitin as a melanogenesis inhibitor. *Food Chem.* **2012**, *135*, 993–998. [CrossRef] [PubMed]
22. Skrivan, M.; Englamaierová, M. The deposition of carotenoids and α-tocopherol in hen eggs produced under a combination of sequential feeding and grazing. *Anim. Feed Sci. Technol.* **2014**, *190*, 79–86. [CrossRef]
23. Rakonjac, S.; Bogosavljevic-Boskovic, S.; Pavlovski, Z.; Skrbic, Z.; Doskovic, V.; Petrovic, M.D.; Petricevic, V. Laying hen rearing Systems: A review of Chemicals composition and hygienic conditions of eggs. *World Poult. Sci. J.* **2014**, *70*, 151–163. [CrossRef]
24. Kelly, E.R.; Plat, J.; Haenen, G.R.M.M.; Kijlstra, A.; Berendschot, T.T.J.M. The effect of modified eggs and egg-yolk based bevegare on serum lutein and zeaxanthin concentrations and macular pigment optical density: Results from a randomized trial. *PLoS One* **2014**, *9*, e92659. [CrossRef] [PubMed]
25. Bovier, E.R.; Renzi, L.M.; Hammond, B.R. A doucle-blind, placebo-controlled study on the effects of lutein and zeaxathin on neural processing speed and efficiency. *PLoS One* **2014**, *9*, e108178. [CrossRef] [PubMed]
26. Glynn, E.L.; Fry, C.S.; Drummond, M.J.; Timmerman, K.L.; Dhanani, S.; Volpi, E.; Rasmussen, B.R. Excess leucine intake enhances muscle anabolic signalig but not net proteína anabolism in young men and women. *J. Nutr.* **2010**, *140*, 1970–1976. [CrossRef] [PubMed]
27. Hida, A.; Hasegawa, Y.; Mekata, Y.; Usuda, M.; Masuda, Y.; Kawano, H.; Kawano, Y. Effects of egg white protein supplementation on muscle strength and serum free amino acid concentrations. *Nutrients* **2012**, *4*, 1504–1517. [CrossRef] [PubMed]
28. Nakamura, Y.; Iso, H.; Kita, Y.; Ueshima, H.; Okada, K.; Konishi, M.; Inoue, M.; Tsugane, S. Egg consumption, serum total cholesterol concentrations and coronary heart disease incidence: Japan Health Center-based prospective study. *Br. J. Nutr.* **2006**, *96*, 921–928. [CrossRef] [PubMed]
29. Weggemans, R.M.; Zock, P.L.; Katan, M.B. Dietary cholesterol from eggs increases the ratio of total cholesterol to high-density lipoprotein cholesterol in humans: A meta-analysis. *Am. J. Clin. Nutr.* **2001**, *73*, 885–891. [PubMed]
30. Djousse, L.; Graziano, J.M. Egg consumption and risk of heart failure in the Physicians Health Study. *Circulation* **2008**, *117*, 512–516. [CrossRef] [PubMed]
31. Spence, J.D.; Jenkins, D.J.; Davignon, J. Egg yolk consumption and carotid plaque. *Atherosclerosis* **2012**, *224*, 469–473. [CrossRef] [PubMed]

32. Wang, Z.; Klipfell, E.; Bennett, B.J.; Koeth, R.; Levison, B.S.; DuGar, B.; Feldstein, A.E.; Britt, E.B.; Fu, X.; Chung, Y.M.; *et al.* Gut flora metabolism of phosphatidylcholine promotes cardiovascular disease. *Nature* **2011**, *472*, 57–63. [CrossRef] [PubMed]

33. Tran, N.L.; Barraj, L.M.; Heilman, J.M.; Scrafford, C.G. Egg consumption and cardiovascular disease among diabetic individuals: A systematic review. *Diabetes Metab. Syndr. Obes.* **2014**, *7*, 121–137. [CrossRef] [PubMed]

34. Hu, F.B.; Stampfer, M.J.; Rimm, E.B.; Manson, J.E.; Ascherio, A.; Colditz, G.A.; Rosner, B.A.; Spiegelman, D.; Speizer, F.E.; Sacks, F.M.; *et al.* A prospective study of egg consumption and risk of cardiovascular disease in men and women. *JAMA-J. Am. Med. Assoc.* **1999**, *281*, 1387–1394. [CrossRef]

35. Rong, Y.; Chen, L.; Zhu, T.; Song, Y.; Yu, M.; Shan, Z.; Sands, A.; Hu, F.B. Egg consumption and risk of coronary heart disease and stroke: Dose-response meta-analysis of prospective cohort studies. *Br. Med. J.* **2013**, *346*, 8539–8551. [CrossRef]

36. McNamara, D.J. The impact of egg limitations on coronary heart disease risk: Do the numbers add up? *J. Am. Coll. Nutr.* **2000**, *19*, 540–548. [CrossRef]

37. Masson, L.F.; McNeill, G.; Avenell, A. Genetic variation and the lipid response to dietary intervention: A systematic review. *Am. J. Clin. Nutr.* **2003**, *77*, 1098–1111. [PubMed]

38. Djousse, L.; Graziano, J.M. Egg consumption in relation to cardiovascular disease and mortality: The Physicians' Health Study. *Am. J. Clin. Nutr.* **2008**, *87*, 964–969. [PubMed]

39. Katz, D.L.; Evans, M.A.; Nawaz, H.; Njike, V.Y.; Chan, W.; Comerford, B.P.; Hoxley, M.L. Egg consumption and endothelial function: A randomized controlled crossover trial. *Int. J. Cardiol.* **2005**, *99*, 65–70. [CrossRef] [PubMed]

40. McNamara, D.J. Dietary cholesterol and atherosclerosis. *Biochim. Biophys. Acta* **2000**, *1529*, 310–320. [CrossRef] [PubMed]

41. Nakamura, Y.; Okamura, T.; Tamaki, S.; Kadowaki, T.; Hayakawa, T.; Kita, Y.; Okayama, A.; Ueshima, H. Egg consumption, serum cholesterol, and cause-specific and all-cause mortality: The National Integrated Project for Prospective Observation of Non-communicable disease and its trends in the aged, 1980 (NIPPON DATA80). *Am. J. Clin. Nutr.* **2004**, *80*, 58–63. [PubMed]

42. Mutungui, G.; Ratliff, J.; Puglisi, M.; Torres-Gonzalez, M.; Vaishnav, U.; Leite, J.O.; Quann, E.; Volek, J.S.; Fernandez, M.L. Dietary cholesterol from eggs increases plasma HDL cholesterol in overweight men consuming a carbohydrate-restricted diet. *J. Nutr.* **2008**, *138*, 272–276. [PubMed]

43. Njike, V.; Faridi, Z.; Dutta, S.; Gonzalez-Simon, A.J.; Katz, D.L. Daily egg consumption in hyperlididemic adults-effects on endothelial function and cardiovascular risk. *Nutr. J.* **2010**, *9*, 28–36. [CrossRef] [PubMed]

44. Qureshi, A.I.; Suri, F.K.; Ahmed, S.; Nasar, A.; Divani, A.A.; Kirmani, J.F. Regular egg consumption does not increase the risk of stroke and cardiovascular diseases. *Med. Sci. Monit.* **2007**, *13*, CR1–CR18. [PubMed]

45. Scrafford, C.G.; Tan, N.L.; Barraj, L.M.; Mink, P.L. Egg consumption and CHD and stroke and mortality: A prospective study of US adults. *Public Health Nutr.* **2011**, *14*, 261–270. [CrossRef] [PubMed]

46. Shin, J.Y.; Xun, P.; Nakamura, Y.; He, K. Egg consumption in relation to risk cardiovascular disease and diabetes: A systematic review and meta-analysis. *Am. J. Clin. Nutr.* **2013**, *98*, 146–159. [CrossRef] [PubMed]

47. Spence, J.D.; Jenkins, D.J.; Davignon, J. Dietary cholesterol and egg yolks: Not for patients at risk of cardiovascular disease. *Can. J. Cardiol.* **2010**, *26*, 336–339. [CrossRef]

48. Voutilainen, S.; Nurmi, A.; Mursu, J.; Tuomainen, T.P.; Ruusunen, A.; Virtanen, J.K. Regular consumption of eggs does not affect carotid plaque area or risk of acute myocardial infarction in Finnish men. *Atherosclerosis* **2013**, *227*, 186–188. [CrossRef] [PubMed]

49. Zampelas, A. Still questioning the association between egg consumption and the risk of cardiovascular diseases. *Atherosclerosis* **2012**, *224*, 318–319. [CrossRef] [PubMed]

50. Zazpe, I.; Beunza, J.J.; Bes-Rastollo, M.; Warnberg, J.; de la Fuente-Arraliga, C.; Benito, S.; Vázquez, Z.; Martínez-González, M.A.; SUN Project Investigadors. Egg consumption and risk of cardiovascular disease in the SUN Project. *Eur. J. Clin. Nutr.* **2011**, *65*, 676–682. [CrossRef] [PubMed]

51. Baumgartner, S.; Kelly, E.R.; van der Made, S.; Berendschot, T.T.; Constance, H.; Lütjohann, D. The influence of consuming an egg or an egg-yolk buttermilk drink for 12 wk on serum lipids, inflammation, and liver function markers in human volunteers. *Nutrition* **2013**, *29*, 1237–1244. [CrossRef] [PubMed]

52. Patrignani, F.; Vannini, L.; Sado Kamdem, S.L.; Hernando, I.; Marco-Molés, R.; Guerzoni, M.E.; Lanciotti, R. High pressure homogenization *vs.* heat treatment: Safety and functional properties of liquid whole egg. *Food Microbiol.* **2013**, *36*, 63–69. [CrossRef] [PubMed]

53. Official Journal of the European Union. European Commission Regulation (EC) No. 1441/2007 of 5 December 2007 amending Regulation (EC) No. 2073/2005 on microbiological criteria for foodstuffs. *OJEU* **2007**, *L322*, 12–29.

54. Official Journal of the European Union. European Commission Regulation (EC) No. 853/2004 of 24 April 2004 laying down specific rules for on the hygiene of foodstuffs. *OJEU* **2004**, *L139*, 30–62.

55. Official Journal of the European Union. European Commission Regulation (EC) No. 2295/2003 of 23 December 2003 introducing detailed rules for implementing Council Regulation (EEC) No. 1907/1990 on certain marketing standards for eggs. *OJEU* **2003**, *L340*, 16–18.

56. Goetting, V.; Lee, K.A.; Tell, L.A. Pharmacokinetics of veterinary drugs in laying hens and residues in eggs: A review of the literature. *J. Vet. Pharmacol. Ther.* **2011**, *34*, 521–556. [CrossRef] [PubMed]

57. Domingo, J.L. Health risks of human exposure to chemical contaminants through egg consumption: A review. *Food Res. Int.* **2014**, *56*, 159–165. [CrossRef]

58. Piskorska-Pliszczynska, J.; Mikolajczyk, S.; Warenik-Bany, M.; Maszewski, S.; Strucinski, P. Soil as a source of dioxin contamination in eggs from free-range hens on a polish farm. *Sci. Total Environ.* **2014**, *466–467*, 447–454. [CrossRef] [PubMed]

59. Koplin, J.J.; Dharmage, S.C.; Ponsonby, A.L.; Tang, M.L.K.; Lowe, A.J.; Gurrin, L.C.; Osborne, N.J.; Martin, P.E.; Robinson, M.N.; Wake, M.; *et al.* Environmental and demographic risk factors for egg allergy in a population-based study of infants. *Allergy* **2014**, *67*, 1415–1422. [CrossRef]

60. Nwaru, B.I.; Hickstein, L.; Panesar, S.S.; Roberts, G.; Muraro, A.; Sheikh, A. Prevalence of common food allergies in Europe: A systematic review and meta-analysis. *Allergy* **2014**, *69*, 992–1007. [CrossRef] [PubMed]

61. Practicó, A.D.; Mistrello, G.; la Rosa, M.; del Giudice, M.M.; Marseglia, G.; Salpietro, C.; Leonardi, S. Immunotherapy: A new horizon for egg allergy? *Expert Rev. Clin. Immunol.* **2014**, *10*, 677–686. [CrossRef] [PubMed]

62. Álvaro, M.; García-Paba, M.B.; Giner, M.T.; Piquer, M.; Domínguez, O.; Lozano, J.; Jiménez, R.; Machinena, A.; Martín-Mateos, M.A.; Plaza, A.M.; *et al.* Tolerance to egg proteins in egg-sensitized infants without previous consumption. *Allergy* **2014**, *69*, 1350–1356. [PubMed]

63. Tan, J.W.; Joshi, P. Egg allergy: An update. *J. Paediatr. Child Health* **2014**, *50*, 11–15. [CrossRef] [PubMed]

64. Tey, D.; Heine, R.G. Egg allergy in childhood: An update. *Curr. Opin. Allergy Clin. Immunol.* **2009**, *9*, 244–250. [CrossRef] [PubMed]

65. Hasan, S.A.; Wells, R.D.; Davis, C.M. Egg hypersensitivity in review. *Allergy Asthma Proc.* **2013**, *1*, 26–32. [CrossRef]

66. Netting, M.; Makrides, M.; Gold, M.; Quinn, P.; Penttila, I. Heated allergens and introduction of tolerance in food allergic children. *Nutrients* **2013**, *5*, 2028–2046. [CrossRef] [PubMed]

67. Food and Agricultural Organization of the United Nations (FAO). Food Based Dietary Guidelines by Country. Available online: http://www.fao.org/ag/humannutrition/nutritioneducation/fbdg/en/ (accessed on 20 September 2014).

68. International Egg Commission. The Egg Industry 2010. Available online: https://www.internationalegg.com/corporate/eggindustry/index.asp (accessed on 15 September 2014).

69. Wimalawansa, S.J. Rational food fortification programs to alleviate micronutrient deficiencies. *J. Food Process. Technol.* **2013**, *4*, 257–267. [CrossRef]

70. Meynier, A.; Leborgne, C.; Viau, M.; Schuck, P.; Guichardant, M.; Rannou, C.; Anton, M. N-3 fatty acid enriched eggs and production of egg yolk powders: An increased risk of lipid oxidation? *Food Chem.* **2014**, *153*, 94–100. [CrossRef] [PubMed]

71. Sloan, A.E. The top ten functional food trends. *Food Technol.* **2004**, *58*, 28–51.

72. Annunziata, A.; Vecchio, R. Functional foods development in the European market: A consumer perspective. *J. Funct. Food* **2004**, *5*, 66–68.

73. Kotilainen, L.; Rajalahti, R.; Ragasa, C.; Pehu, E. Health enhancing foods: Opportunities for strengthening the sector in developing countries. *Agric. Rural Dev. Dis.* **2006**, *30*, 1–82.

74. Bech-Larsen, T.; Scholderer, J. Europe: Consumer research, market experiences and regulatory aspects. *Trends Food Sci. Technol.* **2007**, *18*, 231–234. [CrossRef]

75. Özen, A.E.; Biblioni, M.M.; Pons, A.; Tur, J.A. Consumption of functional foods in Europe; a systematic review. *Nutr. Hosp.* **2014**, *29*, 470–478. [PubMed]

76. Van Kleef, E.; van Trijp, H.C.M.; Luning, P.; Jongen, W.M.F. Consumer-oriented functional food development: How well do functional disciplines reflect the "voice of the consumer"? *Trends Food Sci. Technol.* **2002**, *13*, 93–101. [CrossRef]

77. Jones, P.J.; Jew, S. Functional food development: Concept to reality. *Trends Food Sci. Technol.* **2007**, *18*, 387–390. [CrossRef]

78. Sahin, N.; Akdemir, F.; Orhan, C.; Kucuk, O.; Hayirli, A.; Sahin, K. Lycopene-enriched quail egg as functional food for humans. *Food Res. Int.* **2008**, *41*, 295–300. [CrossRef]

79. Official Journal of the European Union. European Commission Regulation (EC) No. 116/2010 of 9 February 2010 amending Regulation 1924/2006 of the European Parliament and of the Council with regard to the list of nutrition claims. *OJEU* **2010**, *L37*, 16–34.

80. Hayat, Z.; Cherian, G.; Pasha, T.N.; Khattak, F.M.; Jabbar, M.A. Oxidative stability and lipid components of eggs from flax-fed hens: Effect of dietary antioxidants and storage. *Poult. Sci.* **2010**, *89*, 1285–1292. [CrossRef] [PubMed]

81. Yuan, Y.V. Marine algal constituents. In *Marine Nutraceuticals and Functional Foods*; Barrow, C., Shahidi, F., Eds.; CRC Taylor & Francis Press Inc.: Boca Ratón, FL, USA, 2008; pp. 259–260.

82. Gonzalez-Esquerra, R.; Leeson, S. Effect of feeding hens regular or deodorized menhaden oil on production parameters, yolk fatty acid profile, and sensory quality of eggs. *Poult. Sci.* **2000**, *79*, 1597–1602. [CrossRef] [PubMed]

83. Lawlor, J.B.; Gaudette, N.; Dickson, T.; House, J.D. Fatty acid profile and sensory characteristics of table eggs from laying hens fed diets containing microencapsulated fish oil. *Anim. Feed Sci. Technol.* **2010**, *156*, 97–103. [CrossRef]

84. Plaza, M.; Herrero, M.; Cifuentes, A.; Ibanez, E. Innovative natural functional ingredients from microalgae. *J. Agric. Food Chem.* **2009**, *57*, 7159–7170. [CrossRef] [PubMed]

85. Official Journal of the European Union. European Commission Decision 2009/778/EC of 22 October 2009 concerning the extension of uses of algal oil from the micro-algae Schizochytrium sp. as a novel food ingredient under Regulation (EC) No. 258/97 of the European Parliament and of the Council. *OJEU* **2009**, *L278*, 56–57.

86. Official Journal of the European Union. European Commission Decision 2009/777/EC of 21 October 2009 concerning the extension of uses of algal oil from the micro-algae *Ulkenia* sp. as a novel food ingredient under Regulation (EC) No. 258/97 of the European Parliament and of the Council. *OJEU* **2009**, *L278*, 54–55.

87. Rizzi, L.; Bochicchio, D.; Bargellini, A.; Parazza, P.; Simioli, M. Effects of dietary microalgae, other lipid sources, inorganic selenium and iodine in yolk *n*-3 fatty acid composition, selenium content and quality of eggs in laying hens. *J. Sci. Food Agric.* **2009**, *89*, 1775–1781. [CrossRef]

88. Official Journal of the European Union. European Commission Regulation (EC) No. 557/2007 of 23 May 2007 laying down detailed rules for implementing Council Regulation (EC) No. 1028/2006 on marketing standards for eggs. *OJEU* **2007**, *L132*, 5–20.

89. Elkin, R.G. Reducing shell egg cholesterol content, I. Overview, genetic approaches, and nutritional strategies. *Worlds Poult. Sci. J.* **2006**, *62*, 665–687. [CrossRef]

90. Elkin, R.G.; Furumoto, E.J.; Thomas, C.R. Assessment of egg nutrient compositional changes and residue in eggs, tissues, and excreta following oral administration of atorvastatin to laying hens. *J. Agric. Food Chem.* **2003**, *51*, 3473–3481. [CrossRef] [PubMed]

91. Elkin, R.G. Reducing shell egg cholesterol content, II. Review of approaches utilizing non-nutritive dietary factors or pharmacological agents and an examination of emerging strategies. *Worlds Poult. Sci. J.* **2007**, *63*, 5–32. [CrossRef]

92. Pesti, G.M.; Bakalli, R.I. Studies on the effect of feeding cupric sulfate pentahydrate to laying hens on eggs cholesterol content. *Poult. Sci.* **1998**, *77*, 1540–1545. [CrossRef] [PubMed]

93. Patterson, P.H.; Cravener, T.L.; Hooge, D.M. The impact of dietary copper source and level on hen performance, egg quality, and egg yolk cholesterol. *Poult. Sci.* **2004**, *83*, 435–436.

94. Pekel, A.Y.; Alp, M. Effects of different dietary copper sources on laying hen performance and egg yolk cholesterol. *J. Appl. Poult. Res.* **2011**, *20*, 506–513. [CrossRef]

95. Chowdhury, S.R.; Chowdhury, S.D.; Smith, T.K. Effects of dietary garlic on cholesterol metabolism of laying hens. *Poult. Sci.* **2002**, *81*, 1856–1862. [CrossRef] [PubMed]

96. Sotelo, A.; González, L. Huevo en polvo con bajo contenido de colesterol. Características nutricias y sanitarias del producto. *Arch. Latinoam. Nutr.* **2000**, *50*, 134–141. [PubMed]

97. Martucci, E.T.; Borges, S.V. Extraction of cholesterol from dehydrated egg yolk with acetone: Determination of the practical phase equilibrium and simulation of the extraction process. *J. Food Eng.* **1997**, *32*, 365–373. [CrossRef]

98. Froning, G.W. Egg products industry and future perspectives. In *Egg Bioscience and Biotechnology*; Mine, Y., Ed.; John Willey & Sons, Inc.: Ontario, Canada, 2008; pp. 307–320.

99. Sun, Y.; Yang, H.L.; Zhong, X.M.; Zhang, L.; Wang, W. Ultrasonic-assisted enzymatic degradation of cholesterol in egg yolk. *Innov. Food Sci. Emerg. Technol.* **2011**, *12*, 505–508. [CrossRef]

100. Aihara, H.; Watabane, K.; Nakamura, R. Degradation of cholesterol in egg yolk by *Rhodoccocus equi* No. 23. *J. Food Sci.* **1998**, *53*, 659–660. [CrossRef]

101. Christodoulou, S.; Hung, T.V.; Trewhell, M.A.; Black, R.G. Enzymatic degradation of egg yolk cholesterol. *J. Food Prot.* **1994**, *57*, 908–912.

102. Lv, C.; Tang, Y.; Wang, L.; Wenming, J.L.; Chen, Y.; Yang, S.; Wang, W. Bioconversion of yolk cholesterol by extra-cellular cholesterol oxidase from *Brevibacterium* sp. *Food Chem.* **2002**, *77*, 457–463. [CrossRef]

103. Valcarce, G.; Nusblat, A.; Florin-Christensen, J.; Nudel, B.C. Bioconversion of egg cholesterol to pro-vitamin D sterols with *Tetrahymena thermophila*. *J. Food Sci.* **2002**, *67*, 2405–2409. [CrossRef]

104. Manohar, B.; Basappa, C.; Rao, D.N.; Divakar, S. Response surface on cholesterol reduction in egg yolk using β-cyclodextrin. *Eur. Food Res. Technol.* **1998**, *206*, 189–192.

105. Chiu, S.H.; Chung, T.W.; Giridhar, R.; Wu, W.T. Immobilization of β-cyclodextrin in chitosan beads for separation of cholesterol from egg yolk. *Food Res. Int.* **2004**, *37*, 217–233. [CrossRef]

106. Garcia-Rojas, E.E.; Reis Coimbra, J.S.D.; Minin, L.A.; Freitas, J.F. Cholesterol removal in liquid egg yolk using high methoxyl pectins. *Carbohydr. Polym.* **2007**, *69*, 72–78. [CrossRef]

107. García-Rojas, dos Reis Coimbra, J.S.; Minim, L.A. Adsorption of egg yolk cholesterol using a hydrophobic absorbent. *Eur. Food Res. Technol.* **2006**, *223*, 705–709. [CrossRef]

108. Hsieh, R.J.; Snyder, D.P.; Ford, E.W. Method for Removing Cholesterol and Fat from Egg Yolk by Chelation and Reduced-Cholesterol Egg Product. U.S. Patent 5,302,405 A, 12 April 1994.

109. Jackeschky, M. Dietary Low Cholesterol Whole Egg or Egg Yolk Product. U.S. Patent 6,177,120 B1, 23 January 2001.

110. Kijowski, M.; Lombardo, S.P. Enhanced Cholesterol Extraction from Egg Yolk. U.S. Patent 6,093,434 A, 25 July 2000.

111. Laca, A.; Paredes, B.; Rendueles, M.; Díaz, M. Egg yolk granules: Separation, characteristics and applications in food industry. *LWT-Food Sci. Technol.* **2014**, *59*, 1–5. [CrossRef]

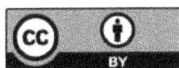

19

nutrients

MDPI

Review

Egg Phospholipids and Cardiovascular Health

Christopher N. Blesso

Department of Nutritional Sciences, University of Connecticut, Storrs, CT 06269, USA;
christopher.blesso@uconn.edu; Tel.: +860-486-9049; Fax: +860-486-3674

Received: 3 March 2015; Accepted: 3 April 2015; Published: 13 April 2015

Abstract: Eggs are a major source of phospholipids (PL) in the Western diet. Dietary PL have emerged as a potential source of bioactive lipids that may have widespread effects on pathways related to inflammation, cholesterol metabolism, and high-density lipoprotein (HDL) function. Based on pre-clinical studies, egg phosphatidylcholine (PC) and sphingomyelin appear to regulate cholesterol absorption and inflammation. In clinical studies, egg PL intake is associated with beneficial changes in biomarkers related to HDL reverse cholesterol transport. Recently, egg PC was shown to be a substrate for the generation of trimethylamine N-oxide (TMAO), a gut microbe-dependent metabolite associated with increased cardiovascular disease (CVD) risk. More research is warranted to examine potential serum TMAO responses with chronic egg ingestion and in different populations, such as diabetics. In this review, the recent basic science, clinical, and epidemiological findings examining egg PL intake and risk of CVD are summarized.

Keywords: atherosclerosis; cardiovascular disease; egg; HDL; phosphatidylcholine; phospholipids; sphingomyelin; TMAO

1. Introduction

Cardiovascular disease (CVD) claims upwards of 17 million lives worldwide each year [1]. In the United States, more than one third of adults suffer from some form of CVD which accounts for approximately one out of three deaths [2]. Atherosclerosis is a key contributor to CVD and is characterized by the hardening and thickening of the artery wall caused by accumulation of fatty plaque. Atherosclerosis is an insidious and progressive chronic inflammatory disease that takes decades to develop in humans [3]. Atherosclerosis is not only an inflammatory disease characterized by infiltration of immune cells, but also a lipid disorder; subendothelial accumulation of lipids derived from plasma lipoproteins is a key initiator of plaque development [4]. Lipoprotein metabolism is therefore critical to the development of atherosclerosis [5]. Lipoproteins have evolved to facilitate the extracellular transport of water-insoluble lipids in multicellular organisms [6]. Apolipoprotein B-containing lipoproteins that originate from the liver, such as very-low-density lipoprotein (VLDL) and low-density lipoprotein (LDL), contribute to the CVD process. In contrast, high-density lipoprotein (HDL) improves CVD through its ability to remove excess lipid from the artery and transport it back to the liver for excretion from the body, a pathway termed "reverse cholesterol transport" (RCT) [7]. The atheroprotective effect of HDL is mainly attributed to its role in RCT, with plasma HDL-cholesterol (HDL-C) considered to be a surrogate metric for this pathway [8]. The relationship between blood cholesterol and CVD is well-established, with the lowering of LDL-cholesterol (LDL-C) levels being the primary target of preventive therapy [9]. There has also been considerable interest in studying the relationship between dietary cholesterol intake and CVD risk [10]. Eggs are one of the richest sources of cholesterol in the diet. However, numerous large-scale epidemiological studies have failed to find any association between the intake of eggs and CVD risk [11–13]. This lack of association may be related to the other factors found in eggs that may influence CVD risk, such as the antioxidant carotenoids lutein and zeaxanthin [14]. Besides being an important contributor of dietary cholesterol in the Western diet, eggs are also a rich source of phospholipids (PL) [15]. Dietary PL have emerged as a potential source of bioactive lipids that may have widespread effects on pathways related to inflammation, cholesterol metabolism, and HDL function. The aim of this review is to summarize the recent basic science, clinical, and epidemiological research examining egg PL intake and CVD risk.

2. Phospholipid Content and Composition of the Chicken Egg

PL are key components of all biological membranes and are abundantly found in the diet, primarily as glycerophospholipid and sphingolipid classes. Dietary glycerophospholipids are made up of two fatty acids (FA), a glycerol backbone, a phosphate group, and a polar organic molecule (choline, serine, inositol, or ethanolamine) (Figure 1A). Dietary glycerophospholipids are primarily absorbed in the gastrointestinal (GI) tract as lysophospholipids and free FA after pancreatic phospholipase A_2 (PLA$_2$) hydrolyzes the fatty acyl bond at the *sn*-2 position [16]. Glycerophospholipids are absorbed into the GI tract with high efficiency, for example, >90% of phosphatidylcholine (PC) is absorbed [17]. Dietary sphingolipids are primarily in the form of sphingomyelin (SM) [18], which consists of a ceramide (a FA linked to a long-chain sphingoid base through an amide linkage) with a phosphorylcholine head group (Figure 1B). Digestion of SM in the intestine is slow and incomplete, with initial hydrolysis of SM to ceramide by alkaline sphingomyelinase and subsequent hydrolysis to sphingosine by neutral ceramidase [19]. Both ceramide and sphingosine can be absorbed into intestinal mucosal cells [19]. Chicken eggs contain approximately 28% of total lipids by weight as PL, with the remaining 66% as triglycerides (TG) and 5% as cholesterol [20]. The average large egg contains approximately 1.3 g of PL [15,21], which are almost exclusively found in the yolk. A typical Western diet contains about 2–8 g of dietary PL per day [22]. Estimates of average egg intake in the U.S. [23] indicate that egg-derived PL contributes 10%–40% (or 0.8 g) of daily consumed PL. The major PL species found in egg include PC, phosphatidylethanolamine (PE), SM, and phosphatidylinositol (PI) [24]. The typical PL composition of egg is shown in Table 1, which reveals PC as the predominant species making up almost three quarters of the total PL. The typical FA compositions of egg PL species vary [25,26] and are shown in Table 1. These FA compositions can be influenced somewhat by modifying the dietary FA intake of the hen [25,27,28]. Egg PC typically consists primarily of palmitic acid (16:0) and oleic acid (18:1) at the *sn*-1 and *sn*-2 positions, respectively. The major PC molecular species include PC (16:0/18:1), PC (22:6/16:0), and PC (22:6/16:1) [28,29]. Egg PE consists primarily of saturated FA such as stearic acid (18:0) at the *sn*-1 position, with a balanced mixture of unsaturated FA at the *sn*-2 position. The major PE molecular species include PE (16:0/18:1), PE (18:0/18:1), PE (18:0/18:2), and PE 18:0/20:4 [28–30]. Egg SM contains primarily saturated FA with palmitic acid (16:0) and stearic acid (18:0) making up ~80% of SM FA.

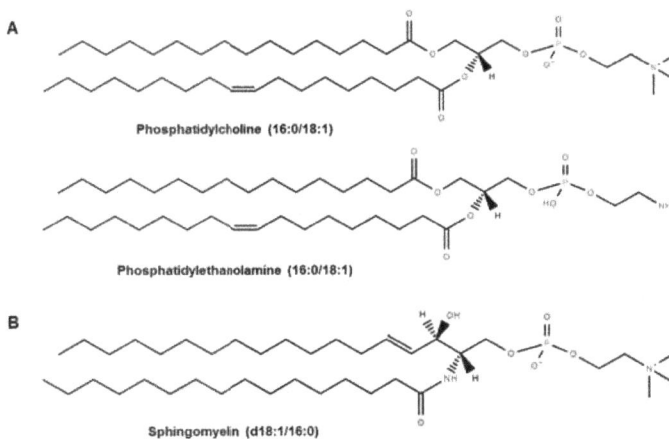

Figure 1. Structures of major phospholipids in egg yolk. Major molecular species of egg glycerophospholipids (**A**) and sphingomyelin (**B**). Lipid structures were drawn using Lipid MAPS tools [31].

3. Egg Phospholipids and Lipid Absorption

Inhibition of luminal cholesterol absorption is an attractive target to lower blood cholesterol and reduce CVD risk. Cholesterol absorption is widely recognized to influence serum lipids [32]. Pharmacological agents, such as ezetimibe, have been developed to reduce intestinal cholesterol absorption as a means of lowering serum cholesterol and CVD risk [33]. Large intakes of dietary lecithin have long been known to influence serum cholesterol levels in humans [34]. Meta-analysis of soy lecithin trials has suggested that the unsaturated FA component was primarily responsible for the hypocholesterolemic effects observed in early studies [35]. However, recent studies with more saturated sources of PL, such as egg, show that intact PL strongly influence lipid absorption through molecular interactions. Dietary phospholipids are known to inhibit cholesterol absorption when added in significant amounts to the diet (as reviewed by Cohn *et al.* [22]). Animal studies have shown that egg PL, such as PC and SM, reduce cholesterol and FA absorption by possibly interfering with lipid mobilization from mixed micelles [36–39].

Table 1. Typical Composition of Egg Phospholipids.

Egg PL Composition [24]						
Egg Yolk	PC	PE	LysoPC	SM	LysoPE	PI
Concentration (mg/100 g yolk)	5840	1500	270	190	90	330
Percentage of total PL (%)	71.1	18.3	3.3	2.3	1.1	4.0

Egg PC FA Composition [25]							
Position	16:0	16:1	18:0	18:1	18:2	20:4	22:6
sn-1	62.8	1.4	27.2	6.5	0.8	Trace	-
sn-2	6	1	2	56	24.5	5.6	2.9
Total	31	1.2	14.1	33.4	13.4	3.3	1.9

Egg PE FA Composition [25]						
Position	16:0	18:0	18:1	18:2	20:4	22:6
sn-1	34.2	51.2	10.5	0.3	Trace	-
sn-2	7	4.3	32.1	17.5	23.9	11
Total	16.4	28.3	21.5	10.2	14	6.8

Egg SM FA Composition Adapted from [26]									
16:0	18:0	18:1	20:0	22:0	22:1	23:0	23:1	24:0	24:1
68	10	1	4	6	1	2	-	3	6

Abbreviations: FA, fatty acid; LysoPC, lysophosphatidylcholine; LysoPE, lysophosphatidylethanolamine; PC, phosphatidylcholine; PE, phosphatidylethanolamine; PI, phosphatidylinositol; PL, phospholipid; SM, sphingomyelin.

Although biliary PC is a critical emulsifier of dietary lipids and aids in their digestion and absorption in the GI tract, excess luminal PC appears to inhibit lipid absorption. Young and Hui [40] showed that hydrolysis of surface PC by pancreatic PLA_2 is required for proper pancreatic lipase/colipase digestion of TG and absorption of cholesterol and FA from lipid emulsions. With high PL concentrations in lipid emulsions (>0.3 PL/TG molar ratio), pancreatic lipase/colipase hydrolysis of TG was impaired and cholesterol absorption into rat IEC-6 intestinal cells was diminished [40]. Furthermore, micellar PC was shown to inhibit dietary cholesterol absorption into Caco-2 cells, which was reversed by conversion to lysophosphatidylcholine by pancreatic PLA_2 [41]. PC-enriched micelles appear to impede diffusion across the unstirred water layer of the intestine [42,43]. Thus, digestion of surface PC appears to be necessary for proper absorption of lipids from both lipid emulsions and micelles. Jiang *et al.* [36] showed that duodenal infusion of a lipid emulsion containing egg PC significantly reduced cholesterol absorption by ~20% in lymph duct cannulated rats. The influence of PC on cholesterol absorption appears to be dependent on FA saturation, as egg PC inhibited the absorption of cholesterol into lymphatics greater than the more unsaturated soy PC in the same study. Soy PC infusion actually increased cholesterol and FA absorption compared to no PC control lipid emulsion. Furthermore, hydrogenated egg PC had a greater effect on cholesterol and TG absorption than egg PC. PC that is saturated at the *sn*-1 position is known to be a poor substrate for pancreatic PLA_2 hydrolysis [44]. Thus, it appears that the saturation of egg PC makes it more effective at inhibiting cholesterol absorption than more unsaturated PC, such as soy PC.

SM and other sphingolipids have been shown to dose-dependently reduce the absorption of cholesterol, TG, and FA in rodents [37–39]. SM interacts with cholesterol with high affinity and appears to alter its micellar solubilization. The amide portion of SM can interact with the hydroxyl group of cholesterol through hydrogen bonding [45]. Furthermore, the strength of association appears to be influenced by SM FA chain length and saturation [38]. Ceramide and sphingosine, which are products of SM digestion, also appear to reduce lipid absorption into intestinal cells through hydrogen bonding with the hydroxyl group of cholesterol [46] and possibly through interactions with the carboxylic acid group of FA [39]. Sphingosine can form complexes with cholesterol and limit uptake via the cholesterol transporter Niemann-Pick C1 like 1 (NPC1L1) [46]. Duivenvoorden *et al.* [39] supplemented the diets of APOE*3Leiden mice with different types of sphingolipids (including SM, ceramide, and sphingosine) and examined their effects on plasma lipids. Dietary sphingolipids dose-dependently lowered plasma cholesterol and TG in Western-type diet-fed mice through an inhibition of luminal FA and cholesterol absorption. While egg SM makes up only about 2% of total PL in egg yolk [24], this amount may still influence cholesterol absorption. Feeding of 0.2% and 0.4% egg SM to Western-type diet-fed APOE*3Leiden mice resulted in plasma cholesterol reductions of >20% [39]. Dried egg powder contains about 0.25% SM by weight, so this could potentially have an impact on inhibiting blood cholesterol changes that would normally occur from ingesting the amount of cholesterol found in the yolk. Milk SM has been shown to be a more potent inhibitor of cholesterol and FA absorption when compared to egg SM [38]. The greater inhibitory effect of milk SM on lipid absorption appears to be associated with its greater saturation and longer chain-length of its fatty acyl group, which may allow for stronger hydrophobic interactions [38]. Milk SM primarily consists of very long-chain FA (22:0, 23:0, 24:0), whereas egg SM consists primarily of the long-chain FA palmitic acid (16:0) [38].

Feeding of dietary PE has been shown to lower serum cholesterol in rats [47,48]. Mono- and di-unsaturated PE may influence cholesterol absorption like SM, as it has been shown to display a similar affinity to cholesterol as SM [49,50]. Both 1-palmitoyl-2-oleoyl-*sn*-glycero-3-phosphoethanolamine (POPE) [49] and 1-stearoyl-2-linoleoyl-*sn*-glycero-3-phosphoethanolamine (SLPE) [50], major PE molecular species in egg yolk [30], have been shown to interact with cholesterol in monolayers to a similar degree as SM; this suggests an important role for PE in lipid raft formation at the inner membrane leaflet of cells where it is most abundant. Due to the high affinity for cholesterol observed with certain PE species, dietary PE from egg may influence the absorption of luminal cholesterol similar to dietary SM.

4. Egg Phospholipids and Hepatic Lipid Metabolism

In animal models, egg PL appear to influence hepatic lipid metabolism through effects on cholesterol and bile acid synthesis, FA oxidation, and lipoprotein secretion [51–53]. Hepatic lipid levels are often shown to be reduced by dietary PL in animals, and this may be due to indirect effects via inhibition of intestinal lipid absorption and direct effects on hepatic nuclear receptors that regulate lipid metabolism. Feeding rats an egg yolk-enriched diet (~5% egg PL by weight) for 12 weeks lowered serum and hepatic lipids, and increased fecal sterol excretion compared to a cholesterol and fat-matched control group [51]. These changes were related to lower hepatic expression of cholesterol biosynthesis genes and increased expression of bile acid synthesis genes.

Peroxisome proliferator-activated receptor-α (PPARα) is a nuclear receptor abundantly expressed in the liver, where it functions as a key regulator of hepatic FA metabolism through transcriptional control of beta oxidation-related genes [52]. *In vitro* and rodent studies suggest that PC, specifically the 16:0 and 18:1-containing species PC (16:0/18:1), is a natural agonist of hepatic PPARα. Chakravarthy *et al.* [52] showed that portal vein infusion of PC (16:0/18:1) reduced hepatic steatosis in C57BL/6 mice and induced PPARα-dependent gene expression; although, this effect was not observed with intraperitoneal administration. Furthermore, incubation of PC (16:0/18:1) with the Hepa 1–6 mouse hepatoma cell line induced PPARα-target genes involved in FA oxidation. PC (16:0/18:1) was found to be a minor PL species in the liver which suggests it acts as a signaling molecule in this organ. Thus, this data suggests that providing PC (16:0/18:1) in the diet may affect hepatic PPARα activation if sufficient amounts reach the liver, as this is only a minor PL species in this organ [52]. Interestingly, PC (16:0/18:1) is the major PC species in eggs [29]. However, Cohn and colleagues [54] showed that feeding C57BL/6 mice a high fat diet supplemented with egg PC (1.25% by weight) for 3 weeks did not alter hepatic lipids and expression of a PPARα target gene (acyl-CoA oxidase) compared to control high fat diet. In contrast, feeding mice a hydrogenated form of egg PC, which contained only saturated FA, significantly lowered hepatic lipid levels [54]. Hydrogenated egg PC is associated with a greater inhibition of lipid absorption in rodents compared to natural egg PC [36]. Thus, it appears that at least in mice, the effects of short-term feeding of PC on hepatic lipids may related to its interference with lipid absorption, rather than modulation of PPARα.

Rye and colleagues [53] studied the effects of egg SM on hepatic lipid metabolism in Western-type diet-fed C57BL/6 mice. Egg SM feeding (0.6% of diet by weight) for 18 days was shown to reduce hepatic lipid levels and increase fecal cholesterol output compared to control mice. Although egg SM feeding substantially reduced hepatic lipids and led to a ~30% reduction in cholesterol absorption, it did not affect plasma cholesterol or TG levels. Sphingoid bases have been shown to activate PPARα transcriptional activity *in vitro* [55]. However, egg SM feeding of Western-type diet-fed mice reduced the hepatic expression of PPARα-target genes involved in FA oxidation [53]. The reduced hepatic lipid levels in egg SM-fed mice coincided with significantly lower hepatic expression of genes involved in cholesterol and FA metabolism [53].

The choline moiety of PL also appears to influence hepatic lipid metabolism and lipoprotein production. PC and SM are both sources of choline in the Western diet. Choline is an essential nutrient and is not synthesized in adequate amounts to meet the needs of humans [56]. Dietary choline is considered especially important for maintaining a healthy liver [57]. Methionine- and choline-deficient diets (MCD) are well-known inducers of liver injury in mice and are used as a model of nonalcoholic steatohepatitis [58]. This combined nutrient deficiency causes hepatic lipid accumulation by enhancing lipid uptake and reducing VLDL secretion [58]. In humans, a single-nucleotide polymorphism in the PC-synthesizing enzyme, phosphatidylethanolamine *N*-methyltransferase (PEMT), is associated with greater risk for non-alcoholic fatty liver disease (NAFLD) [59]. Dietary choline may also influence more advanced stages of liver disease, as low intake of choline was shown to be associated with increased hepatic fibrosis in postmenopausal women with NAFLD [60].

While there has been no reports specifically examining the effects of dietary egg PE on hepatic lipid metabolism, feeding soy PE to rats has been shown to lower hepatic cholesterol levels [47]. Soy PE consists of primarily PE (16:0/18:2), PE (18:2/18:2), and PE (16:0/18:1) molecular species [30].

5. Egg Phospholipids and HDL Metabolism

Therapies aimed at increasing plasma HDL-C may be beneficial for preventing CVD. Plasma HDL-C has been shown to be inversely related to the extent of atherosclerosis [61]. According to data from large prospective cohort studies, it can be estimated that for every 1 mg/dL (0.0259 mmol/L) increase in HDL-C, there is an approximate 2–3% reduction in CVD risk [62]. Strong experimental evidence confirms that atherosclerosis is directly alleviated by HDL [63–65]. HDL is thought to improve CVD outcomes largely by its ability to remove cholesterol from the artery via RCT. Regular egg yolk consumption has been shown to increase plasma HDL-C and increase the mean size of HDL particles in healthy [66], overweight [67], and metabolic syndrome (MetS) populations [68]. These increases in HDL-C and HDL size may be due to the high intake of egg PL.

PL feeding has been associated with increases in HDL-C in animal and human studies [69,70]. PL content of HDL has been shown to be a major factor in its ability to accept cholesterol from cells during the initial stages of RCT [71,72]. Dietary PC has been observed to preferentially incorporate into HDL particles after ingestion. Zierenberg and Grundy [17] examined the metabolic fate of ^{3}H/^{14}C-labeled polyunsaturated PC in men. Soybean PC was labeled in its FA (^{14}C) and choline moiety (^{3}H), given orally at a dose of 1 g, and then blood was collected from 6–24 h post-ingestion. The ^{4}C and ^{3}H radiolabels preferentially incorporated into plasma lipoproteins compared to red blood cells, with higher specific activity appearing in plasma HDL than in apoB-containing lipoproteins. This increased appearance of radiolabeled PC in plasma HDL may be explained by the exchange of chylomicron-PC to HDL in circulation or direct secretion of PC into nascent intestinally-derived HDL. Tall *et al.* [73] examined the incorporation of oral ^{3}H/^{14}C-labeled polyunsaturated PC into HDL subclasses. Major peaks in radiolabel specific activity appeared after 5–8 h in the PL fraction of several HDL subclasses, in the order of HDL$_{2a}$ (1.11–1.12 g/mL) > HDL$_3$ (1.19 g/mL) > HDL$_{2b}$ (1.07–1.09 g/mL). Thus, the results suggest that the HDL$_{2a}$ subclass is the major HDL acceptor of oral PL, but all HDL subclasses appear to incorporate dietary PL to some extent. Plasma HDL-PL content has been shown to increase postprandially after egg yolk feeding [74]. Thus, dietary egg PL appears in serum HDL after meals and may impact HDL function.

Clinical studies where subjects were fed egg yolks demonstrated improvements in other markers of RCT besides HDL-C, such as plasma lecithin-cholesterol acyltransferase (LCAT) activity [68,75,76] and serum cholesterol efflux capacity [77]. Recently, HDL cholesterol efflux capacity has emerged as a significant predictor of heart disease status, even after adjusting for plasma HDL-C and its major protein, apolipoprotein (apo) A-I [78]. PL-enrichment of HDL with either PC or SM improves its ability to mobilize cholesterol from cells [71,72]. The first component of RCT, involving cellular cholesterol mobilization, relies on apo A-I and HDL particle interactions to promote cholesterol efflux by a variety of passive and active mechanisms [79]. Important factors in HDL cellular cholesterol efflux include cholesterol mobilization via ABC transporters (ATP-binding cassette transporters A1 and G1) and scavenger receptor B1 (SR-B1), desorption of free cholesterol via aqueous diffusion, and esterification of cholesterol by LCAT [79]. Preferred acceptors for ABCG1 and SR-B1 are larger HDL particles containing PL [71,72]. Egg yolk feeding was shown to increase HDL-PE and decrease HDL-TG [77]. Interestingly, egg ingestion shifted HDL-SM towards molecular species that more closely resembled egg SM, suggesting that egg SM may be incorporated into HDL [77]. Thus, increasing dietary intake of egg PL may change HDL-PL content and this could explain the increases in serum cholesterol efflux capacity and enlargement in HDL particle size observed with egg yolk intake in humans [68,77]. The increases in HDL-C associated with egg PL intake may reflect a greater capacity for RCT.

6. Egg Phospholipids and Inflammation

In addition to effects on lipid metabolism, dietary intake of egg PL may also reduce inflammation. Consuming three eggs per day for 12 weeks resulted in a reduction in plasma C-reactive protein (CRP) and an increase in adiponectin in overweight men; changes which were not observed with yolk-free egg substitute [80]. Egg consumption has also led to improvements in circulating plasma inflammatory markers in adults with MetS [81]. In combination with moderate carbohydrate restriction, the addition of three eggs per day led to decreases in plasma TNFα and serum amyloid A in men and women with MetS, whereas no changes were observed in subjects consuming a yolk-free egg substitute [81]. Egg yolk contains a significant amount of choline as PC. Dietary choline intake has been shown to be inversely associated with serum inflammation markers in healthy adults [82]. Choline administration to mice has been shown to significantly reduce plasma TNFα and enhance survival in response to an endotoxin challenge [83]. Choline seems to act through nicotinic acetylcholine receptor subunit α7 (α7nAChR) activation, which has a tonic inhibitory effect on immune cell inflammatory responses [83,84]. Some studies have suggested that dietary PC may reduce inflammation in the GI tract [85,86]. Therapeutic usage of oral PC (>1 g daily) in ulcerative colitis is well-documented and improves inflammation [85,86]. This GI anti-inflammatory effect of PC may be of significance to MetS, as there is evidence linking GI inflammation to the development of obesity and insulin resistance in animal models [87]. Furthermore, intestinal inflammation is associated with impaired formation of intestinally-derived nascent HDL in Crohn's disease [88,89].

7. Egg Phospholipids and Trimethylamine *N*-Oxide (TMAO) Formation

Recently, Hazen and colleagues [90] used unbiased metabolomics to identify three metabolites of dietary PC (choline, TMAO, and betaine) which were predictors of CVD in a large clinical cohort. The presumed atherogenic factor, TMAO, is a known metabolite of dietary choline. Dietary choline can undergo catabolism in the GI tract by gut microflora to form the gas trimethylamine (TMA), which is absorbed and rapidly oxidized to TMAO in the liver by the hepatic enzyme flavin containing monooxygenase 3 (FMO3) [91,92]. Hazen and colleagues [90] showed that feeding apoE$^{-/-}$ mice diets rich in either choline (0.5% or 1% wt/wt) or TMAO (0.12% wt/wt) for 20 weeks resulted in increased aortic root lesion size despite no changes in traditional CVD risk biomarkers. Highlighting the role of gut microflora in this process, TMAO formation from dietary PC and the atherogenic effect of choline feeding were abolished when the mice were germ-free or co-administered broad spectrum antibiotics to deplete gut bacteria. Additionally, the plasma levels of TMAO in mice and humans were associated with the expression of hepatic FMO3. Thus, formation of blood TMAO subsequent to dietary PC intake requires intact gut microflora and may be influenced by hepatic FMO3 expression. Interestingly, TMAO levels do not appear to be strongly influenced by genetic factors in humans [93], suggesting that diet and gut microflora primarily determine differences in plasma TMAO levels between individuals. TMAO formation was also shown to be formed from the consumption of another dietary trimethylamine compound, carnitine [94]. Subsequently, the relationship between TMAO and CVD was confirmed in a larger prospective cohort [95]. The investigators suggested that the atherogenic effect of TMAO is due to inhibition of RCT and increased macrophage scavenger receptor expression, resulting in enhanced foam cell formation [96]. Increases in plasma TMAO that occurred after carnitine and choline feeding of mice were associated with impaired RCT at the stage of bile acid production [94]. TMAO was also shown to induce the scavenger receptors CD36 and SR-A in macrophages [90,94].

Notably, it was shown that healthy participants who consumed a dietary PC challenge (hard-boiled eggs and deuterium (d9)-labeled PC) had acute increases in plasma TMAO in a gut microflora-dependent manner [95]. Furthermore, Zeisel and colleagues [97] performed a small, double-blind, randomized dose-response study where healthy subjects (*n* = 6) consumed a breakfast with 0, 1, 2, 4 or 6 egg yolks and levels of plasma TMAO were measured at pre- and post-breakfast time intervals (up to 24 h). Egg intake dose-dependently increased mean plasma TMAO area under the curve (AUC) values, with TMAO response peaks occurring 6–8 h after ingestion. Interestingly, there were >4-fold differences in plasma TMAO levels between subjects at similar dosages, potentially due to differences in gut microflora or hepatic FMO3 activity. Regardless of the large interindividual variation in plasma TMAO, each subject displayed an increase in plasma TMAO when increasing the number of egg yolks consumed. Collectively, these two studies demonstrate that acute intake of PC from egg may influence postprandial plasma TMAO levels in humans. The effect of chronic egg intake on TMAO levels has not been examined yet. Findings from chronic egg intake studies would be more meaningful than acute egg feedings in regards to atherosclerosis risk, since it is a disease that takes decades to develop. Chronic egg intake could influence gut microflora composition and this would presumably impact TMAO formation from choline, such as that observed with chronic exposure to carnitine [94]. It remains to be seen whether there is an "optimal" egg dose, where the RCT-promoting aspects or other HDL-promoting effects outweigh any possible TMAO effects on RCT and CVD risk. It will also be important to determine whether chronic or acute egg intake in humans affects the expression of scavenger receptors in peripheral blood mononuclear cells (PBMCs). Although egg ingestion may increase plasma TMAO to some extent, it potentially may not reach the threshold level needed to affect scavenger receptor expression.

The majority of luminal PC available for absorption comes from the endogenously-derived PL found in bile (10–20 g/day) [98]. Biliary PC, however, does not seem to be a major contributor to TMAO levels, as plasma TMAO is low in the absence of large amounts of dietary choline [90]. It is unclear why the large amounts of biliary PC normally found in the intestine do not result in very high levels of plasma TMAO regardless of dietary PC intake. High amounts of dietary PC, particularly saturated PC [44], may overwhelm pancreatic PLA_2 activity since it is known to be less efficient than other lipases [16]. Intact PC digestion in $PLA_2^{-/-}$ mice demonstrates additional enzymes in the intestine are capable of phospholipase activity [99]. Ileal phospholipase B acts in the distal intestinal mucosa to hydrolyze PC [100]. Thus, a large dietary PL load may result in greater amounts of intact PC reaching the distal parts of the intestine, where more bacteria reside and can contribute to the PC-TMA-TMAO pathway.

Daily egg intake has not been shown to be associated with CVD risk in healthy populations [11–13]. In contrast, several large cohort studies have found a positive association between egg intake and CVD in diabetics [11,12,101,102]. Consequently, patients with diabetes may be discouraged from eating eggs. These relationships are suggested to be caused by components found in the egg yolk, such as cholesterol and saturated fat [101]. It is also possible that the PC-TMA-TMAO pathway is more important or altered in diabetes. Serum TMAO levels have been shown to be elevated in those with type 2 diabetes [103]. This may be related to the kidney dysfunction that is often seen with diabetes, as TMAO levels can build up in the blood if they are not cleared by the kidneys. Regardless of kidney function, however, TMAO is a strong predictor of all-cause mortality risk [104,105]. If the plasma TMAO response to egg intake is increased in diabetics relative to non-diabetics, that may explain the consistent link between egg intake and CVD in diabetics. Further research is warranted to see if plasma TMAO response to egg intake is altered in insulin-resistant or diabetic humans.

8. Conclusions

Egg PL are important contributors to the overall dietary PL intake in the Western diet. Based on pre-clinical studies, egg PC and SM appear to regulate lipid absorption, hepatic lipid metabolism, and inflammation. In clinical studies, egg PL intake is associated with beneficial changes in serum biomarkers related to HDL function. However, the recent evidence linking acute ingestion of eggs with postprandial increases in plasma TMAO warrants concern. More research needs to be done to examine TMAO responses to chronic egg intake and in different populations, such as diabetics. It will be critical determine if the perceived benefits of egg PL intake on CVD risk markers outweigh the risk of potential TMAO formation (Figure 2).

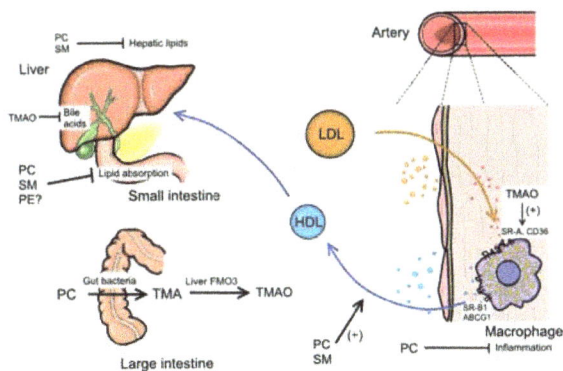

Figure 2. Potential pathways egg phospholipids could influence atherosclerosis. Egg phospholipids may lessen risk for cardiovascular disease (CVD) via reducing lipid absorption (PC, SM), reducing hepatic lipids (PC, SM), increasing HDL cholesterol efflux (PC, SM), and reducing inflammation (PC). Egg PC may also influence CVD risk via gut microflora-dependent catabolism to TMA and liver conversion to TMAO. TMAO may increase CVD risk via increasing macrophage scavenger receptors and decreasing RCT via reduced bile acid synthesis. Abbreviations: ABCG1, ATP-binding cassette transporter G1; CD36, Cluster of Differentiation 36; FMO3, flavin containing monooxygenase 3; HDL, high-density lipoprotein; LDL, low-density lipoprotein; PC, phosphatidylcholine; PE, phosphatidylethanolamine; SM, sphingomyelin; SR-A, scavenger receptor A; SR-B1, scavenger receptor B1; TMA, trimethylamine; TMAO, trimethylamine *N*-oxide.

Conflicts of Interest: The author declares no conflict of interest.

References

1. World Health Organization. *Global Status Report on Noncommunicable Diseases 2010*; World Health Organization: Geneva, Switzerland, 2011.

2. Roger, V.L.; Go, A.S.; Lloyd-Jones, D.M.; Adams, R.J.; Berry, J.D.; Brown, T.M.; Carnethon, M.R.; Dai, S.; de Simone, G.; Ford, E.S.; *et al.* Heart disease and stroke statistics—2011 update: A report from the american heart association. *Circulation* **2011**, *123*, e18–e209. [CrossRef]

3. Ross, R. Atherosclerosis—An inflammatory disease. *N. Engl. J. Med.* **1999**, *340*, 115–126. [CrossRef] [PubMed]

4. Tabas, I.; Williams, K.J.; Boren, J. Subendothelial lipoprotein retention as the initiating process in atherosclerosis: Update and therapeutic implications. *Circulation* **2007**, *116*, 1832–1844. [CrossRef] [PubMed]

5. Williams, K.J.; Tabas, I. The response-to-retention hypothesis of early atherogenesis. *Arterioscler. Thromb. Vasc. Biol.* **1995**, *15*, 551–561. [CrossRef] [PubMed]

6. Davis, R.A. Evolution of processes and regulators of lipoprotein synthesis: From birds to mammals. *J. Nutr.* **1997**, *127*, 795S–800S. [PubMed]

7. Fielding, C.J.; Fielding, P.E. Molecular physiology of reverse cholesterol transport. *J. Lipid Res.* **1995**, *36*, 211–228. [PubMed]

8. Singh, I.M.; Shishehbor, M.H.; Ansell, B.J. High-density lipoprotein as a therapeutic target: A systematic review. *JAMA* **2007**, *298*, 786–798. [CrossRef] [PubMed]

9. Expert Panel on Detection, Evaluation, and Treatment of High Blood Cholesterol in Adults. Executive summary of the third report of the national cholesterol education program (NCEP) expert panel on detection, evaluation, and treatment of high blood cholesterol in adults (adult treatment panel III). *JAMA* **2001**, *285*, 2486–2497.

10. Fernandez, M.L.; Calle, M. Revisiting dietary cholesterol recommendations: Does the evidence support a limit of 300 mg/d? *Curr. Atheroscler. Rep.* **2010**, *12*, 377–383. [CrossRef] [PubMed]

11. Hu, F.B.; Stampfer, M.J.; Rimm, E.B.; Manson, J.E.; Ascherio, A.; Colditz, G.A.; Rosner, B.A.; Spiegelman, D.; Speizer, F.E.; Sacks, F.M.; *et al.* A prospective study of egg consumption and risk of cardiovascular disease in men and women. *JAMA* **1999**, *281*, 1387–1394. [CrossRef]

12. Qureshi, A.I.; Suri, F.K.; Ahmed, S.; Nasar, A.; Divani, A.A.; Kirmani, J.F. Regular egg consumption does not increase the risk of stroke and cardiovascular diseases. *Med. Sci. Monit.* **2007**, *13*, CR1–CR8. [PubMed]

13. Nakamura, Y.; Iso, H.; Kita, Y.; Ueshima, H.; Okada, K.; Konishi, M.; Inoue, M.; Tsugane, S. Egg consumption, serum total cholesterol concentrations and coronary heart disease incidence: Japan public health center-based prospective study. *Br. J. Nutr.* **2006**, *96*, 921–928. [CrossRef] [PubMed]

14. Handelman, G.J.; Nightingale, Z.D.; Lichtenstein, A.H.; Schaefer, E.J.; Blumberg, J.B. Lutein and zeaxanthin concentrations in plasma after dietary supplementation with egg yolk. *Am. J. Clin. Nutr.* **1999**, *70*, 247–251. [PubMed]

15. Weihrauch, J.L.; Son, Y.S. Phospholipid content of foods. *JAOCS* **1983**, *60*, 1971–1978.

16. Carey, M.C.; Small, D.M.; Bliss, C.M. Lipid digestion and absorption. *Annu. Rev. Physiol.* **1983**, *45*, 651–677. [CrossRef] [PubMed]

17. Zierenberg, O.; Grundy, S.M. Intestinal absorption of polyenephosphatidylcholine in man. *J. Lipid Res.* **1982**, *23*, 1136–1142. [PubMed]

18. Vesper, H.; Schmelz, E.M.; Nikolova-Karakashian, M.N.; Dillehay, D.L.; Lynch, D.V.; Merrill, A.H., Jr. Sphingolipids in food and the emerging importance of sphingolipids to nutrition. *J. Nutr.* **1999**, *129*, 1239–1250. [PubMed]

19. Ohlsson, L.; Hertervig, E.; Jonsson, B.A.; Duan, R.D.; Nyberg, L.; Svernlov, R.; Nilsson, A. Sphingolipids in human ileostomy content after meals containing milk sphingomyelin. *Am. J. Clin. Nutr.* **2010**, *91*, 672–678. [CrossRef] [PubMed]

20. Kovacs-Nolan, J.; Phillips, M.; Mine, Y. Advances in the value of eggs and egg components for human health. *J. Agric. Food Chem.* **2005**, *53*, 8421–8431. [CrossRef] [PubMed]

21. U.S. Department of Agriculture, A.R.S. *USDA National Nutrient Database for Standard Reference, Release 26. Nutrient Data Laboratory Home Page*; USDA: Washington, DC, USA, 2013.

22. Cohn, J.S.; Kamili, A.; Wat, E.; Chung, R.W.; Tandy, S. Dietary phospholipids and intestinal cholesterol absorption. *Nutrients* **2010**, *2*, 116–127. [CrossRef] [PubMed]
23. U.S. Department of Agriculture. *The World Agricultural Supply and Demand Estimates Report (Wasde)*; USDA: Washington, DC, USA, 2015.
24. Zhao, Y.Y.; Xiong, Y.; Curtis, J.M. Measurement of phospholipids by hydrophilic interaction liquid chromatography coupled to tandem mass spectrometry: The determination of choline containing compounds in foods. *J. Chromatogr. A* **2011**, *1218*, 5470–5479. [CrossRef] [PubMed]
25. Schreiner, M.; Hulan, H.W.; Razzazi-Fazeli, E.; Bohm, J.; Iben, C. Feeding laying hens seal blubber oil: Effects on egg yolk incorporation, stereospecific distribution of omega-3 fatty acids, and sensory aspects. *Poult. Sci.* **2004**, *83*, 462–473. [CrossRef] [PubMed]
26. Ramstedt, B.; Leppimaki, P.; Axberg, M.; Slotte, J.P. Analysis of natural and synthetic sphingomyelins using high-performance thin-layer chromatography. *Eur. J. Biochem.* **1999**, *266*, 997–1002. [CrossRef] [PubMed]
27. Baucells, M.D.; Crespo, N.; Barroeta, A.C.; Lopez-Ferrer, S.; Grashorn, M.A. Incorporation of different polyunsaturated fatty acids into eggs. *Poult. Sci.* **2000**, *79*, 51–59. [CrossRef] [PubMed]
28. Shinn, S.; Liyanage, R.; Lay, J.; Proctor, A. Improved fatty acid analysis of conjugated linoleic acid rich egg yolk triacylglycerols and phospholipid species. *J. Agric. Food Chem.* **2014**, *62*, 6608–6615. [CrossRef] [PubMed]
29. Pacetti, D.; Boselli, E.; Hulan, H.W.; Frega, N.G. High performance liquid chromatography-tandem mass spectrometry of phospholipid molecular species in eggs from hens fed diets enriched in seal blubber oil. *J. Chromatogr. A* **2005**, *1097*, 66–73. [CrossRef] [PubMed]
30. Zhou, L.; Zhao, M.; Ennahar, S.; Bindler, F.; Marchioni, E. Determination of phosphatidylethanolamine molecular species in various food matrices by liquid chromatography-electrospray ionization-tandem mass spectrometry (LC-ESI-MS2). *Anal. Bioanal. Chem.* **2012**, *403*, 291–300. [CrossRef] [PubMed]
31. Sud, M.; Fahy, E.; Subramaniam, S. Template-based combinatorial enumeration of virtual compound libraries for lipids. *J. Cheminform.* **2012**, *4*, 23. [CrossRef] [PubMed]
32. Hegsted, D.M.; McGandy, R.B.; Myers, M.L.; Stare, F.J. Quantitative effects of dietary fat on serum cholesterol in man. *Am. J. Clin. Nutr.* **1965**, *17*, 281–295. [PubMed]
33. Lipka, L.J. Ezetimibe: A first-in-class, novel cholesterol absorption inhibitor. *Cardiovasc. Drug Rev.* **2003**, *21*, 293–312. [CrossRef] [PubMed]
34. Steiner, A.; Domanski, B.; Seegal, D. Effect of feeding of "soya lecithin" on serum cholesterol level of man. *Exp. Biol. Med. (Maywood)* **1944**, *55*, 236–238. [CrossRef]
35. Knuiman, J.T.; Beynen, A.C.; Katan, M.B. Lecithin intake and serum cholesterol. *Am. J. Clin. Nutr.* **1989**, *49*, 266–268. [PubMed]
36. Jiang, Y.; Noh, S.K.; Koo, S.I. Egg phosphatidylcholine decreases the lymphatic absorption of cholesterol in rats. *J. Nutr.* **2001**, *131*, 2358–2363. [PubMed]
37. Noh, S.K.; Koo, S.I. Egg sphingomyelin lowers the lymphatic absorption of cholesterol and alpha-tocopherol in rats. *J. Nutr.* **2003**, *133*, 3571–3576. [PubMed]
38. Noh, S.K.; Koo, S.I. Milk sphingomyelin is more effective than egg sphingomyelin in inhibiting intestinal absorption of cholesterol and fat in rats. *J. Nutr.* **2004**, *134*, 2611–2616. [PubMed]
39. Duivenvoorden, I.; Voshol, P.J.; Rensen, P.C.; van Duyvenvoorde, W.; Romijn, J.A.; Emeis, J.J.; Havekes, L.M.; Nieuwenhuizen, W.F. Dietary sphingolipids lower plasma cholesterol and triacylglycerol and prevent liver steatosis in APOE*3Leiden mice. *Am. J. Clin. Nutr.* **2006**, *84*, 312–321. [PubMed]
40. Young, S.C.; Hui, D.Y. Pancreatic lipase/colipase-mediated triacylglycerol hydrolysis is required for cholesterol transport from lipid emulsions to intestinal cells. *Biochem. J.* **1999**, *339*, 615–620. [CrossRef] [PubMed]
41. Homan, R.; Hamelehle, K.L. Phospholipase A2 relieves phosphatidylcholine inhibition of micellar cholesterol absorption and transport by human intestinal cell line Caco-2. *J. Lipid Res.* **1998**, *39*, 1197–1209. [PubMed]
42. Rodgers, J.B.; O'Connor, P.J. Effect of phosphatidylcholine on fatty acid and cholesterol absorption from mixed micellar solutions. *Biochim. Biophys. Acta* **1975**, *409*, 192–200. [CrossRef] [PubMed]
43. Rampone, A.J.; Machida, C.M. Mode of action of lecithin in suppressing cholesterol absorption. *J. Lipid Res.* **1981**, *22*, 744–752. [PubMed]
44. Kinkaid, A.; Wilton, D.C. Comparison of the catalytic properties of phospholipase A2 from pancreas and venom using a continuous fluorescence displacement assay. *Biochem. J.* **1991**, *278*, 843–848. [PubMed]

45. Ohvo-Rekila, H.; Ramstedt, B.; Leppimaki, P.; Slotte, J.P. Cholesterol interactions with phospholipids in membranes. *Prog. Lipid Res.* **2002**, *41*, 66–97. [CrossRef] [PubMed]
46. Garmy, N.; Taieb, N.; Yahi, N.; Fantini, J. Interaction of cholesterol with sphingosine: Physicochemical characterization and impact on intestinal absorption. *J. Lipid Res.* **2005**, *46*, 36–45. [CrossRef] [PubMed]
47. Imaizumi, K.; Mawatari, K.; Murata, M.; Ikeda, I.; Sugano, M. The contrasting effect of dietary phosphatidylethanolamine and phosphatidylcholine on serum lipoproteins and liver lipids in rats. *J. Nutr.* **1983**, *113*, 2403–2411. [PubMed]
48. Imaizumi, K.; Sekihara, K.; Sugano, M. Hypocholesterolemic action of dietary phosphatidylethanolamine in rats sensitive to exogenous cholesterol. *J. Nutr. Biochem.* **1991**, *2*, 251–254. [CrossRef]
49. Shaikh, S.R.; Brzustowicz, M.R.; Gustafson, N.; Stillwell, W.; Wassall, S.R. Monounsaturated PE does not phase-separate from the lipid raft molecules sphingomyelin and cholesterol: Role for polyunsaturation? *Biochemistry* **2002**, *41*, 10593–10602. [CrossRef] [PubMed]
50. Grzybek, M.; Kubiak, J.; Lach, A.; Przybylo, M.; Sikorski, A.F. A raft-associated species of phosphatidylethanolamine interacts with cholesterol comparably to sphingomyelin. A Langmuir-Blodgett monolayer study. *PLoS ONE* **2009**, *4*, e5053. [CrossRef] [PubMed]
51. Yang, F.; Ma, M.; Xu, J.; Yu, X.; Qiu, N. An egg-enriched diet attenuates plasma lipids and mediates cholesterol metabolism of high-cholesterol fed rats. *Lipids* **2012**, *47*, 269–277. [CrossRef] [PubMed]
52. Chakravarthy, M.V.; Lodhi, I.J.; Yin, L.; Malapaka, R.R.; Xu, H.E.; Turk, J.; Semenkovich, C.F. Identification of a physiologically relevant endogenous ligand for PPARalpha in liver. *Cell* **2009**, *138*, 476–488. [CrossRef] [PubMed]
53. Chung, R.W.; Kamili, A.; Tandy, S.; Weir, J.M.; Gaire, R.; Wong, G.; Meikle, P.J.; Cohn, J.S.; Rye, K.A. Dietary sphingomyelin lowers hepatic lipid levels and inhibits intestinal cholesterol absorption in high-fat-fed mice. *PLoS ONE* **2013**, *8*, e55949. [CrossRef] [PubMed]
54. Tandy, S.; Chung, R.W.; Kamili, A.; Wat, E.; Weir, J.M.; Meikle, P.J.; Cohn, J.S. Hydrogenated phosphatidylcholine supplementation reduces hepatic lipid levels in mice fed a high-fat diet. *Atherosclerosis* **2010**, *213*, 142–147. [CrossRef] [PubMed]
55. Murakami, I.; Wakasa, Y.; Yamashita, S.; Kurihara, T.; Zama, K.; Kobayashi, N.; Mizutani, Y.; Mitsutake, S.; Shigyo, T.; Igarashi, Y. Phytoceramide and sphingoid bases derived from brewer's yeast saccharomyces pastorianus activate peroxisome proliferator-activated receptors. *Lipids Health Dis.* **2011**, *10*, 150. [CrossRef] [PubMed]
56. Zeisel, S.H. Choline: An essential nutrient for humans. *Nutrition* **2000**, *16*, 669–671. [CrossRef] [PubMed]
57. Corbin, K.D.; Zeisel, S.H. Choline metabolism provides novel insights into nonalcoholic fatty liver disease and its progression. *Curr. Opin. Gastroenterol.* **2012**, *28*, 159–165. [CrossRef] [PubMed]
58. Rinella, M.E.; Elias, M.S.; Smolak, R.R.; Fu, T.; Borensztajn, J.; Green, R.M. Mechanisms of hepatic steatosis in mice fed a lipogenic methionine choline-deficient diet. *J. Lipid Res.* **2008**, *49*, 1068–1076. [CrossRef] [PubMed]
59. Song, J.; da Costa, K.A.; Fischer, L.M.; Kohlmeier, M.; Kwock, L.; Wang, S.; Zeisel, S.H. Polymorphism of the PEMT gene and susceptibility to nonalcoholic fatty liver disease (NAFLD). *FASEB J.* **2005**, *19*, 1266–1271. [CrossRef] [PubMed]
60. Guerrerio, A.L.; Colvin, R.M.; Schwartz, A.K.; Molleston, J.P.; Murray, K.F.; Diehl, A.; Mohan, P.; Schwimmer, J.B.; Lavine, J.E.; Torbenson, M.S.; *et al.* Choline intake in a large cohort of patients with nonalcoholic fatty liver disease. *Am. J. Clin. Nutr.* **2012**, *95*, 892–900. [CrossRef] [PubMed]
61. Linsel-Nitschke, P.; Tall, A.R. HDL as a target in the treatment of atherosclerotic cardiovascular disease. *Nat. Rev. Drug Discov.* **2005**, *4*, 193–205. [CrossRef] [PubMed]
62. Gordon, D.J.; Probstfield, J.L.; Garrison, R.J.; Neaton, J.D.; Castelli, W.P.; Knoke, J.D.; Jacobs, D.R., Jr.; Bangdiwala, S.; Tyroler, H.A. High-density lipoprotein cholesterol and cardiovascular disease. Four prospective american studies. *Circulation* **1989**, *79*, 8–15. [CrossRef] [PubMed]
63. Nissen, S.E.; Tsunoda, T.; Tuzcu, E.M.; Schoenhagen, P.; Cooper, C.J.; Yasin, M.; Eaton, G.M.; Lauer, M.A.; Sheldon, W.S.; Grines, C.L.; *et al.* Effect of recombinant APOA-I Milano on coronary atherosclerosis in patients with acute coronary syndromes: A randomized controlled trial. *JAMA* **2003**, *290*, 2292–2300. [CrossRef] [PubMed]
64. Sacks, F.M.; Rudel, L.L.; Conner, A.; Akeefe, H.; Kostner, G.; Baki, T.; Rothblat, G.; de la Llera-Moya, M.; Asztalos, B.; Perlman, T.; *et al.* Selective delipidation of plasma HDL enhances reverse cholesterol transport *in vivo.* *J. Lipid Res.* **2009**, *50*, 894–907. [CrossRef] [PubMed]

65. Badimon, J.J.; Badimon, L.; Fuster, V. Regression of atherosclerotic lesions by high density lipoprotein plasma fraction in the cholesterol-fed rabbit. *J. Clin. Investig.* **1990**, *85*, 1234–1241. [CrossRef] [PubMed]

66. Herron, K.L.; Vega-Lopez, S.; Conde, K.; Ramjiganesh, T.; Roy, S.; Shachter, N.S.; Fernandez, M.L. Pre-menopausal women, classified as hypo- or hyperresponders, do not alter their LDL/HDL ratio following a high dietary cholesterol challenge. *J. Am. Coll. Nutr.* **2002**, *21*, 250–258. [CrossRef] [PubMed]

67. Mutungi, G.; Ratliff, J.; Puglisi, M.; Torres-Gonzalez, M.; Vaishnav, U.; Leite, J.O.; Quann, E.; Volek, J.S.; Fernandez, M.L. Dietary cholesterol from eggs increases plasma HDL cholesterol in overweight men consuming a carbohydrate-restricted diet. *J. Nutr.* **2008**, *138*, 272–276. [PubMed]

68. Blesso, C.N.; Andersen, C.J.; Barona, J.; Volek, J.S.; Fernandez, M.L. Whole egg consumption improves lipoprotein profiles and insulin sensitivity to a greater extent than yolk-free egg substitute in individuals with metabolic syndrome. *Metabolism* **2013**, *62*, 400–410. [CrossRef] [PubMed]

69. O'Brien, B.C.; Corrigan, S.M. Influence of dietary soybean and egg lecithins on lipid responses in cholesterol-fed guinea pigs. *Lipids* **1988**, *23*, 647–650. [CrossRef] [PubMed]

70. Burgess, J.W.; Neville, T.A.; Rouillard, P.; Harder, Z.; Beanlands, D.S.; Sparks, D.L. Phosphatidylinositol increases HDL-C levels in humans. *J. Lipid Res.* **2005**, *46*, 350–355. [CrossRef] [PubMed]

71. Yancey, P.G.; de la Llera-Moya, M.; Swarnakar, S.; Monzo, P.; Klein, S.M.; Connelly, M.A.; Johnson, W.J.; Williams, D.L.; Rothblat, G.H. High density lipoprotein phospholipid composition is a major determinant of the bi-directional flux and net movement of cellular free cholesterol mediated by scavenger receptor BI. *J. Biol. Chem.* **2000**, *275*, 36596–36604. [CrossRef] [PubMed]

72. Sankaranarayanan, S.; Oram, J.F.; Asztalos, B.F.; Vaughan, A.M.; Lund-Katz, S.; Adorni, M.P.; Phillips, M.C.; Rothblat, G.H. Effects of acceptor composition and mechanism of ABCG1-mediated cellular free cholesterol efflux. *J. Lipid Res.* **2009**, *50*, 275–284. [CrossRef] [PubMed]

73. Tall, A.R.; Blum, C.B.; Grundy, S.M. Incorporation of radioactive phospholipid into subclasses of high-density lipoproteins. *Am. J. Physiol.* **1983**, *244*, E513–E516. [PubMed]

74. Dubois, C.; Armand, M.; Mekki, N.; Portugal, H.; Pauli, A.M.; Bernard, P.M.; Lafont, H.; Lairon, D. Effects of increasing amounts of dietary cholesterol on postprandial lipemia and lipoproteins in human subjects. *J. Lipid Res.* **1994**, *35*, 1993–2007. [PubMed]

75. Mutungi, G.; Waters, D.; Ratliff, J.; Puglisi, M.; Clark, R.M.; Volek, J.S.; Fernandez, M.L. Eggs distinctly modulate plasma carotenoid and lipoprotein subclasses in adult men following a carbohydrate-restricted diet. *J. Nutr. Biochem.* **2010**, *21*, 261–267. [CrossRef] [PubMed]

76. Herron, K.L.; Lofgren, I.E.; Sharman, M.; Volek, J.S.; Fernandez, M.L. High intake of cholesterol results in less atherogenic low-density lipoprotein particles in men and women independent of response classification. *Metabolism* **2004**, *53*, 823–830. [CrossRef] [PubMed]

77. Andersen, C.J.; Blesso, C.N.; Lee, J.; Barona, J.; Shah, D.; Thomas, M.J.; Fernandez, M.L. Egg consumption modulates HDL lipid composition and increases the cholesterol-accepting capacity of serum in metabolic syndrome. *Lipids* **2013**, *48*, 557–567. [CrossRef] [PubMed]

78. Khera, A.V.; Cuchel, M.; de la Llera-Moya, M.; Rodrigues, A.; Burke, M.F.; Jafri, K.; French, B.C.; Phillips, J.A.; Mucksavage, M.L.; Wilensky, R.L.; *et al.* Cholesterol efflux capacity, high-density lipoprotein function, and atherosclerosis. *N. Engl. J. Med.* **2011**, *364*, 127–135. [CrossRef] [PubMed]

79. Oram, J.F.; Vaughan, A.M. ATP-binding cassette cholesterol transporters and cardiovascular disease. *Circ. Res.* **2006**, *99*, 1031–1043. [CrossRef] [PubMed]

80. Ratliff, J.C.; Mutungi, G.; Puglisi, M.J.; Volek, J.S.; Fernandez, M.L. Eggs modulate the inflammatory response to carbohydrate restricted diets in overweight men. *Nutr. Metab. (Lond.)* **2008**, *5*, 6. [CrossRef]

81. Blesso, C.N.; Andersen, C.J.; Barona, J.; Volk, B.; Volek, J.S.; Fernandez, M.L. Effects of carbohydrate restriction and dietary cholesterol provided by eggs on clinical risk factors in metabolic syndrome. *J. Clin. Lipidol.* **2013**, *7*, 463–471. [CrossRef] [PubMed]

82. Detopoulou, P.; Panagiotakos, D.B.; Antonopoulou, S.; Pitsavos, C.; Stefanadis, C. Dietary choline and betaine intakes in relation to concentrations of inflammatory markers in healthy adults: The ATTICA study. *Am. J. Clin. Nutr.* **2008**, *87*, 424–430. [PubMed]

83. Parrish, W.R.; Rosas-Ballina, M.; Gallowitsch-Puerta, M.; Ochani, M.; Ochani, K.; Yang, L.H.; Hudson, L.; Lin, X.; Patel, N.; Johnson, S.M.; *et al.* Modulation of tnf release by choline requires alpha7 subunit nicotinic acetylcholine receptor-mediated signaling. *Mol. Med.* **2008**, *14*, 567–574. [CrossRef] [PubMed]

84. Tracey, K.J. Reflex control of immunity. *Nat. Rev. Immunol.* **2009**, *9*, 418–428. [CrossRef] [PubMed]

85. Hartmann, P.; Szabo, A.; Eros, G.; Gurabi, D.; Horvath, G.; Nemeth, I.; Ghyczy, M.; Boros, M. Anti-inflammatory effects of phosphatidylcholine in neutrophil leukocyte-dependent acute arthritis in rats. *Eur. J. Pharmacol.* **2009**, *622*, 58–64. [CrossRef] [PubMed]

86. Stremmel, W.; Braun, A.; Hanemann, A.; Ehehalt, R.; Autschbach, F.; Karner, M. Delayed release phosphatidylcholine in chronic-active ulcerative colitis: A randomized, double-blinded, dose finding study. *J. Clin. Gastroenterol.* **2010**, *44*, e101–e107. [PubMed]

87. Ding, S.; Lund, P.K. Role of intestinal inflammation as an early event in obesity and insulin resistance. *Curr. Opin. Clin. Nutr. Metab. Care* **2011**, *14*, 328–333. [CrossRef] [PubMed]

88. Field, F.J.; Watt, K.; Mathur, S.N. TNF-alpha decreases ABCA1 expression and attenuates HDL cholesterol efflux in the human intestinal cell line Caco-2. *J. Lipid Res.* **2010**, *51*, 1407–1415. [CrossRef] [PubMed]

89. Van Leuven, S.I.; Hezemans, R.; Levels, J.H.; Snoek, S.; Stokkers, P.C.; Hovingh, G.K.; Kastelein, J.J.; Stroes, E.S.; de Groot, E.; Hommes, D.W. Enhanced atherogenesis and altered high density lipoprotein in patients with Crohn's disease. *J. Lipid Res.* **2007**, *48*, 2640–2646. [CrossRef] [PubMed]

90. Wang, Z.; Klipfell, E.; Bennett, B.J.; Koeth, R.; Levison, B.S.; Dugar, B.; Feldstein, A.E.; Britt, E.B.; Fu, X.; Chung, Y.M.; *et al.* Gut flora metabolism of phosphatidylcholine promotes cardiovascular disease. *Nature* **2011**, *472*, 57–63. [CrossRef] [PubMed]

91. Al-Waiz, M.; Mikov, M.; Mitchell, S.C.; Smith, R.L. The exogenous origin of trimethylamine in the mouse. *Metabolism* **1992**, *41*, 135–136. [CrossRef] [PubMed]

92. Lang, D.H.; Yeung, C.K.; Peter, R.M.; Ibarra, C.; Gasser, R.; Itagaki, K.; Philpot, R.M.; Rettie, A.E. Isoform specificity of trimethylamine N-oxygenation by human flavin-containing monooxygenase (FMO) and p450 enzymes: Selective catalysis by FMO3. *Biochem. Pharmacol.* **1998**, *56*, 1005–1012. [CrossRef] [PubMed]

93. Hartiala, J.; Bennett, B.J.; Tang, W.H.; Wang, Z.; Stewart, A.F.; Roberts, R.; McPherson, R.; Lusis, A.J.; Hazen, S.L.; Allayee, H. Comparative genome-wide association studies in mice and humans for trimethylamine N-oxide, a proatherogenic metabolite of choline and L-carnitine. *Arterioscler. Thromb. Vasc. Biol.* **2014**, *34*, 1307–1313. [CrossRef] [PubMed]

94. Koeth, R.A.; Wang, Z.; Levison, B.S.; Buffa, J.A.; Org, E.; Sheehy, B.T.; Britt, E.B.; Fu, X.; Wu, Y.; Li, L.; *et al.* Intestinal microbiota metabolism of L-carnitine, a nutrient in red meat, promotes atherosclerosis. *Nat. Med.* **2013**, *19*, 576–585. [CrossRef] [PubMed]

95. Tang, W.H.; Wang, Z.; Levison, B.S.; Koeth, R.A.; Britt, E.B.; Fu, X.; Wu, Y.; Hazen, S.L. Intestinal microbial metabolism of phosphatidylcholine and cardiovascular risk. *N. Engl. J. Med.* **2013**, *368*, 1575–1584. [CrossRef] [PubMed]

96. Tang, W.H.; Hazen, S.L. The contributory role of gut microbiota in cardiovascular disease. *J. Clin. Investig.* **2014**, *124*, 4204–4211. [CrossRef] [PubMed]

97. Miller, C.A.; Corbin, K.D.; da Costa, K.A.; Zhang, S.; Zhao, X.; Galanko, J.A.; Blevins, T.; Bennett, B.J.; O'Connor, A.; Zeisel, S.H. Effect of egg ingestion on trimethylamine-N-oxide production in humans: A randomized, controlled, dose-response study. *Am. J. Clin. Nutr.* **2014**, *100*, 778–786. [CrossRef] [PubMed]

98. Northfield, T.C.; Hofmann, A.F. Biliary lipid output during three meals and an overnight fast. I. Relationship to bile acid pool size and cholesterol saturation of bile in gallstone and control subjects. *Gut* **1975**, *16*, 1–11. [CrossRef] [PubMed]

99. Richmond, B.L.; Boileau, A.C.; Zheng, S.; Huggins, K.W.; Granholm, N.A.; Tso, P.; Hui, D.Y. Compensatory phospholipid digestion is required for cholesterol absorption in pancreatic phospholipase A(2)-deficient mice. *Gastroenterology* **2001**, *120*, 1193–1202. [CrossRef] [PubMed]

100. Takemori, H.; Zolotaryov, F.N.; Ting, L.; Urbain, T.; Komatsubara, T.; Hatano, O.; Okamoto, M.; Tojo, H. Identification of functional domains of rat intestinal phospholipase B/lipase. Its cDNA cloning, expression, and tissue distribution. *J. Biol. Chem.* **1998**, *273*, 2222–2231. [CrossRef] [PubMed]

101. Djousse, L.; Gaziano, J.M. Egg consumption in relation to cardiovascular disease and mortality: The Physicians' Health Study. *Am. J. Clin. Nutr.* **2008**, *87*, 964–969. [PubMed]

102. Tanasescu, M.; Cho, E.; Manson, J.E.; Hu, F.B. Dietary fat and cholesterol and the risk of cardiovascular disease among women with type 2 diabetes. *Am. J. Clin. Nutr.* **2004**, *79*, 999–1005. [PubMed]

103. Tang, W.H.; Wang, Z.; Shrestha, K.; Borowski, A.G.; Wu, Y.; Troughton, R.W.; Klein, A.L.; Hazen, S.L. Intestinal microbiota-dependent phosphatidylcholine metabolites, diastolic dysfunction, and adverse clinical outcomes in chronic systolic heart failure. *J. Card. Fail.* **2015**, *21*, 91–96. [CrossRef] [PubMed]

104. Tang, W.H.; Wang, Z.; Fan, Y.; Levison, B.; Hazen, J.E.; Donahue, L.M.; Wu, Y.; Hazen, S.L. Prognostic value of elevated levels of intestinal microbe-generated metabolite trimethylamine-*N*-oxide in patients with heart failure: Refining the gut hypothesis. *J. Am. Coll. Cardiol.* **2014**, *64*, 1908–1914. [CrossRef] [PubMed]
105. Tang, W.H.; Wang, Z.; Kennedy, D.J.; Wu, Y.; Buffa, J.A.; Agatisa-Boyle, B.; Li, X.S.; Levison, B.S.; Hazen, S.L. Gut microbiota-dependent trimethylamine *N*-oxide (TMAO) pathway contributes to both development of renal insufficiency and mortality risk in chronic kidney disease. *Circ. Res.* **2015**, *116*, 448–455. [CrossRef] [PubMed]

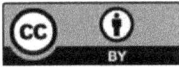

nutrients

MDPI

Article

One Egg per Day Improves Inflammation When Compared to an Oatmeal-Based Breakfast without Increasing Other Cardiometabolic Risk Factors in Diabetic Patients

Martha Nydia Ballesteros [1], Fabrizio Valenzuela [1], Alma E. Robles [1], Elizabeth Artalejo [1], David Aguilar [2], Catherine J. Andersen [2], Herlindo Valdez [3] and Maria Luz Fernandez [2,*]

[1] Centro de Investigacion y Desarrollo (CIAD), Hermosillo, Sonora, 83304, Mexico; nydia@ciad.mx (M.N.B.); fabe_vi@hotmail.com (F.V.); melina@ciad.mx (A.E.R.); eartalejo@ciad.mx (E.A.)
[2] Department of Nutritional Sciences, University of Connecticut, Storrs, CT 06269, USA; david_178@hotmail.com (D.A.); candersen@fairfield.edu (C.J.A.)
[3] Hospital Ignacio Chavez, Hermosillo, Sonora, 83190, Mexico; herlindov@yahoo.com.mx
* Author to whom correspondence should be addressed; maria-luz.fernandez@uconn.edu; Tel.: +1-860-486-5547; Fax: +1-860-486-3674.

Received: 3 April 2015; Accepted: 5 May 2015; Published: 11 May 2015

Abstract: There is concern that egg intake may increase blood glucose in patients with type 2 diabetes mellitus (T2DM). However, we have previously shown that eggs reduce inflammation in patients at risk for T2DM, including obese subjects and those with metabolic syndrome. Thus, we hypothesized that egg intake would not alter plasma glucose in T2DM patients when compared to oatmeal intake. Our primary endpoints for this clinical intervention were plasma glucose and the inflammatory markers tumor necrosis factor (TNF)-α and interleukin 6 (IL-6). As secondary endpoints, we evaluated additional parameters of glucose metabolism, dyslipidemias, oxidative stress and inflammation. Twenty-nine subjects, 35–65 years with glycosylated hemoglobin (HbA1c) values <9% were recruited and randomly allocated to consume isocaloric breakfasts containing either one egg/day or 40 g of oatmeal with 472 mL of lactose-free milk/day for five weeks. Following a three-week washout period, subjects were assigned to the alternate breakfast. At the end of each period, we measured all primary and secondary endpoints. Subjects completed four-day dietary recalls and one exercise questionnaire for each breakfast period. There were no significant differences in plasma glucose, our primary endpoint, plasma lipids, lipoprotein size or subfraction concentrations, insulin, HbA1c, apolipoprotein B, oxidized LDL or C-reactive protein. However, after adjusting for gender, age and body mass index, aspartate amino-transferase (AST) ($p < 0.05$) and tumor necrosis factor (TNF)-α ($p < 0.01$), one of our primary endpoints were significantly reduced during the egg period. These results suggest that compared to an oatmeal-based breakfast, eggs do not have any detrimental effects on lipoprotein or glucose metabolism in T2DM. In contrast, eggs reduce AST and TNF-α in this population characterized by chronic low-grade inflammation.

Keywords: diabetes; eggs; lipoproteins; TNF-α; IL-6; glucose; inflammation

1. Introduction

Epidemiological studies report controversies on the effects of dietary cholesterol and egg intake on the risk for heart disease in patients with diabetes [1,2]. There is also uncertainty regarding the associations between dietary cholesterol and the development of diabetes [3,4]. While some epidemiological studies report a correlation between dietary cholesterol and diabetes risk [5,6], others fail to find this relationship [3,7]. Thus, there is a need for randomized clinical trials to fully understand the effects of egg intake on plasma glucose and markers of heart disease risk in patients diagnosed with type 2 diabetes mellitus (T2DM). Individuals with T2DM are characterized by having impaired glucose metabolism, atherogenic dyslipidemia [8], and chronic low-grade inflammation [9], therefore, recommended foods for diabetic patients should either improve, or have no detrimental effect on biomarkers associated with these conditions.

Oatmeal is recognized as a heart-healthy breakfast due to the effects of β-glucan on reducing plasma LDL cholesterol (LDL-C) [10]. Oatmeal has also been shown to decrease blood glucose in 14 patients with uncontrolled T2DM [11]. In contrast, eggs are identified as a food that might raise plasma LDL-C [12], or that could potentially alter glucose metabolism and lead to diabetes [13].

It has been documented that the Latino population has a genetic predisposition for developing T2DM [14]. In Mexico, 35.7 and 37.2% of adults ≥20 years old are overweight and obese, respectively—a dramatic increase from 2006 (26 and 29%) [15]. This obesity epidemic, combined with the genetic predisposition of Latinos for developing T2DM, contributes to one of the highest incidences of diabetes worldwide [16], with the northern state of Sonora having one of the greatest rates of diabetes in the country [17].

We aimed to compare two breakfasts with perceived differences in effects on heart disease risk, eggs and oatmeal, by conducting a randomized, crossover clinical trial in subjects with T2DM. We evaluated the effects of consuming one egg per day for a relatively extended period (five weeks) *versus* 1/2 cup (40 g) of oatmeal per day on plasma glucose and inflammatory markers, our primary endpoints. Our secondary endpoints included plasma lipids, markers of oxidative stress, and parameters of glucose metabolism, such as glycosylated hemoglobin (HbA1c). We hypothesized that eating one egg per day would not adversely affect primary or secondary endpoints when compared to an oatmeal breakfast. We further hypothesized that eggs would reduce inflammatory markers in this population, likely due to the presence of highly bioavailable carotenoids [18]. Due to the high rate of diabetes, in combination with the fact that Mexico is one of the countries that consumes most eggs per capita (approx. one egg/person/day) [19], we chose our intervention population from the city of Hermosillo, Sonora to conduct this clinical trial.

2. Experimental Section

2.1. Experimental Design

We recruited 33 subjects (aged 35–65 years) diagnosed with T2DM to participate in this randomized crossover design study in the city of Hermosillo, Mexico. Based on the standard deviation from our previous studies where we observed changes in inflammatory markers and using a Z value of 1.96 (95% confidence interval), we estimated that 25 subjects would be sufficient to observe differences between groups [20,21]. We aimed to recruit 35 subjects to allow for attrition. The study took place between June–December 2013, from the first subject who was enrolled to study completion by the last enrolled participant. The exclusion criteria were uncontrolled diabetes, retinopathy, heart disease, cancer, or renal problems. In addition, participants had to have HbA1c <9% (74.9 mmol/mol). On an alternating basis, participants were randomly allocated by one of the researchers to consume either one egg/day or 40 g of oatmeal with 2 cups (472 mL) of lactose-free milk/day for 5 weeks. At the end of the first period, subjects had a 3-week washout followed by allocation to the alternate breakfast for an additional 5 weeks. Eggs, oatmeal and lactose-free milk were provided to the subjects every 2 weeks and they returned the uneaten portions, which were recorded by the researchers. Compliance for both breakfasts was 98 ± 2%. Eggs were purchased from Bachoco, Inc. (Hermosillo, Mexico). Eggs weighed an average of 65 g and contained 8 g protein, 6.8 g fat and 0.3 g carbohydrate. The content of cholesterol was 250 mg and lutein was 180 μg as previously determined [22]. Oatmeal (Quaker oatmeal) was purchased from the local super-market. The average consumption was 1/2 measured cup (40 g) consisting of 5.5 g protein, 3.6 g fat, 23.6 g of total carbohydrate; total fiber was 3.2 g and soluble fiber 0.85 g. Subjects were provided with measuring cups for the oatmeal and they were told not to consume oatmeal or eggs during the whole intervention except those provided by the researchers. Subjects were closely monitored by random phone calls to ensure compliance. All analysis for the study, including experimental analysis of primary and secondary endpoints, were conducted by researchers who were blinded to breakfast allocation.

Twenty-nine subjects finished both dietary interventions. Three subjects dropped out of the study due to personal reasons and 1 subject was removed due to non-compliance with the dietary treatments. In order to maintain control of T2DM, all subjects were taking glucose-lowering medications, as prescribed by their physician, including metmorfin ($n = 26$) and insulin ($n = 6$). In addition, 18 subjects were taking blood pressure medication and 9 were on reductase inhibitors. The intervention protocol was approved by the University of Connecticut Institutional Review Board, the Ethical Committee from Centro de Investigacion en Alimentacion y Desarrollo (CIAD), and the Review Board from Hospital Chávez. All subjects gave written informed consent prior to initiating the study. This study is registered at Clinicaltrials.gov (trial # NCT02181244)

2.2. Diet and Exercise Assessment

Diet was assessed by using four 24-h dietary recalls at the end of each breakfast period, which included 2 weekdays and 2 weekend days. Subjects were visited by trained dietitians, who interviewed the subjects to complete all dietary recalls. Nutrient analysis was conducted utilizing ESHA Food Processor II, version 2007, to which typical diets associated with this region in Mexico have been added. Subjects received specific instructions to include all foods and ingredients in their dietary recall, in addition to their respective breakfast foods during the intervention. Participants were instructed to abstain from consuming oatmeal or eggs during the whole 13-week of the intervention, with the exception of treatment foods provided by the researchers. A typical breakfast consisted of either one egg, usually scrambled, accompanied by vegetables and 2 slices of bread or 2 tortillas, or 40 g of oatmeal with 2 cups (472 mL) of lactose-free milk. We provided lactose-free milk to control for potential lactose intolerance, which is very common in adults from Hispanic origin. The average amount of calories consumed for breakfast was 313 kcal/day for the egg period and 335 kcal/day for the oatmeal period. An exercise diary was also provided to subjects to ensure that there were no changes in their activity level during the interventions. Subjects provided 3 exercise dairies at the end of each breakfast period. All participants were very closely monitored by their physician (HV) throughout the whole study to ensure that they did not change their medications. They were also monitored by the researchers to ensure compliance with egg and oatmeal intake, and to ascertain that they did not change the rest of their dietary habits or their level of physical activity during the 13-week intervention.

2.3. Anthropometrics, Body Fat and Blood Pressure

Weight was measured to the nearest 0.1 kg, height was measured to the nearest centimeter, and body mass index (BMI) was calculated as kg/m². Body fat was measured by electric bioimpedance using an Impedimed IMP5™ (Impedimed Pty Ltd, Carlsbad, CA, USA). Blood pressure was measured with an automated blood pressure monitor (Desk Model Sphingomanometer, Model 100, Bannockburn, IL, USA) after a 5 min rest. The average of 3 separate recordings is reported.

2.4. Plasma Lipids, Oxidized-LDL and Apolipoprotein B

Subjects fasted 12 h prior to blood draws. Plasma was separated from red blood cells by centrifugation at 2400× *g* to measure plasma total cholesterol (TC), LDL (LDL-C), HDL (HDL-C) and triglycerides by using the Cobas c-111 Clinical Analyzer (Roche Diagnostics, Indianapolis, IN, USA). Oxidized-LDL was measured by using an ELISA kit from Mercodia (Uppsala, Sweden) and Apolipoprotein B by utilizing an ELISA kit from Abcam (Cambridge, MA, USA).

2.5. Glucose, Insulin and Homeostatic Mode Assessment (HOMA)

Fasting glucose concentrations, one of our primary endpoints, was analyzed by an enzymatic colorimetric method (Roche Diagnostics, Indianapolis, IN, USA). Plasma insulin was determined with an ELISA method (ALPCO Diagnostics, Salem, NH, USA). The homeostasis model assessment

(HOMA) was used to calculate insulin resistance [23]. HbA1c was measured by utilizing an immunoturbidimetric method standardized by the National Glycohemoglobin standardization program (Roche Diagnostics, Indianapolis, IN, USA).

2.6. Determination of Size and Concentrations of VLDL, LDL and HDL Subfractions

Lipoprotein subclass profiles and diameters were measured by proton NMR spectroscopy as previously reported [24]. This method uses characteristic signals broadcast by lipoprotein subclasses of different size.

2.7. Inflammatory Markers, Liver Enzymes and Adiponectin

Alanine aminotransferase (ALT), aspartate aminotransferase (AST), and C-reactive protein (CRP) were measured using the Cobas c-111 Clinical Analyzer. Interleukin-6 (IL-6) and tumor necrosis factor-α (TNF-α), the other two primary endpoints, were measured utilizing ELISA kits (BD Biosciences, San Jose, CA, USA). Adiponectin was measured by using a Quantikine ELISA by RD Systems Inc. (Minneapolis, MN, USA).

2.8. Statistical Analysis

SPSS version 13.2 was used for Statistics. A paired *t*-test was used to evaluate differences in all measured parameters between the oatmeal and the egg periods. Values are reported as mean $\pm$ SD. A *p*-value < 0.05 was considered to be significant. Those parameters that were significantly different by paired *t*-test were further analyzed by using gender, age and initial BMI as covariates.

3. Results

3.1. Flow Chart of the Study

As indicated in Figure 1, we consented 37 patients for this study. Four of them were excluded because they did not meet the inclusion/exclusion criteria. From these four, three had HbA1c levels >9%, and one did not have diabetes as determined by blood glucose levels and glucose tolerance tests. The 33 patients who met the inclusion criteria were randomly allocated to consume eggs (*n* = 16) or oatmeal (*n* = 17). Before the crossover, three patients decided not to continue the study and one was removed by the investigators due to non-compliance. Twenty-nine patients finished the whole intervention. All measured variables presented are for these 33 patients.

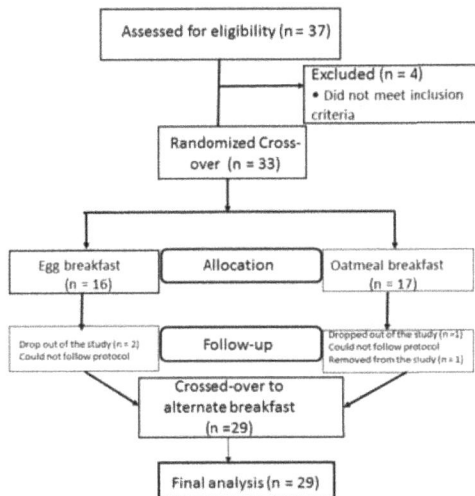

Figure 1. Flow chart of the study.

3.2. Baseline Characteristics

The baseline characteristics of subjects are presented in Table 1. The average age of this population was 53.5 years and the gender distribution was 19 females and 10 males. The mean value for HbA1c was 6.75% (50 mmol/mol) indicating good average glycemic control in this population. Seven subjects were taking statins and 18 subjects were taking hypotensive medications. The majority of subjects (*n* = 27) had plasma TC < 2.5 mmol/L, LDL-C < 1.2 mmol/L, and blood pressure < 130/85 mmHg. Plasma triglycerides were high with a mean 2.2 ± 1.2 mmo/L, typical of a diabetic population.

Table 1. Baseline Characteristics of Subjects *.

Parameter (*n* = 29)	Values
Age (years)	53.5 ± 8.3
Gender (*n* = F/M)	19/10
Total Cholesterol (mmol/L)	4.1 ± 0.7
LDL Cholesterol (mmol/L)	2.3 ± 0.6
Triglycerides (mmol/L)	2.2 ± 1.0
HDL Cholesterol (mmol/L)	1.0 ± 0.2
LDL-C/HDL-C	2.4 ± 1.1
Glucose (mmol/L)	9.0 ± 3.1
Glycosylated Hemoglobin (%) (mmol/L)	6.75 ± 0.89 (50 ± 9.7)

* Values are presented as mean ± SD; *n* = 29.

3.3. Primary end Points

Results for the primary endpoints are presented in Figure 2. There were no differences in plasma glucose concentrations between the egg and oatmeal periods (Figure 2A). Similarly, there was a significant reduction in TNF-α, the other primary endpoints after the egg breakfast period, while IL-6 was, was borderline significant (*p* = 0.051). (Figure 2B).

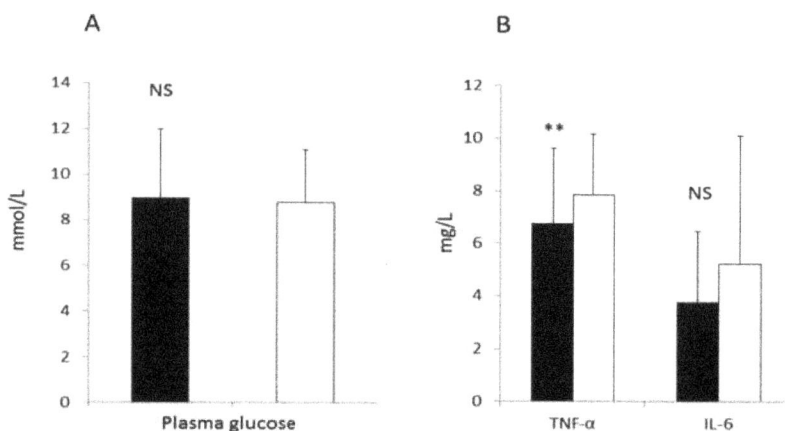

Figure 2. Plasma concentrations of glucose (**A**) and plasma concentrations of interleukin 6 (IL-6) and tumor necrosis factor-α (TNF-α) (**B**) after the egg (dark bar) and the oatmeal (white bar). Mean values for plasma glucose were 9.0 ± 3.0 mmol/L and 8.8 ± 2.3 mmol/L after the oatmeal periods. IL-6 were 3.8 ± 2.7 pg/mL following the egg breakfast (*p* = 0.051) and 5.2 ± 4.8 pg/mL after the oatmeal and for TNF-α were 6.7 ± 2.8 pg/mL after the egg breakfast (*p* = 0.007) and 7.9 ± 2.7 pg/mL after the oatmeal. *Indicates significantly different *p* < 0.05 and ** *p* < 0.01. NS = non-significant.

3.4. Diet

Dietary intake in egg and oatmeal periods is presented in Table 2. Total energy and percent energy from protein were not different between periods. In contrast, percent energy from carbohydrate was higher in the oatmeal period ($p < 0.01$), while percent of energy from total fat, and saturated, monounsaturated and polyunsaturated fatty acids (g) were higher during the egg period ($p < 0.001$). Total and soluble fiber intake was higher during the oatmeal period ($p < 0.01$), while dietary cholesterol was higher during the egg period ($p < 0.01$) (Table 2). Interestingly, intakes of lutein and zeaxanthin, the carotenoids present in eggs, were not different between dietary periods (Table 2).

Table 2. Dietary intake during Egg and Oatmeal Periods *.

Parameter	Egg	Oatmeal	*p* Value
Energy (Kcal)	1629 ± 410	1686 ± 362	0.278
Protein (%)	18.9 ± 3.5	20.0 ± 3.5	0.134
Carbohydrate (%)	50.3 ± 6.5	55.1 ± 7.3	0.010
Total Fat (%)	31.6 ± 5.6	24.7 ± 6.8	<0.0001
SFA (g/day)	21.0 ± 8.9	17.3 ± 9.4	0.043
MUFA (g/day)	17.0 ± 5.3	12.8 ± 6.6	0.006
PUFA (g/day)	8.1 ± 2.4	6.3 ± 2.8	0.009
Total Fiber (g/day)	26.0 ± 10.1	27.5 ± 9.2	0.345
Soluble Fiber (g/day)	5.2 ± 3.3	6.7 ± 3.1	0.008
Insoluble Fiber (g/day)	13.3 ± 5.6	15.2 ± 5.7	0.073
Cholesterol (mg/day)	435.0 ± 119.8	149.4 ± 77	<0.0001
Lutein + Zeaxanthin (μg/day)	1213 ± 1731	1003 ± 1742	0.185
Glycemic Index	49.2 ± 8.7	48.5 ± 7.7	0.752
Glycemic Load	17.3 ± 9.4	17.1 ± 21.3	0.828

* Values are presented as mean ± SD; *n* = 29 subjects.

3.5. Anthropometrics, Blood Pressure, Plasma Lipids, HbA1c and Insulin

There were no significant differences in body weight, body fat, BMI or blood pressure between the egg and oatmeal periods (Table 3). Similarly, body weight was not different from baseline or the washout period (data not shown). While only nine subjects were taking blood pressure medications, all subjects had systolic and diastolic blood pressure < 130/85 mmHg. Similarly, there were no significant differences in TC, LDL-C, HDL-C, triglycerides, LDL-C/HDL-C ratio, apolipoprotein B, Ox-LDL, HbA1c, insulin and insulin resistance measured by HOMA when comparing the egg *versus* oatmeal periods (Table 3). Values for anthropometrics, plasma lipids, glucose and HbA1c were not different between baseline and washout periods ($p > 0.05$) (data not shown).

3.6. Lipoprotein Number and Subclasses

There were no differences in total lipoprotein number or concentrations of lipoprotein subclasses between the egg and the oatmeal periods including the atherogenic lipoproteins large VLDL, IDL and small LDL (Table 4).

3.7. CRP and Liver Enzymes

CRP (6.96 ± 10.15 *vs.* 6.87 ± 8.98 mg/L), adiponectin (6.2 ± 3.2 *vs.* 5.6 ± 2.2 μg/mL), and ALT 24.3 ± 11.7 *vs.* 26.3 ± 13.0 IU/L) were not different when compared at the end of egg and oatmeal periods, respectively. However, AST was significantly reduced following the egg period ($p < 0.05$). Data for liver enzymes is presented in Figure 3.

Table 3. Anthropometrics, Blood Pressure (BP), Plasma Lipids, Oxidized LDL, Apolipoprotein B, Glucose, Glycosylated Hemoglobin, Insulin and HOMA after the Egg and Oatmeal Breakfasts *.

Parameter (*n* = 29)	Egg	Oatmeal
Weight (kg)	82.1 ±17.0	82.1 ± 17.1
BMI (kg/m^2)	30.8 ± 6.4	30.8 ± 6.5
Body Fat (%)	45 ± 9	44 ± 8
Systolic BP (mmHg)	123.5 ± 11.1	123.8 ± 11.3
Diastolic BP (mmHg)	76.1 ± 7.4	76.1 ± 8.0
Total cholesterol (mmol/L)	4.1 ± 1.5	4.0 ± 0.8
LDL cholesterol (mmol/L)	2.5 ± 0.6	2.4 ± 0.6
Triglycerides (mmol/L)	1.48 ± 0.47	1.53 ± 0.55
HDL cholesterol (mmol/L)	1.17 ± 0.23	1.14 ± 0.21
LDL-C/HDL-C	1.99 ± 0.72	1.95 ± 0.68
Apolipoprotein B (mg/L)	90.8 ± 33.9	95 ± 38
Oxidized LDL (U/L)	76.9 ± 25.3	80.6 ± 32.7
Glycosylated Hemoglobin (%)	6.55 ± 0.93	6.60 ± 1.04
Insulin (pmol/L)	101.4 ± 63.2	86.8 ± 50.7
HOMA	3.7 ± 0.7	3.1 ± 0.6

* Values are presented as mean ± SD. There were no significant differences between groups in any of these parameters as measured by paired t-test.

Table 4. Concentrations of VLDL, IDL, LDL, and HDL subclasses after the egg and oatmeal breakfasts *.

Parameter (*n* = 29)	Egg	Oatmeal
Total VLDL Particles (mmo/L)	53.8 ± 27.7	53.1 ± 26.4
Large VLDL (mmol/L)	7.0 ± 4.5	7.6 ± 5.1
Medium VLDL (mmol/L)	21.9 ± 12.3	21.6 ± 13.5
Small VLDL(mmol/L)	24.9 ±17.6	23.8 ± 13.1
Total LDL (mmol/L)	1117 ± 290	1064 ± 253
Large LDL(mmol/L)	189 ± 147	215 ± 141
Small LDL(mmol/L)	775 ± 251	715 ± 230
IDL(mmol/L)	152 ± 89	134 ± 103
Total HDL Particles (µmol/L)	32.7 ± 5.8	33.2 ± 6.3
Large HDL(µmol/L)	3.74 ± 1.88	3.64 ± 1.98
Medium HDL(µmol/L)	8.21 ± 5.33	8.34 ± 5.41
Small HDL(µmol/L)	20.71 ± 3.71	21.17 ± 3.94

* Values are presented as mean ± SD. There were no significant differences between groups in any of these parameters as measured by paired t-test.

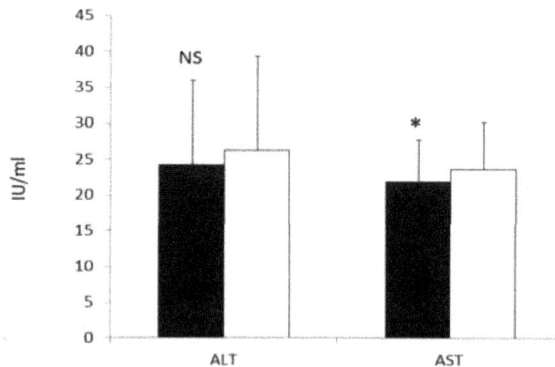

Figure 3. Concentrations of liver enzymes after the egg (dark bar) and the oatmeal (white bar) periods. ALT did not differ between treatments; However, AST was significantly reduced ($p < 0.05$) after the egg period (21.9 ± 5.8 *vs.* 23.7 ± 6.4 IU/L)

4. Discussion

In this very well-controlled randomized, crossover clinical trial, we have demonstrated that consuming 1 egg per day for breakfast during 5 weeks did not alter plasma glucose one of the primary end points. This is a key finding in regards to the current controversies of egg intake affecting plasma glucose levels in individuals with diabetes [3,4]. Further, our results have shown that consuming 1 egg per day could be considered potentially beneficial for this population as documented by the observed reductions in the inflammatory marker, TNF-α, the other primary end point, when compared to consumption of oatmeal.

We have also demonstrated that consuming 1 egg per day for breakfast during 5 weeks did not alter plasma lipids, atherogenic lipoproteins, other parameters of glucose metabolism and CRP when compared to an oatmeal-based breakfast in individuals diagnosed with T2DM. We have previously shown that 4 weeks is sufficient time to see lipid changes following dietary egg challenges [25,26]. For this study, we followed subjects for an additional week, yet still observed no modifications in plasma lipids.

This is one of the first clinical trials in which egg effects on cholesterol and glucose metabolism were determined in a compromised population characterized by having dyslipidemias, insulin resistance and elevated concentrations of plasma inflammatory markers. The results suggest that egg intake (one per day) can be easily incorporated into the diets of patients with T2DM, with no apparent concerns for causing dysregulation of glucose metabolism or formation of atherogenic particles. The beneficial effects on inflammatory markers confirm what we have observed in past studies regarding the effects of eggs in decreasing inflammation in other populations at high risk for heart disease and diabetes, including obesity [20] and metabolic syndrome [21]. In a recent clinical trial, high and low cholesterol diets were compared in 65 individuals with T2DM [27]. Similar to our design, authors used eggs as a source of dietary cholesterol and they reported that the egg diet was more effective in improving glycemic control and the lipid profile by raising HDL-C [27].

Oatmeal has been shown to decrease LDL-C in healthy and hypercholesterolemic individuals [28] in clinical trials, possibly due to the presence of β-glucan, a component present in oats that has been shown to lower cholesterol by disrupting micelle formation and decreasing absorption of dietary cholesterol and bile acids [29]. Thus, it is well recognized that oatmeal is a "heart healthy" food that is recommended for all populations, including diabetic subjects [30]. In contrast, due to the high content of dietary cholesterol, eggs have been identified as a food that should be avoided not only in diseased patients, but also in healthy populations [31]. We have previously demonstrated that consumption of two to three eggs per day for periods between 4 to 12 weeks does not increase the risk profile for heart disease in healthy populations [25,26,32]. Most of our subjects (about 2/3 of the population) do not experience fluctuations in plasma cholesterol following a dietary cholesterol challenge. For those who have increases in plasma total cholesterol, both LDL-C and HDL-C raise with maintenance of the LDL-C/HDL-C ratio [25,26,32]. Further, during weight loss interventions, plasma LDL-C does not change even after consuming three eggs per day during 12 weeks, while HDL-C increases with an improvement of the LDL-C/HDL-C ratio [20,21].

Contrary to the findings of Pearce *et al.* [27], who were using a high protein, energy-restricted diet, our current study found that neither LDL-C nor HDL-C were altered by the egg breakfast when compared to the oatmeal breakfast, an interesting finding due to the documented effect of oatmeal in lowering LDL-C [27]. Although we have previously shown that egg intake increases the formation of large HDL, which has been postulated to promote reverse cholesterol transport [33], and the formation of large LDL, a particle that has been suggested to be less atherogenic [34], we failed to observe any changes in LDL or HDL size between dietary periods in these diabetic patients.

These results indicating a lack of effect of egg and oatmeal consumption on plasma lipids and lipoproteins may be attributable to several factors. In our previous studies, we challenged our subjects with two to three eggs per day [25,26,32], whereas this current study evaluated the effect of consuming only one egg per day; thus, the higher concentrations of both cholesterol and egg phospholipids provided in our previous studies may be related to the formation of the larger lipoprotein particles [34,35]. Another interpretation is that diabetes substantially alters lipoprotein metabolism [36], and consumption of one egg per day was not sufficient to reverse these metabolic abnormalities. Although the number of large and small LDL particles found in this study are similar to those observed in overweight/obese [35] and metabolic syndrome [21,37] populations, the concentrations of intermediate-density lipoprotein (IDL) and large VLDL are higher in this study compared to previous observations in other high-risk populations [21,35,37]. The higher levels of IDL could be associated with the hypertriglyceridemia that is common in diabetes [36], which can lead to the formation of more IDL and large atherogenic VLDL particles.

In addition to maintaining fasting plasma glucose levels, our main finding in this study is that TNF-α and AST were reduced following the 5-week, one-egg-per-day breakfast. Chronic low-grade inflammation is a hallmark of diabetes and diabetic patients are characterized by having elevated concentrations of inflammatory markers [9]; thus, the observed reductions in plasma concentrations of AST and TNF-α following egg intake deserve further consideration, and may be explained by the presence of lutein and zeaxanthin in egg yolk. Although intake of these dietary carotenoids was not different between dietary periods, we have previously shown that plasma concentrations of lutein and zeaxanthin are significantly higher when eggs are the dietary source [38]. This is likely due to the higher bioavailability of egg-derived carotenoids [22]. In addition, lutein and zeaxanthin have been shown to have anti-oxidative and anti-inflammatory properties in cell studies [39], animal models [40] and humans [20,21]. The results from the current study highlight the importance of certain dietary carotenoids that could exert a protective effect against inflammation in those populations characterized by having chronic low-grade inflammation, as is the case of patients with diabetes.

The main strength of this study is that it was a controlled clinical intervention. We performed thorough dietary recalls and ensured that subjects did not change their activity level during the intervention period. We also provided the intervention foods and monitored consumption. In addition, the recruited subjects had good diabetic control as monitored by their HbA1c plasma concentrations, as well as the absence of extreme diabetes complications, which was a key element for subject compliance. Further, we ensured that subjects did not change their medication dose/type during the 13-week intervention. The weaknesses of this study include the short duration of the trial, which might not have been sufficient to determine changes in some of the measured parameters, and the fact that the data cannot be extrapolated for those diabetic patients with uncontrolled diabetes or additional complications associated with T2DM. Another perceived weakness is the lack of blinding of the subjects and that no intention to treat analysis was performed.

5. Conclusions

In this study, we have shown that eggs should not be a concern for those individuals with T2DM when HbA1c levels are well controlled. When compared to an oatmeal breakfast, one egg per day did not result in changes in plasma glucose, our primary end point, LDL-C, triglycerides or in the concentration of atherogenic particles including large VLDL, IDL or small LDL. Further, there were no changes in plasma insulin, HOMA or HbA1c, indicating that eggs can be consumed without any detrimental changes in lipoprotein or glucose metabolism in this population. The most interesting finding, however, was that eggs—possibly due to their content of highly bioavailable lutein and zeaxanthin—reduced inflammation in diabetic subjects when compared to oatmeal intake.

Acknowledgments: Supported by the Egg Nutrition Center from funds received by M.L.F.

Author Contributions: M.N.B. was in charge of recruiting and consenting of all patients, measuring plasma glucose, insulin, HbA1c and adiponectin. She provided substantial input in data analysis and reading the drafts of the manuscript; F.V. participated in subject consenting, monitoring of breakfasts, laboratory measurements and provided input in manuscript drafts; A.E.R. was involved in data collection, scheduling of patients and laboratory analysis; E.A. was responsible for blood drawing, body composition measurements and also participated in data analysis; D.A. and C.J.A. measured plasma lipids, inflammatory markers and liver enzymes, participated in data analysis, and read and revised drafts of the manuscript, H.V. was the physician responsible for patient care, and

Nutrients **2015**, *7*, 3449–3463

referred all subjects who participated in this study; M.L.F. was responsible for designing the experiment, obtaining the funds for conducting the study, supervising experimental design and data collection, conducted statistical analysis of all measured parameters and wrote the manuscript.

Conflicts of Interest: M.L.F. received funding from the Egg Nutrition Center to conduct the human intervention portion of this study. M.N.B., F.V., A.E.R., E.A., D.A., C.J.A., and H.V. declare no conflict of interest.

References

1. Shin, J.Y.; Xun, P.; Nakamura, Y.; He, K. Egg consumption in relation to risk of cardiovascular disease and diabetes: A systematic review and meta-analysis. *Am. J. Clin. Nutr.* **2013**, *98*, 146–159. [CrossRef] [PubMed]
2. Qureshi, A.I.; Suri, M.F.K.; Ajmed, S.; Nasar, A.; Divani, A.A.; Kirmani, J.F. Regular egg consumption does not increase the risk of stroke and cardiovascular diseases. *Med. Sci. Monit.* **2007**, *131*, CR1–CR8.
3. Djousse, L.; Kamineni, A.; Nelson, T.L.; Carnethon, M.; Mozaffarian, D.; Siscovick, D.; Mukamal, K.J. Egg consumption and risk of type 2 diabetes in older adults. *Am. J. Clin. Nutr.* **2010**, *92*, 422–427. [CrossRef] [PubMed]
4. Agrawal, S.; Ebrahim, S. Prevalence and risk factors for self-reported diabetes among adult men and women in India: Findings from a national cross-sectional survey. *Pub. Health Nutr.* **2011**, *15*, 1065–1077. [CrossRef]
5. Radzeviciene, L.; Ostrauskas, R. Egg consumption and the risk of type 2 diabetes mellitus: A case-control study. *Public Health Nutr.* **2012**, *15*, 1437–1441. [CrossRef] [PubMed]
6. Djousse, L.; Gaziano, J.M.; Buring, J.E.; Lee, I.M. Egg consumption and risk of type 2 diabetes in men and women. *Diabetes Care* **2009**, *32*, 295–300. [CrossRef] [PubMed]
7. Zazpe, I.; Beunza, J.J.; Bes-Rastrollo, M.; Basterra-Gortari, F.J.; Mari-Sanchis, A.; Martínez-González, M.Á.; SUN Project Investigators. Egg consumption and risk of type 2 diabetes in a Mediterranean cohort: The SUN Project. *Nutr. Hosp.* **2013**, *28*, 105–111.
8. Ng, D.S. Diabetic dyslipidemia: From evolving pathophysiological insight to emerging therapeutic targets. *Can. J. Diabetes* **2013**, *37*, 319–326. [CrossRef] [PubMed]
9. Kontoangelos, K.; Papageorgiuo, C.C.; Raptis, A.E.; Tsiotra, P.; Boutati, E.; Lambadiari, V.; Papadimitriou, G.N.; Rabavilas, A.D.; Dimitriadis, G.; Raptis, S.A. Cytokines, diabetes mellitus and psychopathology: A challenging combination. *Neuro Endocrinol. Lett.* **2014**, *35*, 159–169. [PubMed]
10. Thongoun, P.; Pavadhgul, P.; Burmrungpert, A.; Satitvipawee, P.; Harjani, Y.; Kurilich, A. Effect of oat consumption on lipid profiles in hypercholesterolemic adults. *J. Med. Assoc. Thai.* **2013**, *96* (Suppl. 5), S25–S32. [PubMed]
11. Lammert, A.; Kratzch, J.; Selhorst, J.; Humpert, P.M.; Bierhaus, A.; Birck, R.; Kusterek, K.; Hammes, H.P. Clinical benefit of a short term dietary oatmeal intervention in patients with type 2 diabetes and severe insulin resistance: A pilot study. *Exp. Clin. Endocrinol. Diabetes* **2008**, *116*, 132–134. [CrossRef] [PubMed]
12. Chakrabarty, G.; Biiljani, R.L.; Mahapatra, S.C.; Mehta, N.; Lakshmy, R.; Vashist, S.; Manchanda, S.C. The effect of ingestion of egg on serum lipid profile in healthy young free-living subjects. *Indian J. Physiol. Pharmacol.* **2002**, *46*, 492–498. [PubMed]
13. Li, Y.; Zhou, C.; Zhou, X.; Li, L. Egg consumption of cardiovascular diseases and diabetes: A meta-analysis. *Atherosclerosis* **2013**, *229*, 524–530. [CrossRef] [PubMed]
14. Pullinger, C.R.; Goldfind, I.D.; Tanyolac, S.; Movseyan, I.; Faynbaym, M.; Durlach, V.; Chiefan, E.; Foti, D.P.; Malloy, M.J.; Brunette, A.; *et al.* Evidence that an HMGA1 gene variant associates with type 2 diabetes, body mass index and high density lipoprotein cholesterol in a Hispanic-American population. *Metab. Syndr. Rel. Disord.* **2014**, *12*, 25–30. [CrossRef]
15. Gutiérrez, J.P.; Rivera-Dommarco, J.; Shamah-Levy, T.; Villalpando-Hernandez, S.; Romero-Martinez, M.; Hernandez-Avila, M. *Encuesta Nacional de Salud y Nutrición 2012. Resultados Nacionales*; Instituto Nacional de Salud Pública (MX): Cuernavaca, México, 2012.
16. Gonzalez-Villalpando, C.; Davila-Ce rvantes, C.A.; Zamora-Macorra, M.; Trejo-Valdivia, B.; Gonzalez-Villalpando, M.E. Incidence of type II diabetes in Mexico. Results of the Mexico City Diabetes study after 18 years follow-up. *Salud Publica Mex.* **2014**, *56*, 11–17.
17. Albarran, N.B.; Ballesteros, M.N.; Morales, G.G.; Ortega, M.I. Dietary behavior and type 2 diabetes care. *Patient Educ. Couns.* **2006**, *6*, 191–199. [CrossRef]

18. Chung, H.Y.; Rasmussen, H.M.; Johnson, E.J. Lutein bioavailability is higher from lutein-enriched eggs than from supplements and spinach in men. *J. Nutr.* **2004**, *134*, 1887–1893. [PubMed]
19. Thurnham, D.I. Macular zeaxanthins and lutein—A review of dietary sources and bioavailability and some relationships with macular pigment optical density and age-related macular disease. *Nutr. Res. Rev.* **2007**, *20*, 163–179. [CrossRef] [PubMed]
20. Ratliff, J.; Mutungi, G.; Puglisi, M.; Volek, J.S.; Fernandez, M.L. Eggs modulate the inflammatory response to carbohydrate restricted diets in overweight men. *Nutr. Metab. (Lond.)* **2008**, *5*, 6. [CrossRef]
21. Blesso, C.N.; Andersen, C.J.; Barona, J.; Volk, B.; Volek, J.S.; Fernandez, M.L. Effects of carbohydrate restriction and dietary cholesterol provided by eggs on clinical risk factors of metabolic syndrome. *J. Clin. Lipidol.* **2013**, *7*, 463–471. [CrossRef]
22. Ballesteros, M.N.; Cabrera, R.M.; Saucedo, M.S.; Fernandez, M.L. Intake of two eggs per day increases plasma lutein and zeaxanthin in a pediatric population at high risk for heart disease. *Brit. J. Med. Med. Res.* **2013**, *3*, 2203–2213. [CrossRef]
23. Lorenzo, C.; Hazuda, H.P.; Haffner, S.M. Insulin resistance and excess risk of diabetes in Mexican-Americans: The San Antonio Heart Study. *J. Clin. Endocrinol. Met.* **2012**, *97*, 793–799. [CrossRef]
24. Wood, R.; Volek, J.S.; Liu, Y.; Shachter, N.S.; Contois, J.H.; Fernandez, M.L. Carbohydrate restriction alters lipoprotein metabolism by modifying VLDL, LDL and HDL subfraction distribution and size in overweight men. *J. Nutr.* **2006**, *136*, 384–389. [PubMed]
25. Herron, K.L.; Vega-Lopez, S.; Ramjiganesh, T.; Conde-Knape, K.; Shachter, N.; Fernandez, M.L. Men classified as hypo- or hyper-responders to dietary cholesterol feeding exhibit differences in lipoprotein metabolism. *J. Nutr.* **2003**, *133*, 1036–1042. [PubMed]
26. Greene, C.M.; Zern, T.L.; Wood, R.; Shrestha, S.; Aggarwal, D.; Sharman, M.; Volek, J.S.; Fernandez, M.L. Dietary cholesterol provided by eggs does not result in an increased risk for coronary heart disease in an elderly population. *J. Nutr.* **2005**, *135*, 2793–2798. [PubMed]
27. Pearce, K.L.; Clifton, P.M.; Noakes, M. Egg consumption as part of an energy-restricted high-protein diet improves blood lipid and blood glucose profiles in individuals with type 2 diabetes. *Brit. J. Nutr.* **2011**, *105*, 584–592. [CrossRef] [PubMed]
28. Romero, A.L.; Romero, J.E.; Laviz, S.; Fernandez, M.L. Cookies enriched with Psyllium and oat bran lower plasma LDL-cholesterol in normal and hypercholesterolemic men from Northern Mexico. *J. Am. Coll. Nutr.* **1998**, *17*, 601–608. [CrossRef] [PubMed]
29. Gunness, P.; Gidley, M.J. Mechanisms underlying the cholesterol-lowering properties of soluble dietary fibre polysaccharides. *Food Funct.* **2010**, *1*, 149–155. [CrossRef] [PubMed]
30. Welch, R.W. Can dietary oats promote health? *Br. J. Biomed. Sci.* **1994**, *51*, 260–270. [PubMed]
31. Griffin, J.D.; Lichtenstein, A.H. Dietary cholesterol and plasma lipoprotein profiles: Randomized-controlled trials. *Clin. Nutr. Rep.* **2013**, *2*, 274–282. [CrossRef]
32. Ballesteros, M.N.; Cabrera, R.M.; Saucedo, M.S.; Fernandez, M.L. Dietary cholesterol does not increase biomarkers for chronic disease in a pediatric population at risk from Northern Mexico. *Am. J. Clin. Nutr.* **2004**, *80*, 855–861. [PubMed]
33. Andersen, C.J.; Blesso, C.N.; Lee, J.Y.; Sha, D.; Thomas, M.J.; Fernandez, M.L. Egg consumption modulates HDL composition and increases the cholesterol accepting capacity of serum in metabolic syndrome. *Lipids* **2013**, *48*, 557–567. [CrossRef] [PubMed]
34. Blesso, C.N.; Andersen, C.J.; Barona, J.; Volek, J.; Fernandez, M.L. Whole egg consumption improves lipoprotein profiles and insulin sensitivity in individuals with metabolic syndrome. *Metabolism* **2013**, *62*, 400–410. [CrossRef] [PubMed]
35. Mutungi, G.; Waters, D.; Ratliff, J.; Puglisi, M.J.; Clark, R.M.; Volek, J.S.; Fernandez, M.L. Eggs distinctly modulate plasma carotenoid and lipoprotein subclasses in adult men following a carbohydrate restricted diet. *J. Nutr. Biochem.* **2010**, *21*, 261–267. [CrossRef] [PubMed]
36. Feingold, K.R.; Grunfeld, C.; Pang, M.; Doemler, W.; Krauss, R.M. LDL subclass phenotypes and triglyceride metabolism in non-insulin-dependent diabetes. *Arterioscler. Thromb. Vasc. Biol.* **1992**, *12*, 1496–1502. [CrossRef]
37. Al-Sarraj, T.; Saadi, H.; Volek, J.S.; Fernandez, M.L. Carbohydrate restriction favorably alters lipoprotein metabolism in Emirati subjects classified with the metabolic syndrome. *Nutr. Met. Cardiovasc. Dis.* **2010**, *20*, 720–726. [CrossRef]

38. Blesso, C.N.; Andersen, C.J.; Bolling, B.; Fernandez, M.L. Egg intake improves carotenoid status by increasing HDL cholesterol in adults with metabolic syndrome. *Food Funct.* **2013**, *4*, 213–221. [CrossRef] [PubMed]

39. Kim, J.H.; Na, H.J.; Kim, C.K.; Kim, J.Y.; Ha, K.S.; Lee, H.; Chung, H.T.; Kwon, H.J.; Kwon, Y.G.; Kim, Y.M. The non-provitamin A carotenoid, lutein, inhibits NF-kappaB-dependent gene expression through redox-based regulation of the phosphatidylinositol3-kinase/PTEN/Akt and NF-kappaB-inducing kinase pathways: Role of H(2)O(2) in NF-kappaB activation. *Free Radic. Biol. Med.* **2008**, *45*, 885–896. [CrossRef] [PubMed]

40. Kim, J.E.; Leite, J.O.; DeOgburn, R.; Smyth, J.A.; Clark, R.M.; Fernandez, M.L. A lutein-enriched diet prevents cholesterol accumulation and decreases oxidized LDL and inflammatory cytokines in the aorta of guinea pigs. *J. Nutr.* **2011**, *141*, 1458–1463. [CrossRef] [PubMed]

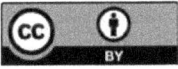

nutrients

MDPI

Article

Egg Yolk Protein Delays Recovery while Ovalbumin Is Useful in Recovery from Iron Deficiency Anemia

Yukiko Kobayashi *, Etsuko Wakasugi, Risa Yasui, Masashi Kuwahata and Yasuhiro Kido

Laboratory of Nutrition Science, Graduate School of Life and Environmental Sciences,
Kyoto Prefectural University, Shimogamo, Sakyo, Kyoto 606-8522, Japan; hgjwj757@yahoo.co.jp (E.W.);
kbysykk@gmail.com (R.Y.); kuwahata@kpu.ac.jp (M.K.); kido@kpu.ac.jp (Y.K.)
* Author to whom correspondence should be addressed; yukicoba@kpu.ac.jp; Tel./Fax: +81-75-703-6017.

Received: 7 April 2015; Accepted: 4 June 2015; Published: 15 June 2015

Abstract: Protein is a main nutrient involved in overall iron metabolism *in vivo*. In order to assess the prevention of iron deficiency anemia (IDA) by diet, it is necessary to confirm the influence of dietary protein, which coexists with iron, on iron bioavailability. We investigated the usefulness of the egg structural protein in recovery from IDA. Thirty-one female Sprague-Dawley rats were divided into a control group (n = 6) fed a casein diet (4.0 mg Fe/100 g) for 42 days and an IDA model group (n = 25) created by feeding a low-iron casein diet (LI, 0.4 mg Fe/100 g) for 21 days and these IDA rats were fed normal iron diet with different proteins from eggs for another 21 days. The IDA rats were further divided into four subgroups depending on the proteins fed during the last 21 days, which were those with an egg white diet (LI-W, 4.0 mg Fe/100 g, n = 6), those with an ovalbumin diet (LI-A, 4.0 mg Fe/100 g, n = 7), those with an egg yolk-supplemented diet (LI-Y, 4.0 mg Fe/100 g, n = 6), and the rest with a casein diet (LI-C, 4.0 mg Fe/100 g, n = 6). In the LI-Y group, recovery of the hematocrit, hemoglobin, transferrin saturation level and the hepatic iron content were delayed compared to the other groups ($p < 0.01, 0.01, 0.01$, and 0.05, respectively), resulting in no recovery from IDA at the end of the experimental period. There were no significant differences in blood parameters in the LI-W and LI-A groups compared to the control group. The hepatic iron content of the LI-W and LI-A groups was higher than that of the LI-C group ($p < 0.05$). We found that egg white protein was useful for recovery from IDA and one of the efficacious components was ovalbumin, while egg yolk protein delayed recovery of IDA. This study demonstrates, therefore, that bioavailability of dietary iron varies depending on the source of dietary protein.

Keywords: dietary protein; iron deficiency anemia; egg-yolk protein; ovalbumin

1. Introduction

Protein is one of the main nutrients involved in all aspects of *in vivo* iron metabolism including iron absorption, transport, hematopoiesis and storage [1,2]. Thus, adequate intake of not only iron, but also protein, is important in the maintenance of normal iron metabolism. Dietary protein differs in the composition of amino acids and the amino acid score by the food origin. Moreover, peptides, which are the digestive form of proteins, are thought to modulate biological functions, and have recently been shown to have various physiological functions. In assessing prevention of iron deficiency anemia (IDA) by diet, it is therefore necessary to confirm the influence and biological use of dietary protein, which coexists with iron, on iron absorption.

Of the three major nutrients (carbohydrate, protein, and lipid), protein has been reported to have the greatest influence on iron absorption [3–6]. For example, Cook *et al.* reported that soybean protein inhibited iron absorption more than egg white protein by a factor of about 5 [7]. Although the whole egg is a food that contains a large amount of iron [8], it is often cited as a food that inhibits iron absorption [9–11]. The majority of iron in eggs is found in the yolk. Although it has been reported that the absorptivity of iron from egg origin is low [12,13], iron absorption was shown to increase and contribute to a delay in the decrease in hemoglobin concentration in an iron-deficient state where iron demands were high [14]. The mineral absorption promoting effect of casein phosphopeptide (CPP) of milk origin is well known from the past researches [15–17]. Although a number of studies have examined the influence of dietary protein on iron absorption, there are few reports on the contribution of dietary protein in the iron deficient state that is accompanied by abnormal iron metabolism [3–17].

We previously examined the effects of various dietary protein sources consumed simultaneously with dietary iron on recovery from IDA. Our previous research showed the possibility that egg white contributes to prompt recovery from IDA compared to soybeans. Furthermore, we showed that the protein form resulted in an increase in serum iron and maturation of red blood cells compared to the peptide form, because the protein form maintained its iron-reducing characteristics in the digestive tract, compared to the peptide form [18]. In the present study, therefore, we investigated the usefulness of the egg structural protein for recovery from IDA.

2. Experimental Section

2.1. Animal Experimental Protocol

This experimental study was approved by the ethics committee of Kyoto Prefectural University, and performed in accordance with the Guidelines for Animal Experimentation at Kyoto Prefectural University. Thirty-one 4-week-old female Sprague-Dawley rats were used in this study (Japan SLC, Inc., Hamamatsu, Japan). The rats were individually housed in stainless steel cages at a controlled temperature of 22–24 °C, a relative humidity of 40%–60%, and a light cycle of 12 h with free access to distilled water (the iron content of the distilled water was previously measured). Body weight and food intake were recorded at the same time everyday.

The 31 rats were divided into two groups on the basis of body weight. The first group (C group, *n* = 6, weighing 106–112 g) was fed a control diet for 42 days. The second group (base LI group, *n* = 25, weighing 94–121 g) was fed a low-iron diet for 21 days to induce IDA. IDA rats were then divided into four subgroups based on weight and hemoglobin concentration such that the mean values of these parameters for each subgroup were the same. Each subgroup was fed either an egg white diet (LI-W group, *n* = 6, weighing 155–195 g), an ovalbumin diet (LI-A group, *n* = 7, weighing 153–177 g), an egg-yolk supplemented diet (LI-Y group, *n* = 6, weighing 158–184 g), or the control diet (LI-C group, *n* = 6, weighing 163–182 g) for another 21 days. The compositions of the diets used in the experiments are shown in Table 1. All diets were prepared according to the AIN-76 formulation with one modification (the addition of choline chloride). The low-iron diet contained 0.4 mg Fe/100 g without any ferrous citrate in the mineral mixture. The amount of protein and lipids within all experimental diets was adjusted to be equal to that of the control diet. During the pair- feeding period, the LI-W, LI-A and LI-Y groups were provided with the same amount of diet that was freely provided to the LI-C group, on the following day.

Table 1. Composition of experimental diet.

	Control Diet	Low Iron Diet	Egg White Diet	Ovalbumin Diet	Egg York Diet
	(g/kg)				
Casein [a]	200	200	-	-	171
Egg White powder [b]	-	-	214	-	-
Ovalbumin [c]	-	-	-	211	-
Egg York powder [d]	-	-	-	-	81
α-starch	457	457	447	448	455
Sucrose	228	228	224	225	228
Mixed oil [e]	50	50	50	50	

Table 1. *Cont.*

	Control Diet	Low Iron Diet	Egg White Diet	Ovalbumin Diet	Egg York Diet
			(g/kg)		
Vitamin mixture [f]			10		
Mineral mixture [g]			35		
Cellose			20		
			(mg/kg)		
Iron (III) Citrate	204	-	205	196	163
Iron content	39.6	4.4	40.0	39.9	40.0

[a] 13.73 gN/100 g. [b] 12.97 gN/100 g. [c] 13.10 gN/100 g. [d] 4.91 gN/100 g. [e] Rapeseed oil/soybean oil ratio = 7/3. [f] AIN-76 vitamin mixture (per g mixture): vitamin A, 400 IU; vitamin D_3, 100 IU; vitamin E, 5 mg; vitamin K_3, 0.005 mg; vitamin B_1, 0.6 mg; vitamin B_2, 0.6 mg; vitamin B_6, 0.7 mg; vitamin B_{12}, 0.001 mg; D-biotin, 0.02 mg; folic acid, 0.2 mg; calcium pantothenate, 1.6 mg; nicotinic acid, 3 mg; choline chloride, 200 mg; sucrose, 0.968 g. [g] AIN-76 mineral mixture (g/kg mixture): calcium phosphate dibasic, 500.0; sodium chloride, 74.0; potassium citrate, 220.0; potassium sulfate, 52.0; magnesium oxide, 24.0; manganese carbonate, 3.5; zinc carbonate, 1.6; cupric carbonate, 0.3; potassium iodate, 0.01; sodium selenite, 0.0066; chromium potassium sulfate, 0.55; sucrose, 124.03.

Blood was drawn from the tail vein of all of the animals every 4 days during the experimental period. At the end of each study period, the rats were euthanized under ether anesthesia during the early phase of the light cycle in a non-fasted state, and blood samples drawn from the inferior vena cava were collected in tubes with heparin. Samples from the liver and small intestinal mucosa (upper side, 1/4th) were also collected.

2.2. Blood Constituent Analysis

The blood hemoglobin concentration was measured using Hemoglobin B test Wako (Wako Pure Chemical Industries, Osaka, Japan). The hematocrit level was measured after centrifugation of the blood at 12,000 rpm for 5 min at 4 °C. Red blood cell (RBC) counts were determined using a Thoma hemacytometer following a 1:200 dilution with Hayem's solution in a pipette. Mean cell volume (MCV), mean corpuscular hemoglobin (MCH) and mean cell hemoglobin concentration (MCHC) were calculated as follows:

$$\text{MCV (pg)} = \text{Hb (g/dL)/RBC} (\times 10^6/\mu L) \times 10 \tag{1}$$

$$\text{MCH (fL)} = \text{Ht (\%)/RBC} (\times 106/\mu L) \times 10 \tag{2}$$

$$\text{MCHC (\%)} = \text{Hb (g/dL)/Ht (\%)} \times 100 \tag{3}$$

Serum iron and unsaturated iron binding capacity (UIBC) were measured using Detaminer Fe and UIBC (Kyowa Medix Co., Ltd., Tokyo, Japan) with an automatic biochemical analyzer (CL-8000; Shimadzu Corp., Kyoto, Japan). Total iron binding capacity and serum transferrin saturation were calculated as follows:

$$\text{Total iron binding capacity} = \text{serum iron} + \text{UIBC} \tag{4}$$

$$\text{Serum transferrin saturation} = \text{serum iron/Total iron binding capacity} \times 100 \tag{5}$$

2.3. Estimation of Gene Expression

Total RNA was isolated from the homogenized mucosa and liver samples using the Total RNA Isolation mini kit (Agilent Technologies, Inc., Santa Clara, CA, USA), and converted to cDNA using a reverse transcriptase enzyme ReverTra Ace (Toyobo Co., Ltd., Osaka, Japan) according to the manufacturer's instructions. Each target DNA fragment was amplified using the respective TaqMan gene expression assay kits and a real-time polymerase chain reaction (PCR) system using cDNA as a template. Real-time PCR for gene expression analysis was performed using DNA Engine Opticon and Opticon Monitor software (Bio-Rad Laboratories, Inc., Hercules, CA, USA). TaqMan primer pairs/probes for gene analysis were obtained using a TaqMan Gene Expression Assay

(Applied Biosystems, Inc., Carlsbad, CA, USA). Assay IDs were Rn00565927_m1, Rn00591187_m1 and Rn00667869_m1 for DMT1, Ferroportin and β-actin, respectively. Reactions were performed with 10 μL of Premix EX Taq (Takara Bio, Inc., Ohtsu, Japan), 1 μL of the primer pairs/probes sets and 3 μL of cDNA in a final volume of 20 μL. After heating the test sample at 96 °C for 10 s, 50 PCR cycles were performed as follows: 95 °C for 7 s, 60 °C for 30 s, and 72 °C for 20 s. The cycle thresholds of the genes of interest were compared with the housekeeping gene β-actin to determine relative changes in expression.

2.4. Iron Content of Hepatic Tissue

Liver samples were perfused with saline, and treated by the wet ash method using a microwave extraction system (Ethos; Milestone Srl., Sorisole, Italy). The ash was suspended in dilute hydrochloric acid solution after evaporation, and left to dry. Iron concentrations were measured by polarizing Zeeman-effect atomic absorption spectrometry (Z-6100; Hitachi, Ltd., Tokyo, Japan) after suitable dilution. We determined that the coefficient of variation was 0.04. Iron concentrations were expressed on a wet-weight basis.

2.5. Statistical Analysis

Data were presented as means ± standard error (SEM). Before assessing the different variables, we carried out a Bartlett test to check the normal distribution of the variables. Data that fit the normal distribution were compared by 1–way analysis of variance (ANOVA) followed by the Tukey-Kramer test (Table 2, Figures 1 and 2), or Student's t test (Table 2). The level of significance was set at $p < 0.05$.

Table 2. Body weight gain, food intake and blood parameters on the day 21 and day 42 after the start of study.

A. day 21				
	Base LI	C	Student's *t*-test*p* value	
Body weight gain (g/day)	3.0 ± 0.1	3.4 ± 0.2	0.138	
Food intake (g/day)	11.7 ± 0.1 [a]	12.7 ± 0.4 [b]	0.034	
Hematocrit level (%)	33.0 ± 0.7 [a]	47.1 ± 1.2 [b]	<0.001	
Hemogrobin concentration (g/dL)	9.7 ± 0.3 [a]	15.4 ± 0.7 [b]	<0.001	

B. day 42						
	LI-W	LI-A	LI-Y	LI-C	C	ANOVA*p* value
Body weight gain (g/day)	1.4 ± 0.3	1.5 ± 0.1	1.3 ± 0.1	1.5 ± 0.2	1.7 ± 0.1	0.196
Food intake (g/day)	10.9 ± 0.0 [a]	10.9 ± 0.0 [a]	10.9 ± 0.0 [a]	10.9 ± 0.0 [a]	11.9 ± 0.5 [b]	0.006
Hematocrit level (%)	49.9 ± 1.5 [a]	49.3 ± 1.0 [a]	44.4 ± 3.2 [b]	48.5 ± 2.8 [a]	50.7 ± 1.0 [a]	0.002
Hemogrobin concentration (g/dL)	18.0 ± 0.6 [a]	17.8 ± 0.6 [a]	15.0 ± 0.6 [b]	17.4 ± 1.0 [a]	18.2 ± 0.5 [a]	<0.001
Red blood cell counts ($\times 10^6$/μL)	14.8 ± 1.1	13.0 ± 1.5	13.5 ± 1.3	14.1 ± 1.8	15.8 ± 2.2	0.072
Mean cell volume * (fL)	12.0 ± 0.4 [ab]	13.8 ± 1.8 [a]	11.2 ± 1.1 [b]	12.4 ± 0.7 [ab]	11.7 ± 2.0 [ab]	0.013
Mean corpuscular hemoglobin ** (pg)	33.2 ± 1.0 [a]	38.4 ± 4.0 [b]	33.3 ± 4.5 [a]	34.4 ± 2.0 [a]	31.6 ± 4.7 [a]	0.043
Mean cell hemogrobin concentration *** (%)	36.0 ± 1.6 [ab]	39.0 ± 1.1 [ab]	33.7 ± 1.4 [a]	31.4 ± 0.3 [ab]	36.0 ± 0.6 [b]	0.022

Normal rats fed low iron diet (base LI, *n* = 25) for 21 days or control diet (C, *n* = 6) for 42 days. Base LI group divided four subgroups, were fed either an egg white diet (LI-W, *n* = 6), an ovalbumin diet (LI-A, *n* = 7), an egg york-supplemented diet (LI-Y, *n* = 6) or control diet (LI-C, *n* = 6) for another 21 days. Values are mean ± SEM. Values with an unlike letter were significant: $p < 0.05$. * Mean cell volume (pg) = Hb (g/dL)/RBC ($\times 10^6$/μL) × 10, ** Mean corpuscular hemoglobin (fL) = Ht (%)/RBC ($\times 10^6$/μL) × 10, *** Mean cell hemogrobin concentration (%) = Hb (g/dL)/Ht (%) × 100.

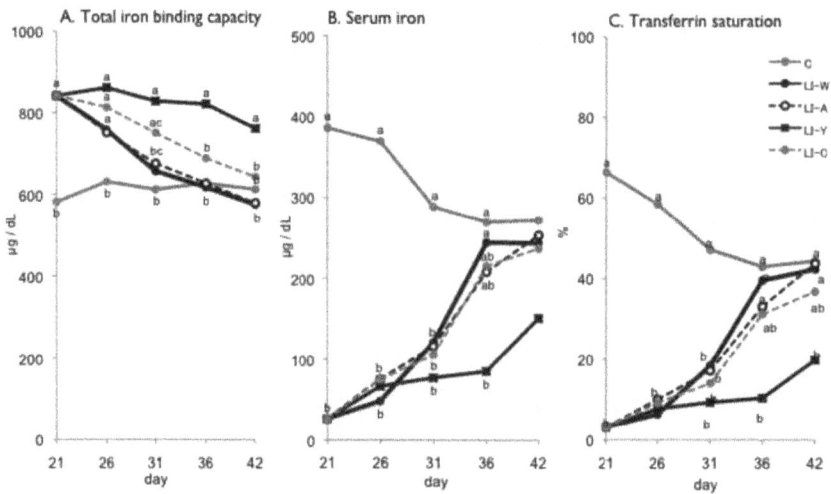

Figure 1. Total iron binding capacity (**A**); serum iron (**B**); transferrin saturation (**C**) on day 21, 26, 31, 36 and 42 after start of experimental period. Iron deficiency anemia rats, fed low iron diet for 21 days, divided four subgroups, was fed either an egg white diet (LI-W, *n* = 6), an ovalbumin diet (LI-A, *n* = 7), an egg york diet (LI-Y, *n* = 6) or a control diet (LI-C, *n* = 6) and normal rats fed the control diet (C, *n* = 6) for 42 days. Values were represented as mean. Values with an unlike letter were significant: $p < 0.05$.

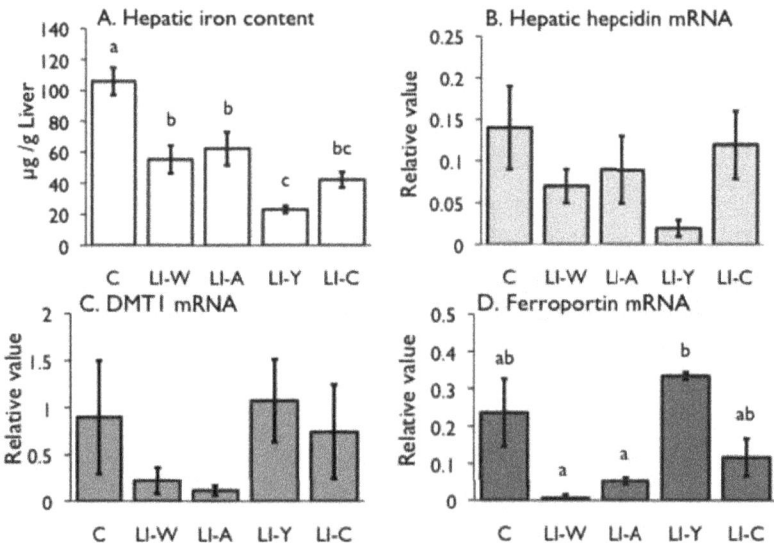

Figure 2. Iron content (**A**) and hepcidin mRNA expression (**B**) in the liver, and iron transporter DMT1 (**C**) and Ferroportin (**D**) mRNA expression in small intestines on day 42 after start of study. Iron deficiency anemia rats, fed low iron diet for 21 days, divided four subgroups, was fed either an egg white diet (LI-W, *n* = 6), an ovalbumin diet (LI-A, *n* = 7), an egg york diet (LI-Y, *n* = 6) or a control diet (LI-C, *n* = 6) and normal rats fed the control diet (C, *n* = 6) for 42 days. The cycle thresholds of the genes of interest were compared with the housekeeping gene β-actin to determine relative changes in expression. Values were represented as means ± SEM. Values with unlike letter were significant: $p < 0.05$.

3. Results

3.1. Body Weight Gain, Food Intake and Blood Parameters

Body weight gain, food intake and blood parameters on day 21 and day 42 after the start of the study are shown in Table 2. There was no significant difference in body weight gain or food intake between the two base groups on day 21. The hematocrit level and hemoglobin concentration of the base LI group (LI-W, LI-A, LI-Y and LI-C group) were lower than those of the C group on day 21 (hematocrit: 33.0 ± 0.7 *vs.* $47.1 \pm 1.2\%$; $p < 0.001$, hemoglobin: 9.7 ± 0.3 *vs.* 15.4 ± 0.7 g/dL; $p < 0.001$), confirming that the base LI group had developed IDA. On day 42 after the start of the study, the hematocrit level and hemoglobin concentration of the LI-Y group were significantly lower than that of the other four groups (Table 2, hematocrit: LI-Y 44.4 ± 3.2 *vs.* C 50.7 ± 1.0 and LI-C $48.5 \pm 2.8\%$; $p < 0.05$, LI-Y *vs.* LI-A 49.3 ± 1.0 and LI-W $49.9 \pm 1.5\%$; $p < 0.01$, hemoglobin: LI-Y 15.0 ± 0.6 *vs.* LI-W 18.0 ± 0.6, LI-A 17.8 ± 0.6, LI-C 17.4 ± 1.0 and C 18.2 ± 0.5 g/dL; $p < 0.01$ for all); however, no statistical difference was found among the LI-W, LI-A, LI-C, and C groups. The MCV of the LI-Y group was significantly lower than that of the LI-A group ($p < 0.05$) and the MCH of the LI-A group was higher than that of the other four groups ($p < 0.05$). There were no significant differences in body weight gain, food intake, RBC and MCHC among four groups of base LI.

3.2. The Changes in the Total Iron Binding Capacity, Serum Iron and Transferrin Saturation Level of the Groups

Figure 1 shows the changes in the total iron binding capacity, serum iron and transferrin saturation level of the groups on days 21, 26, 31, 36 and 42 after the study. On day 21, the base LI group (LI-W, LI-A, LI-Y and LI-C group) exhibited lower serum iron and transferrin saturation and higher total iron binding capacity compared to the C group ($p < 0.01$ for all). The total iron binding capacity, serum iron and transferrin saturation level of the base LI group fed the diets containing iron were gradually restored. The total iron binding capacity of the LI-Y group was statistically higher than that of the C group from day 21 to day 42 ($p < 0.01$ for all). From day 21 to day 31, the total iron binding capacity of the LI-C group was higher than that of the C group ($p < 0.01$ for all); however, there were no significant differences between the LI-W, LI-A and C groups on day 31. There were also no statistical differences among the LI-W, LI-A and LI-C groups after day 21, until day 42 (Figure 1A). The serum iron level of the LI-Y group was statistically lower than that of the C group from day 21 to day 36 ($p < 0.01$ for all). There were no significant differences among the LI-W, LI-A, LI-C and C groups on day 36 and no significant differences between LI-W, LI-A and LI-C after day 21 to the end of the experiment (Figure 1B). The transferring saturation level of LI-Y group was statistically lower than that of the C group from day 21 to day 42 ($p < 0.01$ for all). There were no significant differences among the LI-W, LI-A, LI-C and C groups on day 36 (Figure 1C).

3.3. The Hepatic Iron Content and the mRNA Expression Level of Liver and Mucos

The hepatic iron content of the base LI group (LI-W: 55.2 ± 9.0, LI-A: 62.3 ± 10.8, LI-Y: 23.2 ± 2.2 and LI-C: 42.2 ± 4.9 µg/g liver) was much lower than that of the C group (73.7 ± 20.3 µg/g liver) on day 42. The iron content of hepatic tissue of the LI-W and LI-A groups was dramatically increased compared with that of the LI-Y group ($p < 0.05$), and higher than that of the LI-C group but no significant differences were observed among the three groups (Figure 2A). A correlation between the mRNA expression level of hepatic hepcidin and hepatic iron content was observed in both groups (Figure 2B–D). The hepcidin mRNA expression level of the LI-Y group was lower compared with the other groups, but no significant difference was shown among five groups (Figure 2B). The DMT1 mRNA expression levels of the LI-W, LI-A and LI-C groups were lower than those of the C group. In contrast, the mRNA expression level of the LI-Y group was increased compared with the C group, but there were no statistical differences between the C and the other groups (Figure 2C). The pattern of expression levels of ferroportin mRNA was similar to the DMT1 mRNA expression levels (Figure 2D).

4. Discussion

In the present study, we examined the usefulness of egg constitutive proteins on recovery of IDA. Our results provided new finding that egg yolk protein delayed recovery of IDA while ovalbumin was useful in recovery of IDA, and that the bioavailability of dietary iron varies depending on dietary protein source.

Although the iron content of all diets was equivalent, the transitions of total iron binding capacity, transferring saturation level, and serum iron in the LI-Y group of IDA rats, which were fed the diet containing egg yolk, showed delayed recovery compared with the other groups, and resulted in no recovery at the end of the experimental period. Moreover, the blood properties and hepatic iron content of the LI-Y group were lower than those of the other groups on day 42. These data suggest that egg yolk resulted in delayed recovery from IDA. On the other hand, the mRNA expression of hepatic hepcidin, which regulates iron absorption in the gut [19,20], was decreased in the LI-Y group compared to the other diet groups, and it correlated with hepatic iron content. The mRNA expression of ferroportin and DMT1, which are transporters of iron absorption in the small intestine [21,22], were up-regulated in the LI-Y group compared to the C group, suggesting that in this group, iron storage was insufficient and iron absorption was promoted by homeostasis. Nevertheless, expression of the iron transporters was up-regulated. One reason for the lack of recovery from IDA in the Li-Y group may be that the absolute quantity of dietary iron transported in the small intestines was low. A previous study reported that intake of egg yolk protein decreased the apparent absorption of iron, calcium and magnesium compared with casein and soy protein in normal rats [23]. Most of the iron in egg yolk is combined with phosvitin of phosphate protein. Phosvitin is known to have a very high binding capacity for divalent metals, especially iron [24]. It was observed that the amount of insoluble iron in the small intestines of rats fed the diet containing phosvitin was higher than that in rats fed diets without phosvitin [25]. In the present study, feeding the diet containing egg yolk may have delayed recovery from IDA because the iron in the egg yolk iron and/or other dietary iron may have strongly combined with phosvitin, and formed an insoluble iron complex in the small intestine. Since phosvitin is a resistant protein [26], it is possible that the insoluble iron complex was excreted from the body without being used *in vivo*. These findings suggest, therefore, that iron from eggs is not readily used *in vivo*, and ingredients from egg yolk reduce the bioavailability of dietary iron. In cases of IDA, the choice of egg yolk as the source of protein and iron should be avoided.

Conversely, at the end of the experimental period, the blood parameters of the LI-W group, which was fed egg white, the LI-A group, which was fed ovalbumin, and the LI-C group, which was fed casein, were not significantly different from those of the control group, suggesting that IDA improved in these groups. The hepatic iron content of the LI-W, LI-A, and LI-C groups was significantly lower than the C group, however, and iron storage was not recovered in these groups despite receiving the standard amount of dietary iron given to IDA rats for 3 weeks. The total iron binding capacity of the LI-W and LI-A group was lower than that of the LI-C, but was not significantly different from the C group. In addition, the hepatic iron content of the LI-W and LI-A groups was higher than that of the LI-C group, but there were no significant differences among the three groups. These findings show that IDA of the LI-W and LI-A groups, which were fed egg white protein, was promptly recovered due to inhibition of transferrin production at an early stage compared with the LI-C group, which was fed casein protein. We conclude, therefore, that the egg white protein contributed to an improvement in the iron deficient state compared to casein protein. These results are in agreement with our previous reports [18]. If iron absorption in the LI-C group, which was fed casein protein, was promoted by CPP, this raises the possibility that egg white protein has the absorption promoting effect on iron that exceeds CPP. On the other hand, a previous study reported that the specific amino acid that accelerated iron absorption exists in animal protein, such as red meat [27]. These results suggest that the mechanism for promotion of recovery from IDA by egg white protein differs from the rise in iron absorption caused by red meat, since the existence of this amino acid in egg has not been reported even though eggs are from animal sources. Moreover, we assume that the component of egg white protein active in recovery of IDA was ovalbumin, because there were no significant differences in changes in blood parameters and in hepatic iron content between the LI-W and LI-A groups. Albumin possesses a large number of negative carboxylate sites ($-CO_2^-$) on the surface of the molecule, many clustered in groups of three or more [28]. These sites are suitable for binding iron (III) [29]. Indeed, albumin has been demonstrated to be a sufficiently powerful ligand for binding iron (III) even when transferrin is not fully saturated [30]. Therefore, the combination of dietary iron and albumin in the lumen may form a soluble complex that is advantageous for iron absorption.

Despite the fact that the amount of stored iron in the LI-W, LI-A, and LI-C groups was not restored, the ferroportin and DMT1 mRNA levels in the small intestine significantly decreased in these groups compared with the C group. Accordingly, iron absorption by the transporters was suppressed in the LI-W, LI-A, and LI-C groups, even though they were in an iron-deficient state. It is known that the expression of the iron transporter ferroportin is down-regulated by secretion of hepcidin [31]; however, there was no correlation between hepatic iron content and the level of hepatic hepcidin and ferroportin mRNA expression in this study. Thus, these findings raise the possibility of the presence of another mechanism for regulation of ferroportin expression in the absence of secretion of hepcidin.

One of the limitations of the present study is that we did not directly measure the rate of iron absorption as the trend of dietary iron in the intestine is one of clues to comprehend the usefulness of the dietary iron for the recovery of IDA. In order to elucidate the effects of egg protein on the promotion of iron absorption, further studies should be conducted to investigate iron balance. Moreover, our findings suggest that phosvitin, contained within egg yolk protein, likely reduces the bioavailability of dietary iron. Further research is required to investigate the role of egg yolk phosvitin in the recovery of IDA and its possible usefulness in iron removal therapy. Although the results obtained in this study have some implications for public health, it is necessary to keep in mind that the iron bioavailability varies with different cooking processes, especially of egg yolk.

5. Conclusions

We demonstrated that the origin of dietary protein influenced iron absorption and maturation of red blood cells without affecting iron transport and hematogenesis in recovery from IDA. In particular, we showed that egg white protein was useful for recovery from IDA, and one of the efficacious components was ovalbumin and egg yolk protein delayed recovery of IDA. This study demonstrates, therefore, that bioavailability of dietary iron varies depending on the source of dietary protein. Further analysis of the mechanism for IDA recovery by ovalbumin may lead to the development of a new diet therapy for IDA such as thalassaemias, that does not include iron loading. Conversely, egg yolk protein may be useful in iron removal therapy without the need for medicine and may potentially be used in the treatment of diseases such as haemochromatosis, which require control of iron absorption.

Acknowledgments: We would like to thank Kaoru Yoshida (Kyoto Koka Women's University, Japan) for her technical support. This work was supported by Grant-in-Aids for Young Scientists B (No. 19700593 and No. 21700764) from the Japan Society for the Promotion of Science.

Author Contributions: Design of study (Y.K.; Y.K.), experiment (Y.K.; E.W.; R.Y.), analysis (Y.K.; E.W.; R.Y.), interpretation of date (Y.K.; E.W.; R.Y.; K.M.; Y.K.), preparation of manuscript (Y.K.; Y.K.).

Conflicts of Interest: The authors declare no conflict of interest.

References

1. Geissler, C.; Singh, M. Iron, meat and health. *Nutrients* **2011**, *3*, 283–316. [CrossRef] [PubMed]
2. Andrew, N.C. Forging a field: The golden age of iron biology. *Blood* **2008**, *112*, 219–223. [CrossRef] [PubMed]
3. Monsen, E.R.; Cook, J.D. Food iron absorption in human subjects. V. Effects of the major dietary constituents of semisynthetic meal. *Am. J. Clin. Nutr.* **1979**, *32*, 804–808. [PubMed]
4. Miller, J.; Nnanna, I. Bioavailability of iron in cooked egg yolk for maintenance of hemoglobin levels in growing rats. *J. Nutr.* **1983**, *133*, 1169–1175.

5. Hurrell, R.F.; Lynch, S.R.; Trinidad, T.P.; Dassenko, S.A.; Cook, J.D. Iron absorption in humans as influenced by bovine milk protein. *Am. J. Clin. Nutr.* **1989**, *49*, 546–552. [PubMed]

6. Hurrell, R.F.; Lynch, S.R.; Trinidad, T.P.; Dassenko, S.A.; Cook, J.D. Iron absorption in humans: Bovine serum albumin compared with beef muscle and egg white. *Am. J. Clin. Nutr.* **1988**, *47*, 102–107. [PubMed]

7. Cook, J.D.; Morck, T.A.; Lynch, S.R. The inhibitory effect of soy products on nonheme iron absorption in man. *Am. J. Clin. Nutr.* **1981**, *34*, 2622–2629. [PubMed]

8. Watkins, B.A. *The Nutritive Value of the Egg*; Stadelman, W.J., Cotterill, O.J., Eds.; Food Products Press: Binghamton, NY, USA, 1995; pp. 177–194.

9. Callender, S.T.; Marney, S.R., Jr.; Warner, G.T. Eggs and iron absorption. *Br. J. Haematol.* **1970**, *19*, 657–665. [CrossRef] [PubMed]

10. Fritz, J.C.; Pla, G.W.; Roberts, T.; Boehne, J.W.; Hove, E.L. Biological availability in animals of iron from common dietary sources. *J. Agric. Food. Chem.* **1970**, *18*, 647–651. [CrossRef] [PubMed]

11. Peters, T., Jr.; Apt, L.; Ross, J.F. Effect of phosphates upon iron absorption studied in normal human subjects and in an experimental model using dialysis. *Gastroenterology* **1971**, *61*, 315–322. [PubMed]

12. Morris, E.R.; Greene, F.E. Utilization of the iron of egg yolk for hemoglobin formation by the growing rat. *J. Nutr.* **1972**, *102*, 901–908. [PubMed]

13. Miller, J.; McNeal, L.S. Bioavailability of egg yolk iron measured by hemoglobin regeneration in anemic rats. *J. Nutr.* **1983**, *113*, 1169–1175. [PubMed]

14. Uehara, M.; Endo, Y.; Suzuki, K.; Goto, S. Effects of dietary eggs on tissue iron and copper levels and hepatic metalloenzyme activity in iron-deficient rats. *Jpn. J. Nutr. Diet.* **1986**, *44*, 203–208. [CrossRef]

15. Sato, R.; Noguchi, T.; Naito, H. Casein phosphopeptide (CPP) enhances calcium absorption from the ligate segment of rat small intestine. *J. Nutr. Sci. Vitaminol.* **1986**, *32*, 67–76. [CrossRef] [PubMed]

16. Aît-Oukhatar, N.; Bouhallab, S.; Arhan, P.; Maubois, J.L.; Drosdowsky, M.; Bouglé, D. Iron tissue storage and hemoglobin levels of deficient rats repleted with iron bound to the caseinophosphopeptide 1-25 of beta-casein. *J. Agric. Food. Chem.* **1999**, *47*, 2786–2790. [CrossRef] [PubMed]

17. Bouhallab, S.; Cinga, V.; Aît-Oukhatar, N.; Bureau, F.; Neuville, D.; Arhan, P.; Maubois, J.L.; Bouglé, D. Influence of various phosphopeptides of caseins on iron absorption. *J. Agric. Food Chem.* **2002**, *50*, 7127–7130. [CrossRef] [PubMed]

18. Kobayashi, Y.; Kido, Y.; Nakabou, Y. Effects of dietary protein and peptide on recovery from iron deficiency anemia by rats. *Jpn. J. Nutr. Diet.* **2007**, *65*, 165–171. [CrossRef]

19. Anderson, G.J.; Frazer, D.M. Recent advances in intestinal iron transport. *Curr. Gastroenterol. Rep.* **2005**, *7*, 365–372. [CrossRef] [PubMed]

20. Fuqua, B.K.; Vulpe, C.D.; Anderson, G.J. Intestinal iron absorption. *J. Trace Elem. Med. Biol.* **2012**, *26*, 115–119. [CrossRef] [PubMed]

21. Gunshin, H.; Mackenzie, B.; Berger, U.V.; Gunshin, Y.; Romero, M.F.; Boron, W.F.; Nussberger, S.; Gollan, J.L.; Hediger, M.A. Cloning and characterization of a mammalian proton-coupled metal-iron transporter. *Nature* **1997**, *388*, 482–488. [CrossRef] [PubMed]

22. Donovan, A.; Brownlie, A.; Zhou, Y.; Shepard, J.; Pratt, S.J.; Moynihan, J.; Paw, B.H.; Drejer, A.; Barut, B.; Zapata, A.; et al. Positional cloning of zebrafish ferroportin1 identifies a conserved vertebrate iron exporter. *Nature* **2000**, *403*, 776–781. [PubMed]

23. Ishikawa, S.I.; Tamaki, S.; Arihira, K.; Itoh, M. Egg yolk protein and egg yolk phosvitin inhibit calcium, magnesium, and iron absorption in rats. *J. Food Sci.* **2007**, *72*, S412–S419. [CrossRef] [PubMed]

24. Albright, K.J.; Gordon, D.T.; Cotterill, O.J. Release of iron from phosvitin by heat and food additives. *J. Food Sci.* **1984**, *49*, 78–81. [CrossRef]

25. Sato, R.; Noguchi, T.; Naito, H. The effect of feeding demineralized egg yolk protein on the solubility of intra-intestinal iron. *Nutr. Rep. Int.* **1987**, *36*, 593–602.

26. Goulas, A.; Triplett, E.L.; Taborsky, G. Oligophosphopeptides of varied structural complexity derived from the egg phosphoprotein, phosvitin. *J. Protein Chem.* **1996**, *15*, 1–9. [CrossRef] [PubMed]

27. Hurrell, R.F.; Reddy, M.B.; Juillerat, M.; Cook, J.D. Meat protein fractions enhance nonheme iron absorption in humans. *J. Nutr.* **2006**, *136*, 2808–2812. [PubMed]

28. He, S.M.; Carter, D.C. Atomic structure and chemistry of human serum albumin. *Nature* **1992**, *358*, 209–215. [CrossRef] [PubMed]

29. Hider, R.C. Nature of nontransferrin-bound iron. *Eur. J. Clin. Investig.* **2002**, *33* (Suppl. S1), 50–54. [CrossRef]

Nutrients **2015**, *7*, 4792–4803

30. Van der Heul, C.; van Eijk, H.G.; Wiltink, W.F.; Leijnse, B. The binding of iron to transferrin and to journal serum components at different degrees of saturation with iron. *Clin. Chim. Acta* **1972**, *38*, 347–353. [CrossRef]
31. Mena, N.P.; Esparza, A.; Tapia, V.; Valdés, P.; Núñez, M.T. Hepcidin inhibits apical iron uptake in intestinal cells. *Am. J. Physiol. Gastrointest. Liver Physiol.* **2008**, *294*, G192–G198. [CrossRef] [PubMed]

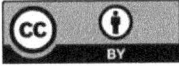

nutrients

MDPI

Review

Egg Consumption and Human Cardio-Metabolic Health in People with and without Diabetes

Nicholas R. Fuller *, Amanda Sainsbury, Ian D. Caterson and Tania P. Markovic

The Boden Institute of Obesity, Nutrition, Exercise & Eating Disorders, Charles Perkins Centre, The University of Sydney, NSW 2006, Australia; amanda.salis@sydney.edu.au (A.S.); ian.caterson@sydney.edu.au (I.D.C.); tania.markovic@bigpond.com (T.P.M.)

* Author to whom correspondence should be addressed; nick.fuller@sydney.edu.au; Tel.: +61-2-8627-1932; Fax: +61-2-8627-0141.

Received: 1 August 2015; Accepted: 26 August 2015; Published: 3 September 2015

Abstract: The guidelines for dietary cholesterol and/or egg intake for both the general population and those at higher risk of cardiovascular disease (for example, people with type 2 diabetes mellitus (T2DM)) differ between countries, and even for different specialist societies in a country. The disparity between these guidelines is at least in part related to the conflicting evidence as to the effects of eggs in the general population and in those with T2DM. This review addresses the effect of eggs on cardiovascular disease (CVD) risk from both epidemiological research and controlled prospective studies, in people with and without cardio-metabolic disease. It also examines the nutritional qualities of eggs and whether they may offer protection against chronic disease. The evidence suggests that a diet including more eggs than is recommended (at least in some countries) may be used safely as part of a healthy diet in both the general population and for those at high risk of cardiovascular disease, those with established coronary heart disease, and those with T2DM. In conclusion, an approach focused on a person's entire dietary intake as opposed to specific foods or nutrients should be the heart of population nutrition guidelines.

Keywords: dietary cholesterol; eggs; type 2 diabetes mellitus; cardiovascular disease

---

1. Introduction

Despite our increased understanding of the pathophysiology of cardiovascular disease, there remains uncertainty regarding the role of dietary cholesterol and eggs in its pathophysiology. The guidelines for dietary cholesterol and/or egg intake for both the general population and those at higher risk of cardiovascular disease (for example, people with type 2 diabetes mellitus (T2DM)) differ between countries, and even for different specialist societies in a country. For example, the National Heart Foundation guidelines recommend that all Australians, including those with T2DM or metabolic syndrome, restrict their egg intake to six eggs or fewer per week [1]; the British Heart Foundation and Diabetes United Kingdom do not have a limit for dietary cholesterol or egg consumption [2]; and the American Diabetes Association (ADA) until very recently had a limit on total cholesterol consumption for both the general population and those with T2DM of 300 mg per day [3], with one egg containing approximately 200 mg cholesterol. This guideline has since been changed and there is no longer a limit on dietary cholesterol intake [4]. The American Heart Foundation and the American College of Cardiology have also abolished their dietary cholesterol restrictions, but another group in the United States, the National Lipid Association (NLA), has since revised their guidelines and is recommending <200 mg per day of dietary cholesterol for those with dyslipidaemia [5–7]. The disparity between these guidelines is at least in part related to the conflicting evidence as to the effects of eggs in the general population and in those with T2DM. This review addresses the effect of eggs on cardiovascular disease (CVD) risk from both epidemiological research and controlled prospective studies, in people with and without cardio-metabolic disease. Cardio-metabolic risk refers to risk factors associated with increased risk of cardiovascular disease and metabolic disease, and these two conditions are in turn related. Metabolic disease or disorders include T2DM, insulin resistance, hypertension and dyslipidaemia. The review also examines the nutritional qualities of eggs and whether they may offer protection against chronic disease.

2. Epidemiological Evidence Suggesting That a High-Egg Diet Is Safe for the General Population But Has Adverse Cardio-Metabolic Effects, Particularly in Those with Diabetes Mellitus

Epidemiological studies to date have indicated very little association between a high egg intake and cardiovascular disease or mortality in the general population; however, evidence suggests an adverse effect in sub-groups of the population, notably in those with diabetes mellitus. A summary of each of the epidemiological studies is provided in Table 1. Some of these studies of longer-term follow up or larger sample size will be reviewed below in greater detail.

Nutrients **2015**, 7, 7399–7420

Table 1. Summary of epidemiological evidence regarding egg consumption, cardiovascular disease, and incidence of diabetes.

Study	Design	Association between Egg Consumption and Cardiovascular Disease	Association between Egg Consumption and Incidence of Diabetes
Framingham Study and Offspring study [8,9]	24 year follow up of 912 and a prospective cohort of 2879 American participants	No association between egg intake and subsequent development of CHD	Intake of eggs associated with incidence of type 2 diabetes with some dietary pattern scores
Italian case-control study [10]	287 cases with AMI and 649 controls, Italian women, conducted over 5 years	No association between egg consumption of greater than 2 eggs/week and nonfatal myocardial infarction	Not reported
Finnish Study [11]	14 year follow up of 5133 Finnish men and women aged 30–69 years	No difference in egg consumption between individuals who developed fatal coronary heart disease and those who did not	Not reported
Oxford Vegetarian Study [12]	14 year follow up of 11,140 English vegetarians and meat eating participants	>6 eggs/week associated with increased mortality from ischemic heart disease	Not reported
Adventist Health Study [13]	6 year follow up of 34,192 vegetarian and non-vegetarian American Seventh Day Adventists	Consuming >2 eggs/week presents no difference in risk of developing CHD compared to consuming <1 eggs/week	Not reported
Nurses Health [14]	14 year follow up of 80,082 American women aged 39–54 years	No association between consumption of up to 1 egg/day and risk of CHD or stroke; higher egg consumption was associated with increased CHD risk in people with diabetes	Not reported
Health Professionals Follow-up [14]	14 year follow up of 37,851 American men aged 40–75 years	No association between consumption of up to 1 egg/day and risk of CHD or stroke; higher egg consumption was associated with increased CHD risk in people with diabetes	Not reported
Japanese case-control study [15]	660 cases with AMI and 1277 controls, Japanese men and women aged 40–79 years	No association between egg intakes up to 4 or more/week and incidence of AMI	Not reported

Table 1. Cont.

Study	Design	Association between Egg Consumption and Cardiovascular Disease	Association between Egg Consumption and Incidence of Diabetes
NIPPON DATA80 [16]	14 year follow up of 5186 women and 4077 men, all Japanese aged 30 years and over	No effect of egg consumption on risk of fatal CHD events; stroke and cancer in men or women consuming ≥2 eggs/day; increased risk of all cause mortality in women for ≥1 egg/day	Not reported
Japan Public Health Centre-based study [17]	21 year follow up of 90,735 Japanese male and female participants aged 40–69 years	Total cholesterol levels were significantly related to an increased risk of CHD, however consumption of eggs almost daily was not associated with CHD risk in middle-aged Japanese men and women	Not reported
Greek EPIC diabetic subgroup [18]	11 year follow up of 1013 Greek adults with diabetes	Positive association with increased egg consumption and cardiovascular mortality in people with diabetes	Not reported
NHANES I [19]	20 year follow up of 9734 American adults aged 25 to 74 years	No significant difference between consuming >6 eggs/week compared to <1 egg/week in any stroke, ischemic stroke or coronary artery disease; consumption of >6 eggs/week was associated with an increased risk of CHD in people with diabetes	Not reported
Physician's Health [20–22]	20 year follow up of 21,327 American male participants aged 40 years and over and 36,295 American women aged 45 years	Egg consumption did not increase CVD risk, but consumption of ≥7/week was associated with a 23% increased risk of all cause mortality and in a separate study of the same cohort, a 28% increase risk of heart failure; consumption of ≤6 eggs/week did not increase the risk of death from all causes	Men who ate 5–6 eggs/week had a 46% higher risk of developing type 2 diabetes than no eggs, and 58% higher for ≥7 eggs/week; women who ate 2–4 eggs a week had a 19% higher risk, and 77% higher for ≥7 eggs/week. In both groups, there was a significantly increased risk of developing type 2 diabetes with increasing egg consumption

Table 1. *Cont.*

Study	Design	Association between Egg Consumption and Cardiovascular Disease	Association between Egg Consumption and Incidence of Diabetes
INTERHEART (A Global Case-Control Study of Risk Factors for Acute Myocardial Infarction) [23]	Global study reporting on 5761 patients who have had a heart attack and 10,646 controls free of heart disease, recruited over 4 years	Western dietary pattern (characterised by higher intakes of fried foods, salty snacks and meat) was shown to be associated with an increased risk of heart attack; no association between eggs and heart attack risk	Not reported
Atherosclerosis Risk in Communities (ARIC) [24]	11 year follow up of 15,792 African American and white American men and women aged 45–64 years	23% increased risk of heart failure for each extra serving of eggs/day, up to 7 eggs/week	Not reported
Insulin Resistance Atherosclerosis Study [25]	Prospective cohort of 880 American individuals with normal glucose tolerance or impaired glucose tolerance	Not reported	High intake of a dietary pattern that included eggs (as well as red meat, low fibre bread and cereal, dried beans, fried potatoes, tomato, vegetables, cheese and cottage cheese, and low in wine) was associated with developing type 2 diabetes
Cardiovascular health study [26]	Prospective study of 3898 American older adults (>65 years) followed for an average of 11.3 years	Not reported	There was no association between egg consumption or dietary cholesterol intake and risk of developing type 2 diabetes
Health ABC Study [27]	9 year follow up of 1941 70–79 years old Americans	Dietary cholesterol and consumption of ≥3 eggs/week was associated with increased CVD risk only in older adults with type 2 diabetes (but not in those without type 2 diabetes)	Not reported
NHANES III [28]	9 year follow up of 20,050 American adults (17 years and over)	No association between egg intake (>7/week compared to <1/week) and CHD mortality	Not reported

Table 1. *Cont.*

Study	Design	Association between Egg Consumption and Cardiovascular Disease	Association between Egg Consumption and Incidence of Diabetes
Chinese cohort study [29]	Data from 2849 Chinese adults (20 years and over)	Not reported	Egg consumption was significantly and positively associated with diabetes risk. The OR of diabetes associated with egg consumption <2/week, 2–6/week, and ≥1/day in the total sample were 1.00, 1.75, 2.28 respectively. These associations were stronger in women compared to men
The SUN Project [30]	6 year follow up of 14,185 Mediterranean university students	No association between egg consumption and the incidence of CVD for the highest (>4 eggs/week) *versus* the lowest (<1 egg/week) category of egg consumption	Not reported
Case-control study [31]	234 Lithuanians aged 35–86 years with a newly confirmed diagnosis of type 2 diabetes according to WHO criteria, and 468 controls	Not reported	Participants who consumed >5 eggs/week had a higher risk (threefold) of type 2 diabetes than those who consumed <1 egg/week
Malmo Diet and Cancer Cohort [32]	Prospective cohort including 27,140 Swedish participants (45–74 years) during a 12 year follow up	Not reported	Highest quintiles of egg intake associated with increased risk of developing type 2 diabetes
Mediterranean cohort—the SUN project [33]	Prospective cohort of 15,956 participants from Spanish population (average age 38.5 years) during 6.6 years (median) follow up	Not reported	Egg consumption was not associated with the development of diabetes, comparing the highest (>4 eggs/week) with the lowest (<1 egg/week) quartile of egg consumption
The Northern Manhattan Study [34]	1429 American adults with carotid ultrasounds followed for 11 years	Egg consumption was inversely associated with carotid intima media thickness. For every additional egg consumed/week, risk of plaque decreased by 11%	Not reported

Table 1. *Cont.*

Study	Design	Association between Egg Consumption and Cardiovascular Disease	Association between Egg Consumption and Incidence of Diabetes
The Kuopio Ischaemic Heart Disease Risk Factor Study [35]	2332 men from Finnish population (42–60 years) during 19.3 years follow-up	Not reported	Higher egg intake was associated with a 38% lower risk of developing type 2 diabetes compared to those in the lowest group of egg intake
Meta-Analysis/Systematic Review regarding egg consumption, cardiovascular disease, and incidence of diabetes			
Cardiovascular diseases and diabetes meta-analysis [36]	14 studies (320,778 participants):11 prospective, 1 case-control and 2 cross-sectional studies. Sample size ranged from 488 to 117,943. Follow-up time from 6.1 to 20 years	Positive dose-response association between egg consumption and risk of CVD. A 19% increased risk of CVD in highest egg consumption compared to lowest egg intake. A sub group (participants with diabetes) found to have a further increased risk of CVD (RR 1.83)	There was a dose-response positive association between egg consumption and risk of diabetes
Dose-response meta-analysis of prospective cohort studies [37]	8 articles with 17 reports (9 for CHD and 8 for stroke)	No significant association found between egg consumption up to 1 egg/day and risk of CHD or stroke. In a subgroup analysis of people with diabetes, higher egg consumption (up to 1 egg/day) associated with a higher risk of CHD but lower risk of haemorrhagic stroke	Not reported
Cardiovascular disease and diabetes systematic review and meta-analysis [38]	22 independent cohorts from 16 studies. Number of participants ranged from 1600 to 90,735. Follow-up time ranged from 5.8 to 20 years	Consuming ≥1 egg/day was not associated with risk of overall CVD, ischemic heart disease, stroke or mortality. In a subgroup population (people with diabetes), those who ate eggs >once a day were 1.69 times more likely to develop CVD co-morbidity	Those who ate ≥1 egg/day (compared to those who never ate eggs) were 42% more likely to develop type 2 diabetes
Tran *et al.* systematic review [39]	8 epidemiological studies that examined the risk of developing type 2 diabetes mellitus. 6 of the studies evaluated egg consumption, whilst 2 of the studies evaluated dietary patterns that included eggs	Not reported	4 of the 8 studies found a significant association between diabetes risk and egg consumption.

Abbreviations: ABC, ageing and body composition; AMI, acute myocardial infarction; ARIC, atherosclerosis risk in communities; CHD, coronary heart disease; CVD, cardiovascular disease; EPIC, European prospective investigation into cancer and nutrition; NHANES, national health and nutrition examination survey; OR, odds ratio; RR, relative risk.

Earlier evidence as to the effect of egg intake on cardio-metabolic outcomes comes from the Framingham study (follow up of 24 years), which aimed to determine factors related to the development of cardiovascular disease. In doing so it addressed the effect of dietary intake (including egg consumption) on circulating cholesterol levels and on the incidence of coronary heart disease in a free living population in Framingham, MA, USA [8]. Egg intake in this population ranged from 0 to 24 eggs per week in males and from 0 to 19 per week in females, with an average egg consumption of 5.9 per week for males and 3.8 per week for females. Results showed no significant association between the number of eggs consumed with all-cause mortality, total coronary heart disease, myocardial infarction, or angina pectoris. Furthermore, a low *versus* high egg consumption had no effect on blood cholesterol level. This finding supported the data from intervention studies conducted at the same time (late 1970s) showing no effect of egg feeding in the general population [40–42]. Importantly, the Framingham study also suggested that focus should be placed on a person's entire dietary intake rather than egg or cholesterol intake alone, because circulating cholesterol distribution curves of the subjects according to tertiles of egg or cholesterol intake were more or less identical. This study has been supported by several other large epidemiological studies conducted later. Hu and colleagues reported on egg consumption and risk of cardiovascular disease in two large prospective cohort studies examining both males from the Health Professionals Follow-up Study ($n = 37,851$) and females from the Nurses' Health Study ($n = 80,082$) [43]. Both studies found a decline in the average egg consumption from 2.3 per week in 1986 to 1.6 eggs per week in 1990 for males, and a decline from 2.8 eggs per week in 1980 to 1.4 eggs per week in 1990 for females. This coincided with the increased emphasis in the USA during that same period [44,45], to restrict dietary cholesterol intake to less than 300 mg per day and limit egg consumption due to the high dietary cholesterol content of eggs. Egg consumption (one egg per day) had no significant association with nonfatal myocardial infarction or mortality from coronary heart disease, or risk of total stroke or its subtypes, whether or not subjects with diabetes or hypercholesterolemia were included in the analyses [43]. However, when examining subgroups of the population, a positive association between a higher egg intake and relative risk of coronary heart disease was found for those with diabetes [43]. Results were similar in the Physicians Health Study ($n = 21,327$), in that egg consumption (<7/week) was not associated with myocardial infarction, stroke or total mortality in male physicians [21]. However, consumption of greater than or equal to seven eggs per week was associated with a greater risk of mortality for this entire cohort of male physicians. This positive correlation to mortality with a higher intake of eggs ($\geq$7 eggs/week) was evident more so in those with diabetes [21]. At the time when the Physicians Health Study was conducted (as well as the majority of the other epidemiological studies), a public health campaign (which was emphasised in the early 1980s) was advising people to limit their cholesterol intake (including their consumption of eggs) [44,45]. Individuals (particularly physicians) consuming a high number of eggs during that time may have been less likely to have been following healthy dietary and lifestyle advice in general. Indeed, in this study [21], male physicians consuming a higher intake of eggs were also following other unhealthy behaviours including reduced frequency of exercise and increased smoking, and had a higher prevalence of diabetes and hypertension [21].

Epidemiological data from studies conducted in Japan [15–17], Italy [10] and Finland [11] and systematic and meta-analytic reviews [37,38] also support the above-mentioned data from the United States (Framingham Study [8], Health Professionals Follow-up Study, Nurses' Health Study [43]) as well as data from other United States studies listed in Table 1 [13,19,28], in that egg consumption showed no significant association with the risk of coronary heart disease or cardiovascular heart disease in the general population. However, again, as seen with some studies conducted in the United States [21,27,43], this result was not consistent when analysing sub-groups of the population, such as in those with self-reported diabetes [17,18]. With respect to egg consumption and incidence of diabetes, again there are inconsistencies. Despite most studies suggesting an increased association of diabetes incidence and egg consumption [20,29,31,32,36,38], some studies show no association between egg consumption and risk of developing T2DM [26,33], with one study even showing a higher egg intake being associated with a 38% lower risk of developing T2DM [35].

While the above-mentioned studies show no overall effect of eggs on CVD (at least up to an intake of six eggs per week), and an increased incidence of T2DM with increased egg consumption, when considering stroke, some of these epidemiological studies have shown a significant inverse relationship between a high egg consumption and reduced risk of total and haemorrhagic stroke, and stroke mortality [19,28,46]. This data provides circumstantial and weak evidence that eggs may have protective effects against certain pathologies.

In summary, there are inconsistencies in the findings between these prospective cohort studies in terms of the risk of CVD and mortality, and incidence of diabetes mellitus. Most studies show no association between egg consumption and CVD risk in a healthy population [8,10,11,13,17,19,28,30,34,47], while others suggest an increased risk of CVD with higher egg consumption (≥7 eggs per week) [12,16,21,24]. With respect to the incidence of diabetes with egg consumption, most studies suggest an increased association of diabetes incidence and egg consumption [20,29,31,32,36,38], some studies show no association between egg consumption and risk of developing T2DM [26,33], and one study shows a protective effect of higher egg intake and incidence of T2DM [35]. Conversely, the risk of stroke appears to be lower with higher egg consumption [19,28,46]. Similar discrepant findings are seen in subgroups of the population and specifically in people with diabetes mellitus, with some studies showing no increased risk in CVD with egg consumption [8,17,28,35], but the majority suggesting that a higher egg intake (usually ≥7 eggs per week) may increase the risk of CVD in this group [18,19,21,27,43]. An important limitation of these epidemiologic studies in general is the presence of confounding factors that have a known effect on coronary artery disease and cardiovascular heart disease that may not have been accounted for. Despite adjusting for some confounding factors in statistical models in the Physicians Health Study, detailed dietary data (total energy intake and saturated fat) and other important variables (markers of insulin resistance and lipids) that predict the onset of cardiovascular disease were not taken into account [21]. Intake of energy, total fat, fruit or wholegrains, as well as body mass index and family history, were only controlled for in a minority of the above-mentioned epidemiological studies [28,43]. These limitations highlight the need for controlled, prospective studies to determine the impact of eggs *per se* on cardio-metabolic health. Importantly, it is now known that dietary cholesterol is not the principal factor affecting circulating cholesterol levels, with the main determining dietary factors being saturated and trans-fat intake [48,49], for which only one [28] of these epidemiological studies adjusted. In this study that adjusted for saturated fat intake [28], there was no increased risk of coronary heart disease mortality or stroke in those eating greater than six eggs per week compared to those eating one to six eggs per week.

3. Controlled Prospective Studies of the Effects of a High Egg Diet on Dietary Cholesterol Intake and Circulating Cholesterol Levels

3.1. The Relationship between Dietary and Circulating Cholesterol

The effect of dietary cholesterol intake on circulating cholesterol level is small. A meta-analysis of cholesterol feeding studies including both healthy populations and populations with cardio-metabolic disease, using a variety of sources of dietary cholesterol (including eggs) showed that for every 100 mg per day increase in dietary cholesterol intake, circulating total cholesterol increased by 0.06 mmol/L, high-density lipoprotein (HDL) increased by 0.008 mmol/L, and the ratio of total to HDL cholesterol increased by 0.020 [50]. One large egg contains approximately 200 mg of dietary cholesterol, so consuming an egg a day would be expected to increase total circulating cholesterol levels by approximately 0.12 mmol/L [50]. While mean changes in lipoproteins in response to dietary cholesterol are small, considerable heterogeneity has been observed in circulating cholesterol responses to dietary cholesterol [51]. For example, there appears to be less efficient absorption of dietary cholesterol in those who have obesity and insulin resistance, when compared to those who are lean and insulin sensitive [52,

53]. However, meta-analyses comparing the effects of dietary cholesterol and fat on circulating lipid and lipoprotein levels reveal that dietary saturated and trans-fat elicit much stronger effects, and taking into consideration their higher percentage energy contribution in the diet relative to dietary cholesterol, saturated and trans-fat are the major contributors to circulating total and low-density lipoprotein (LDL) cholesterol levels [48,49,54]. For every 2.8-gram per day reduction in saturated fat intake, total cholesterol reduces by approximately 0.08 mmol/L. Therefore, while increasing egg intake by one egg per day would be expected to increase total cholesterol by approximately 0.12 mmol/L, a concomitant reduction in saturated fat intake by 6 g per day (the amount of saturated fat in a tablespoon of butter, for example) would be expected to reduce circulating cholesterol levels by a similar amount.

3.2. Studies Conducted in the General Population

Prospective controlled studies conducted in the general population (that is, in those that are relatively healthy without cardio-metabolic disorders) have shown differing effects of egg consumption on CVD risk. There have been numerous cholesterol feeding studies conducted in a free-living general population over the last 50 years and some of these studies are referenced in the following section. However, a summary of only those controlled prospective studies conducted in the general population since the meta-analytic review performed by Weggemans and colleagues [50] is provided in Table 2.

In some studies in which additional cholesterol (in the form of eggs) has been added to peoples' diet under strict control, there have been increases in circulating total and LDL cholesterol noted [55–57], whilst in other such studies there have been no changes [40–42,58–60]. In some studies, circulating HDL cholesterol levels significantly increased with the addition of eggs to the diet [61–63], which was also found in the meta-analytic review of dietary cholesterol feeding in 556 subjects from 17 heterogeneous studies using both eggs and high cholesterol products [50]. However, in that review the authors reported the adverse coronary risk finding of an increase in the ratio of total to HDL cholesterol by 0.02 units [50]. The majority of these studies (15 of 17 of them) involved subjects from an otherwise healthy population without metabolic disorders, but one study included those with type 1 diabetes mellitus (T1DM) and another included subjects with hypercholesterolemia and hyperlipidaemia. While there was a small but statistically significant adverse change in the total to HDL cholesterol ratio overall, five of the 17 studies showed no adverse effects of cholesterol feeding on the lipid profile, six studies showed equivocal effects, and only six studies showed adverse effects. More importantly, this change in lipid profile appeared to be dependent on the quality of the diet prescribed, or background diet of the population group [50,64,65]. This meta-analytic review [50] found that in subjects who were fed a high cholesterol diet and who had a background diet that was low in saturated fats (a polyunsaturated to saturated fat ratio > 0.7), the increase in LDL cholesterol was less apparent than in those studies in subjects in whom the background diet was high in saturated fats (a polyunsaturated to saturated fat ratio ≤ 0.7) [50]. Thus, these observations suggest that a person consuming a higher dietary cholesterol diet in the context of a diet lower in saturated fat is unlikely to experience any adverse effect on circulating lipids.

Table 2. Effect of egg consumption on cholesterol levels in the general population.

Reference	Study Details	Cholesterol/Egg Intake	Effect on Lipids from High Cholesterol or Egg Intake
Greene *et al.* 2005 [66]	42 healthy postmenopausal women and men > 60 years	3 eggs/day for 1 month (compared to egg substitute)	LDL and HDL cholesterol levels increased; LDL:HDL and TC:HDL ratios did not change
Katz *et al.* 2005 [67]	49 healthy adults	2 eggs/day for 6 weeks (compared to oats breakfast)	No effect on total cholesterol or endothelial function
Goodrow *et al.* 2006 [68]	33 adults > 60 years	1 egg/day for 5 weeks (compared to egg substitute)	No increase in total cholesterol, LDL cholesterol or HDL cholesterol levels

Table 2. *Cont.*

Reference	Study Details	Cholesterol/Egg Intake	Effect on Lipids from High Cholesterol or Egg Intake
Harman *et al.* 2008 [69]	45 overweight or obese adults (18–55 years)	2 eggs/day as part of an energy restricted weight loss diet (compared to no eggs/day)	Decreased total and LDL cholesterol
Mutungi *et al.* 2008 [61]	28 overweight or obese men (40–70 years)	3 eggs/week as part of a CHO restricted weight loss diet (compared to egg substitute)	Increased HDL cholesterol; no change in LDL cholesterol levels
Rueda *et al.* 2013 [70]	73 university students	Breakfast with eggs 5 times/week for 14 weeks (compared to breakfast without eggs) Egg breakfast contained 400mg more cholesterol than the breakfast without eggs	No significant differences in total, LDL cholesterol or HDL cholesterol between the two groups
Clayton *et al.* 2015 [71]	25 healthy young adults (18–35 years)	2 eggs per day (compared to a bagel breakfast) for 12 weeks	No impact on total cholesterol, HDL cholesterol or LDL cholesterol levels The egg breakfast led to improvements in triglyceride levels

Abbreviations: CHO, carbohydrate; HDL, high density lipoprotein; LDL, low density lipoprotein; TC, total cholesterol.

Of the more recent studies completed (Table 2), five of the seven studies have shown no adverse effects on the lipid profile following a high egg intake [66–68,70,71] and two have shown improvements in circulating lipids with an increased egg consumption [61,69].

3.3. Studies Conducted in people with High Risk of Cardiovascular Disease, Established Coronary Heart Disease, or with Diabetes Mellitus

In contrast to the variable effects of cholesterol feeding on circulating lipid profiles in the general population (that is, in those that are otherwise healthy and without cardio-metabolic disorders), with some studies showing an increase in the ratio of total to HDL cholesterol and LDL cholesterol, but others showing no adverse effects, in people with a high risk of cardio-metabolic disease the effects of a high egg diet appear generally positive. As there has been only a small number of well-designed studies conducted in such a population (that is, in people with high risk of cardiovascular disease or T2DM, established coronary heart disease, or with diabetes mellitus), these will be reviewed in greater detail. Six of these studies have been conducted in individuals at high risk of cardiovascular disease or T2DM [52,53,72–78], one in those with established coronary heart disease [79], and three in those with T2DM [80–82]. Of these, three studies have shown beneficial effects of a high egg diet on cardio-metabolic risk factors with respect to the comparator or control group [72–75,81,82], five have shown no adverse effect [53,76,78–80], and two have shown a detrimental effect, but only in sub-groups of the population being investigated [52,77]. A summary of each of the controlled prospective studies conducted in people with cardio-metabolic disease is provided in Table 3.

Table 3. Effect of egg consumption on cholesterol levels in those with cardio-metabolic disease, including type 2 diabetes mellitus.

Reference	Study Details	Cholesterol/Egg Intake	Effect on Lipids from Increased Cholesterol or Egg Intake
Edington *et al.* 1987 [76]	168 adults with hyperlipidaemia	2 eggs/week or 7 eggs/week as part of a low fat, high fibre diet for 8 weeks	No change to total, LDL or HDL cholesterol

Table 3. Effect of egg consumption on cholesterol levels in those with cardio-metabolic disease, including type 2 diabetes mellitus.

Reference	Study Details	Cholesterol/Egg Intake	Effect on Lipids from Increased Cholesterol or Egg Intake
Knopp *et al.* 1997 [77]	161 adults with hypercholesterolemia or hyperlipidaemia	2 eggs/day as part of an American Heart Association diet for 6 weeks	Increased LDL and HDL cholesterol levels; Adults with only high cholesterol had only non-significant increases in LDL cholesterol
Knopp *et al.* 2003 [52]	197 adults with insulin resistance	4 eggs/day for 4 weeks	Increased LDL cholesterol; This increase in LDL cholesterol was less in insulin resistant individuals compared to insulin sensitive individuals
Tannock *et al.* 2005 [53]	201 lean insulin-sensitive adults and lean or obese insulin resistant adults	4 eggs/day as part of a low fat diet for 4 weeks	HDL cholesterol increased in all subjects; non HDL cholesterol levels increased in lean insulin-sensitive subjects but not insulin-resistant subjects
Njike *et al.* 2010 [78]	40 adults with hyperlipidemia	3 and then 2 eggs/day (acute and sustained phase) for 6 weeks (compared to sausage/cheese breakfast sandwich and egg substitute)	No change to total, LDL or HDL cholesterol. No detrimental effects on flow mediated dilatation
Pearce *et al.* 2011 [81]	65 adults with type 2 diabetes or impaired glucose tolerance	2 eggs/day as part of an energy restricted, high protein diet for 12 weeks (compared to animal protein substitute)	Increased HDL cholesterol levels
Blesso *et al.* 2013 [73–75] and Andersen *et al.* 2013 [72]	37 adults with metabolic syndrome	3 eggs/day as part of carbohydrate restricted diet for 12 weeks (compared to egg substitute)	No change in total or LDL cholesterol; Increased HDL cholesterol; Increased LDL particle size
Fuller *et al.* 2015 [80]	140 overweight or obese adults with impaired glucose tolerance or type 2 diabetes	2 eggs/day for 6 days/week as part of a 3 month weight maintenance diet (compared to <2 eggs/week)	No difference in change in HDL cholesterol, total cholesterol or LDL cholesterol levels between the two groups
Katz *et al.* 2015 [79]	32 adults with CAD	2 eggs/day for 6 weeks	Daily consumption of eggs showed no adverse effects on total cholesterol levels compared to a high-carbohydrate breakfast

Abbreviations: CAD, coronary artery disease; HDL, high density lipoprotein; LDL, low density lipoprotein.

In a study investigating the effect of high egg intake (three eggs per day) *versus* egg substitute (which is comprised of 99% egg white and contains no cholesterol or fat) in those with metabolic syndrome, improvements in dyslipidemia were noted for both groups when accompanied by a three-month weight reduction program. However, reductions in circulating concentrations of the inflammatory markers tumour necrosis factor alpha (TNF-α) and serum amyloid A (a protein secreted in response to inflammatory stimuli) only occurred in the egg group [74]. Thus the high egg diet had a beneficial effect in reducing inflammation in this population with metabolic syndrome.

One study has been conducted in people with established coronary heart disease, and in contrast to the majority of studies, the primary outcome was endothelial function, assessed by flow-mediated dilatation. The authors found no difference in flow-mediated dilatation or circulating lipid levels between subjects that were following a high egg diet of two eggs per day compared to those following a high carbohydrate breakfast or a breakfast containing egg substitute [79]. One other study in which subjects with hyperlipidaemia were prescribed three eggs during the acute phase and two hard-boiled eggs during the sustained phase for breakfast along with their habitual diet, found no detrimental effects on flow mediated dilatation or lipid profile when compared to baseline levels [78].

In an earlier study in those with either hypercholesterolemia or hyperlipidaemia, subjects followed the National Cholesterol Education Program (NCEP) Step I Diet for six weeks before being randomised to 2 eggs or egg substitute daily [77]. There was no difference between the hypercholesterolemia or hyperlipidaemia egg fed groups for change in LDL cholesterol, when compared to a control group not fed eggs. However, the authors also reported on within group changes and found that there were significant increases in LDL cholesterol relative to baseline in the hyperlipidaemic egg fed group, and significant increases in HDL cholesterol in both the hypercholesterolemia and hyperlipidaemic egg fed groups from baseline to 12 weeks [77]. However, an important limitation of this study is that the group on the high egg diet also had a significantly higher intake of saturated fat compared to the control group not fed eggs [77].

There have been only three controlled, prospective studies investigating the effects of a high egg diet specifically in people with T2DM, and only one study in people with T1DM [83]. This short-term study over three weeks examined cholesterol feeding in both subjects with and without T1DM. There was an increase in the ratio of LDL to HDL cholesterol over a three-week period for those with T1DM only when 800 mg of cholesterol was added to their diet daily (as a liquid supplement containing egg yolk) [83]. One of the studies conducted in subjects with T2DM was accompanied by a weight loss prescription, which may have counteracted any potential detrimental effects of eggs on cardiovascular markers. In that study, there was no difference in LDL cholesterol between the high (two eggs per day) and no egg diet groups, and those on a high egg diet had a significant increase in HDL cholesterol compared to the no egg diet [81]. The other two studies were conducted under weight maintenance conditions. Over the course of a three-month weight maintenance study examining the effects of a high (12 eggs per week) *versus* low-egg (<2 eggs per week) diet [80] in those with impaired glucose tolerance or T2DM, the findings were similar to those reported by Pearce *et al.* in their weight loss study [81]. During this study subjects were required to maintain their weight and activity level, with an emphasis placed on replacing saturated fat with poly- and mono-unsaturated fatty acids in the diet. No adverse changes in circulating lipid profiles were evident when compared to those following a low egg diet [80]. Lastly, in a study comparing the consumption of one egg per day for breakfast *versus* an oatmeal-based breakfast in those with T2DM, there was no difference in fasting plasma glucose between groups after a five-week period. Similarly to the study in subjects with metabolic syndrome [74], there was a significant reduction in the inflammatory marker TNF-α in the one egg per day group [82].

Thus, apart from one small study of short duration (three weeks) which showed an increase in the ratio of LDL to HDL cholesterol with the addition of 800 mg dietary cholesterol daily in people with T1DM, all other studies conducted to date in subjects with cardio-metabolic disease or T2DM, have shown either a positive or no adverse effect on cardiovascular risk factors from a high egg diet.

4. Positive and Negative Nutritional Qualities of Eggs

Eggs are very high in dietary cholesterol, and despite an increase in circulating LDL cholesterol levels seen in some but not all dietary cholesterol feeding studies, eggs do possess nutritional benefits that may have benefits on health outcomes and CVD risk.

Eggs contain carotenoids (lutein and zeaxanthin) recognised for their role in protecting against age-related macular degeneration and cataracts, as well as for their antioxidant and anti-inflammatory properties [75,84]. They provide arginine (a precursor to nitric oxide), which in turn causes blood vessels to dilate, thereby playing a key role in endothelial function [85], and folate, which may reduce the risk of T2DM and cardiovascular disease [86,87], and risk of neural tube defects during pregnancy [88].

Omega-3 fortified eggs may also serve a role in the diet, particularly for people with hypertriglyceridemia and those who avoid fish. Two studies have shown consumption of omega-3 supplemented eggs to be associated with a significant decrease in circulating triglycerides [89,90], consistent with the improvements in triglyceride levels seen with fish or fish oil consumption [91,92].

Eggs are a substantial source of choline, which is a known neurotransmitter involved in cognitive function [93], but dietary phosphatidylcholine is associated with the production of a proatherosclerotic metabolite, trimethylamine-*N*-oxide (TMAO) in a gut-flora dependent manner, and this has been associated with an increased risk of cardiovascular events [94]

However, to date the effect of long term egg intake on TMAO levels has not been assessed. Thus despite the potential for an adverse effect of the cholesterol in eggs on LDL cholesterol, it is conceivable that specific components of eggs could also contribute to favourable health outcomes and reduced CVD risk in people who consume a high egg diet. When eggs are included in the context of a healthy diet, these nutritional benefits could conceivably outweigh any adverse effects of eggs, albeit further well-controlled studies are required to test this.

5. Conclusions

Despite conflicting guidelines between countries regarding dietary cholesterol and specifically egg intake, the evidence suggests that a diet including more eggs than is recommended (at least in some countries) may be used safely as part a healthy diet in both the general population and for those at high risk of cardiovascular disease, those with established coronary heart disease, and those with type 2 diabetes mellitus. The background or intervention diet appears to be a key nutritional component. A high egg diet in the context of a background diet that is low in saturated fats (a polyunsaturated to saturated fat ratio > 0.7), or a diet that replaces saturated fats with poly- and mono-unsaturated fats, is likely to result in positive or no adverse changes in LDL cholesterol, and could be safely advised. Hence, an approach focused on a person's entire dietary intake as opposed to specific foods or nutrients should be the heart of population nutrition guidelines.

Author Contributions: The authors' responsibilities were as follows: N.R.F. performed literature search, analysed data, wrote manuscript and had final responsibility for final content. A.S., I.D.C. and T.P.M analysed data, and assisted with writing the manuscript. All authors read and approved the final manuscript. Food & Nutrition Australia provided published data in the form of position statements for healthcare professionals, which was adapted in table format for the purpose of this review.

Conflicts of Interest: N.R.F., I.D.C. and T.P.M. have received research grants for other clinical trials funded by Australian Egg Corporation Limited, Sanofi-Aventis, Novo Nordisk, Allergan, Roche products, Merck, Sharp & Dohm, and GlaxoSmithKline. I.D.C. was an Executive Steering Committee member for the SCOUT trial, is on the Organising Committee of EXSCEL trial, and has received payment for lectures from iNova Pharmaceuticals, Pfizer Australia, and Servier Laboratories (Australia). T.P.M. acts as an advisory member to the Egg Nutrition Council, Nestle Nutrition and Novo Nordisk and has received payments for lectures from Novo Nordisk and Astra Zeneca. A.S. has received research and fellowship funding from the National Health and Medical Research Council and the University of Sydney, she has received honoraria by Eli Lilly Australia, the Pharmacy Guild of Australia, Novo Nordisk and the Dietitians Association of Australia for conference presentations, and holds shares in a company (Zuman International) that sells her books about adult weight management. No one other than the authors listed on this manuscript had any role in the analysis of the data, or the writing of the manuscript.

References

1. National Heart Foundation of Australia (NHF). Position statement: Dietary fats and dietary cholesterol for cardiovascular health. Available online: http://www.heartfoundation.org.au/SiteCollectionDocuments/Dietary-fats-summary-evidence.pdf (accessed on 25 May 2015).
2. Gray, J.; Griffin, B. Eggs and dietary cholesterol—Dispelling the myth. *Nutr. Bull.* **2009**, *34*, 66–70. [CrossRef]
3. Evert, A.B.; Boucher, J.L.; Cypress, M.; Dunbar, S.A.; Franz, M.J.; Mayer-Davis, E.J.; Neumiller, J.J.; Nwankwo, R.; Verdi, C.L.; Urbanski, P.; *et al.* Nutrition Therapy Recommendations for the Management of Adults With Diabetes. *Diabetes Care* **2013**, *36*, 3821–3842. [CrossRef] [PubMed]
4. US Department of Health and Human Services. *Dietary Guidelines for Americans*; US Department of Health and Human Services: Washington, DC, USA, 2015.
5. National Lipid Association. NLA Recommendations for Patient-Centered Management of Dyslipidemia. Available online: https://www.lipid.org/recommendations (accessed on 20 July 2015).

6.   Jacobson, T.A.; Ito, M.K.; Maki, K.C.; Orringer, C.E.; Bays, H.E.; Jones, P.H.; McKenney, J.M.; Grundy, S.M.; Gill, E.A.; Wild, R.A.; *et al.* National Lipid Association Recommendations for Patient-Centered Management of Dyslipidemia: Part 1-Full Report. *J. Clin. Lipidol.* **2015**, *9*, 129–169. [CrossRef] [PubMed]

7.   National Lipid Association (NLA). National Lipid Association Recommendations for Patient-Centered Management of Dyslipidemia 2015. Available online: https://www.lipid.org/sites/default/files/NLA_Recommendations_Part2_04June15_md.pdf (accessed on 20 July 2015).

8.   Dawber, T.R.; Nickerson, R.J.; Brand, F.N.; Pool, J. Eggs, serum cholesterol, and coronary heart disease. *Am. J. Clin. Nutr.* **1982**, *36*, 617–625. [PubMed]

9.   Imamura, F.; Lichtenstein, A.H.; Dallal, G.E.; Meigs, J.B.; Jacques, P.F. Generalizability of dietary patterns associated with incidence of type 2 diabetes mellitus. *Am. J. Clin. Nutr.* **2009**, *90*, 1075–1083. [CrossRef] [PubMed]

10. Gramenzi, A.; Gentile, A.; Fasoli, M.; Negri, E.; Parazzini, F.; Lavecchia, C. Association between certain foods and risk of acute myocardial infarction in women. *BMJ* **1990**, *300*, 771–773. [CrossRef] [PubMed]

11. Knekt, P.; Reunanen, A.; Jarvinen, R.; Seppanen, R.; Heliovaara, M.; Aromaa, A. Antioxidant vitamin intake and coronary mortality in a longitudinal population study. *Am. J. Epidemiol.* **1994**, *139*, 1180–1189. [PubMed]

12. Appleby, P.N.; Thorogood, M.; Mann, J.I.; Key, T.J.A. The Oxford Vegetarian Study: An overview. *Am. J. Clin. Nutr.* **1999**, *70*, 525S–531S. [PubMed]

13. Fraser, G.E. Associations between diet and cancer, ischemic heart disease, and all-cause mortality in non-Hispanic white California Seventh-day Adventists. *Am. J. Clin. Nutr.* **1999**, *70*, 532S–538S. [PubMed]

14. Rimm, E.B.; Spiegelman, D.; Hu, F.B.; Stampfer, M.J.; Speizer, F.E.; Ascherio, A.; Willett, W.C.; Manson, J.E.; Hennekens, C.H.; Colditz, G.A.; *et al.* A Prospective Study of Egg Consumption and Risk of Cardiovascular Disease in Men and Women. *JAMA* **1999**, *281*, 1387–1394.

15. Sasazuki, S.; Kodama, H.; Kono, S.; Liu, Y.; Miyake, Y.; Tanaka, K.; Tokunaga, S.; Yoshimasu, K.; Washio, M.; Mohri, M.; *et al.* Case-control study of nonfatal myocardial infarction in relation to selected foods in Japanese men and women. *Jpn. Circ. J.* **2001**, *65*, 200–206. [CrossRef] [PubMed]

16. Nakamura, Y.; Okamura, T.; Tamaki, S.; Kadowaki, T.; Hayakawa, T.; Kita, Y.; Okayama, A.; Ueshima, H. Egg consumption, serum cholesterol, and cause-specific and all-cause mortality: The National Integrated Project for Prospective Observation of Non-communicable Disease and Its Trends in the Aged, 1980 (NIPPON DATA80). *Am. J. Clin. Nutr.* **2004**, *80*, 58–63. [PubMed]

17. Nakamura, Y.; Iso, H.; Kita, Y.; Ueshima, H.; Okada, K.; Konishi, M.; Inoue, M.; Tsugane, S. Egg consumption, serum total cholesterol concentrations and coronary heart disease incidence: Japan Public Health Center-based prospective study. *Br. J. Nutr.* **2006**, *96*, 921–928. [CrossRef] [PubMed]

18. Trichopoulou, A.; Psaltopoulou, T.; Orfanos, P.; Trichopoulos, D. Diet and physical activity in relation to overall mortality amongst adult diabetics in a general population cohort. *J. Internal Med.* **2006**, *259*, 583–591. [CrossRef] [PubMed]

19. Qureshi, A.I.; Suri, M.F.K.; Ahmed, S.; Nasar, A.; Kirmani, J.F. Regular egg consumption does not increase the risk of stroke and cardiovascular diseases. *Med. Sci. Monit.* **2007**, *13*, CR1–CR8. [PubMed]

20. Djousse, L.; Gaziano, J.M.; Buring, J.E.; Lee, I.M. Egg Consumption and Risk of Type 2 Diabetes in Men and Women. *Diabetes Care* **2009**, *32*, 295–300. [CrossRef] [PubMed]

21. Djoussé, L.; Gaziano, J.M. Egg consumption in relation to cardiovascular disease and mortality: The Physicians' Health Study. *Am. J. Clin. Nutr.* **2008**, *87*, 964–969. [PubMed]

22. Djoussé, L.; Gaziano, J.M. Egg consumption and risk of heart failure in the physicians' health study. *Circulation* **2008**, *117*, 512–516. [CrossRef] [PubMed]

23. Iqbal, R.; Anand, S.; Ounpuu, S.; Islam, S.; Zhang, X.; Rangarajan, S.; Chifamba, J.; Al-Hinai, A.; Keltai, M.; Yusuf, S. Dietary patterns and the risk of acute myocardial infarction in 52 countries: Results of the INTERHEART study. *Circulation* **2008**, *118*, 1929–1937. [CrossRef] [PubMed]

24. Nettleton, J.A.; Steffen, L.M.; Loehr, L.R.; Rosamond, W.D.; Folsom, A.R. Incident Heart Failure Is Associated with Lower Whole-Grain Intake and Greater High-Fat Dairy and Egg Intake in the Atherosclerosis Risk in Communities (ARIC) Study. *J. Am. Diet. Assoc.* **2008**, *108*, 1881–1887. [CrossRef] [PubMed]

25. Liese, A.D.; Weis, K.E.; Schulz, M.; Tooze, J.A. Food Intake Patterns Associated with Incident Type 2 Diabetes. *Diabetes care* **2009**, *32*, 263. [CrossRef] [PubMed]

26. Djousse, L.; Kamineni, A.; Nelson, T.L.; Carnethon, M.; Mozaffarian, D.; Siscovick, D.; Mukamal, K.J. Egg consumption and risk of type 2 diabetes in older adults. *Am. J. Clin. Nutr.* **2010**, *92*, 422–427. [CrossRef] [PubMed]

27. Houston, D.K.; Ding, J.; Lee, J.S.; Garcia, M.; Kanaya, A.M.; Tylavsky, F.A.; Newman, A.B.; Visser, M.; Kritchevsky, S.B. Dietary fat and cholesterol and risk of cardiovascular disease in older adults: The Health ABC Study. *Nutr. Metab. Cardiovasc. Dis.* **2011**, *21*, 430–437. [CrossRef] [PubMed]

28. Scrafford, C.G.; Tran, N.L.; Barraj, L.M.; Mink, P.J. Egg consumption and CHD and stroke mortality: A prospective study of US adults. *Public Health Nutr.* **2011**, *14*, 261–270. [CrossRef] [PubMed]

29. Shi, Z.; Yuan, B.; Zhang, C.; Zhou, M.; Holmboe-Ottesen, G. Egg consumption and the risk of diabetes in adults, Jiangsu, China. *Nutrition* **2011**, *27*, 194–198. [CrossRef] [PubMed]

30. Zazpe, I.; Beunza, J.J.; Bes-Rastrollo, M.; Warnberg, J.; de la Fuente-Arrillaga, C.; Benito, S.; Vazquez, Z.; Martinez-Gonzalez, M.A.; Investigators SUNP. Egg consumption and risk of cardiovascular disease in the SUN Project. *Eur. J. Clin. Nutr.* **2011**, *65*, 676–682. [CrossRef] [PubMed]

31. Radzevičienė, L.; Ostrauskas, R. Egg consumption and the risk of type 2 diabetes mellitus: A case-control study. *Public Health Nutr.* **2012**, *15*, 1437–1441. [CrossRef] [PubMed]

32. Ericson, U.; Sonestedt, E.; Gullberg, B.; Hellstrand, S.; Hindy, G.; Wirfält, E.; Orho-Melander, M. High intakes of protein and processed meat associate with increased incidence of type 2 diabetes. *Br. J. Nutr.* **2013**, *109*, 1143–1153. [CrossRef] [PubMed]

33. Zazpe, I.; Beunza, J.J.; Bes-Rastrollo, M.; Basterra-Gortari, F.J.; Mari-Sanchis, A.; Martinez-Gonzalez, M.A.; Investigators SUNP. Egg consumption and risk of type 2 diabetes in a Mediterranean cohort; the SUN Project. *Nutricion Hosp.* **2013**, *28*, 105–111.

34. Goldberg, S.; Gardener, H.; Tiozzo, E.; Kuen, C.Y.; Elkind, M.S.V.; Sacco, R.L.; Rundek, T. Egg consumption and carotid atherosclerosis in the Northern Manhattan Study. *Atherosclerosis* **2014**, *235*, 273–280. [CrossRef] [PubMed]

35. Virtanen, J.K.; Mursu, J.; Tuomainen, T.P.; Virtanen, H.E.; Voutilainen, S. Egg consumption and risk of incident type 2 diabetes in men: The Kuopio Ischaemic Heart Disease Risk Factor Study. *Am. J. Clin. Nutr.* **2015**, *101*, 1088–1096. [CrossRef] [PubMed]

36. Li, Y.; Zhou, C.; Zhou, X.; Li, L. Egg consumption and risk of cardiovascular diseases and diabetes: A meta-analysis. *Atherosclerosis* **2013**, *229*, 524–530. [CrossRef] [PubMed]

37. Rong, Y.; Chen, L.; Zhu, T.; Song, Y.; Yu, M.; Shan, Z.; Sands, A.; Hu, F.B.; Liu, L. Egg consumption and risk of coronary heart disease and stroke: Dose-response meta-analysis of prospective cohort studies. *BMJ* **2013**, *346*, e8539. [CrossRef] [PubMed]

38. Shin, J.Y.; Xun, P.; Nakamura, Y.; He, K. Egg consumption in relation to risk of cardiovascular disease and diabetes: A systematic review and meta-analysis. *Am. J. Clin. Nutr.* **2013**, *98*, 146–159. [CrossRef] [PubMed]

39. Tran, N.L.; Barraj, L.M.; Heilman, J.M.; Scrafford, C.G. Egg consumption and cardiovascular disease among diabetic individuals: A systematic review of the literature. *Diabetes Metab. Syndr. Obes. Targets Ther.* **2014**, *7*, 121–137. [CrossRef] [PubMed]

40. Porter, M.W.; Yamanaka, W.; Carlson, S.D.; Flynn, M.A. Effect of dietary egg on serum cholesterol and triglyceride of human males. *Am. J. Clin. Nutr.* **1977**, *30*, 490–495. [PubMed]

41. Flynn, M.A.; Nolph, G.B.; Flynn, T.C.; Kahrs, R.; Krause, G. Effect of dietary egg on human serum cholesterol and triglycerides. *Am. J. Clin. Nutr.* **1979**, *32*, 1051–1057. [PubMed]

42. Slater, G.; Mead, J.; Dhopeshwarkar, G.; Robinson, S.; Alfinslater, R.B. Plasma cholesterol and triglycerides in men with added eggs in diet. *Nutr. Rep. Int.* **1976**, *14*, 249–260.

43. Hu, F.B.; Stampfer, M.J.; Rimm, E.B.; Manson, J.E.; Ascherio, A.; Colditz, G.A.; Rosner, B.A.; Spiegelman, D.; Speizer, F.E.; Sacks, F.R.; *et al.* A prospective study of egg consumption and risk of cardiovascular disease in men and women. *JAMA* **1999**, *281*, 1387–1394. [CrossRef] [PubMed]

44. Davis, C.; Saltos, E. Chapter 2: Dietary recommendations and how they have changed over time. In *America's Eating Habits: Changes and Consequences*; Agriculture Information Bulletin No. (AIB-750); US Department of Agriculture: Washington, DC, USA, 1999.

45. Kritchevsky, D. History of recommendations to the public about dietary fat. *J. Nutr.* **1998**, *128*, 449S–452S. [PubMed]

46. Sauvaget, C.; Nagano, J.; Allen, N.; Grant, E.J.; Beral, V. Intake of animal products and stroke mortality in the Hiroshima/Nagasaki Life Span Study. *Int. J. Epidemiol.* **2003**, *32*, 536–543. [CrossRef] [PubMed]

47. Iqbal, R.; Anand, S.S.; Ounpuu, S.; Islam, S.; Rangarajan, S.; Yusuf, S. Dietary patterns and risk of myocardial infarction in 52 countries: Results of the INTERHEART study. *Circulation* **2007**, *115*, E220–E220. [CrossRef] [PubMed]
48. Howell, W.H.; McNamara, D.J.; Tosca, M.A.; Smith, B.T.; Gaines, J.A. Plasma lipid and lipoprotein responses to dietary fat and cholesterol: A meta-analysis. *Am. J. Clin. Nutr.* **1997**, *65*, 1747–1764. [PubMed]
49. Clarke, R.; Frost, C.; Collins, R.; Appleby, P.; Peto, R. Dietary lipids and blood cholesterol: Quantitative meta-analysis of metabolic ward studies. *Br. Med. J.* **1997**, *314*, 112–117. [CrossRef]
50. Weggemans, R.M.; Zock, P.L.; Katan, M.B. Dietary cholesterol from eggs increases the ratio of total cholesterol to high-density lipoprotein cholesterol in humans: A meta-analysis. *Am. J. Clin. Nutr.* **2001**, *73*, 885–891. [PubMed]
51. McNamara, D.J.; Kolb, R.; Parker, T.S.; Batwin, H.; Samuel, P.; Brown, C.D.; Ahrens, E.H. Heterogeneity of cholesterol homeostasis in man—Response to changes in dietary fat quality and cholesterol quantity. *J. Clin. Investig.* **1987**, *79*, 1729–1739. [CrossRef] [PubMed]
52. Knopp, R.H.; Retzlaff, B.; Fish, B.; Walden, C.; Wallick, S.; Anderson, M.; Aikawa, K.; Kahn, S.E. Effects of insulin resistance and obesity on lipoproteins and sensitivity to egg feeding. *Arterioscler. Thromb. Vasc. Biol.* **2003**, *23*, 1437–1443. [CrossRef] [PubMed]
53. Tannock, L.R.; O'Brien, K.D.; Knopp, R.H.; Retzlaff, B.; Fish, B.; Wener, M.H.; Kahn, S.E.; Chait, A. Cholesterol feeding increases C-reactive protein and serum amyloid A levels in lean insulin-sensitive subjects. *Circulation* **2005**, *111*, 3058–3062. [CrossRef] [PubMed]
54. McNamara, D.J. The impact of egg limitations on coronary heart disease risk: Do the numbers add up? *J. Am. Coll. Nutr.* **2000**, *19*, 540S–548S. [CrossRef] [PubMed]
55. Hegsted, D.M.; Ausman, L.M.; Johnson, J.A.; Dallal, G.E. Dietary fat and serum lipids—An evaluation of the experimental data. *Am. J. Clin. Nutr.* **1993**, *57*, 875–883. [PubMed]
56. Roberts, S.L.; McMurry, M.P.; Connor, W.E. Does egg feeding (*i.e.*, dietary cholesterol) affect plasma cholesterol levels in humans? The results of a double-blind study. *Am. J. Clin. Nutr.* **1981**, *34*, 2092–2099. [PubMed]
57. Sacks, F.M.; Salazar, J.; Miller, L.; Foster, J.M.; Sutherland, M.; Samonds, K.W.; Albers, J.J.; Kass, E.H. Ingestion of egg raises plasma low density lipoproteins in free-living subjects. *Lancet* **1984**, *323*, 647–649. [CrossRef]
58. Greene, C.M.; Waters, D.; Clark, R.M.; Contois, J.H.; Fernandez, M.L. Plasma LDL and HDL characteristics and carotenoid content are positively influenced by egg consumption in an elderly population. *Nutr. Metab.* **2006**, *3*, 6. [CrossRef] [PubMed]
59. Herron, K.L.; Vega-Lopez, S.; Conde, K.; Ramjiganesh, T.; Shachter, N.S.; Fernandez, M.L. Men classified as hypo- or hyperresponders to dietary cholesterol feeding exhibit differences in lipoprotein metabolism. *J. Nutr.* **2003**, *133*, 1036–1042. [PubMed]
60. Vorster, H.H.; Benade, A.J.S.; Barnard, H.C.; Locke, M.M.; Silvis, N.; Venter, C.S.; Smuts, C.M.; Engelbrecht, G.P.; Marais, M.P. Egg intake does not change plasma plasma lipoprotein and coagulation profiles. *Am. J. Clin. Nutr.* **1992**, *55*, 400–410. [PubMed]
61. Mutungi, G.; Ratliff, J.; Puglisi, M.; Torres-Gonzalez, M.; Vaishnav, U.; Leite, J.O.; Quann, E.; Volek, J.S.; Fernandez, M.L. Dietary cholesterol from eggs increases plasma HDL cholesterol in overweight men consuming a carbohydrate-restricted diet. *J. Nutr.* **2008**, *138*, 272–276. [PubMed]
62. Schnohr, P.; Thomsen, O.O.; Hansen, P.R.; Bobergans, G.; Lawaetz, H.; Weeke, T. Egg consumption and high density lipoprotein cholesterol. *J. Internal Med.* **1994**, *235*, 249–251. [CrossRef] [PubMed]
63. Packard, C.J.; McKinney, L.; Carr, K.; Shepherd, J. Cholesterol feeding increases low density lipoprotein synthesis. *J. Clin. Investig.* **1983**, *72*, 45–51. [CrossRef] [PubMed]
64. Hopkins, P.N. Effects of dietary cholesterol on serum cholesterol—A meta-analysis and review. *Am. J. Clin. Nutr.* **1992**, *55*, 1060–1070. [PubMed]
65. Chenoweth, W.; Ullmann, M.; Simpson, R.; Leveille, G. Influence of dietary cholesterol and fat on serum lipids in men. *J. Nutr.* **1981**, *111*, 2069–2080. [PubMed]
66. Greene, C.M.; Zern, T.L.; Wood, R.J.; Shrestha, S.; Aggarwal, D.; Sharman, M.J.; Volek, J.S.; Fernandez, M.L. Maintenance of the LDL cholesterol:HDL cholesterol ratio in an elderly population given a dietary cholesterol challenge. *J. Nutr.* **2005**, *135*, 2793–2798. [PubMed]

67. Katz, D.L.; Evans, M.A.; Nawaz, H.; Njike, V.Y.; Chan, W.; Comerford, B.P.; Hoxley, M.L. Egg consumption and endothelial function: A randomized controlled crossover trial. *Int. J. Cardiol.* **2005**, *99*, 65–70. [CrossRef] [PubMed]

68. Goodrow, E.F.; Wilson, T.A.; Houde, S.C.; Vishwanathan, R. Consumption of One Egg Per Day Increases Serum Lutein and Zeaxanthin Concentrations in Older Adults without Altering Serum Lipid and Lipoprotein Cholesterol Concentrations. *J. Nutr.* **2006**, *136*, 2519–2524. [PubMed]

69. Harman, N.L.; Leeds, A.R.; Griffin, B.A. Increased dietary cholesterol does not increase plasma low density lipoprotein when accompanied by an energy-restricted diet and weight loss. *Eur. J. Nutr.* **2008**, *47*, 287–293. [CrossRef] [PubMed]

70. Rueda, J.M.; Khosla, P. Impact of Breakfasts (with or without eggs) on Body Weight Regulation and Blood Lipids in University Students over a 14-Week Semester. *Nutrients* **2013**, *5*, 5097–5113. [CrossRef] [PubMed]

71. Clayton, Z.S.; Scholar, K.R.; Shelechi, M.; Hernandez, L.M.; Barber, A.M.; Petrisko, Y.J.; Hooshmand, S.; Kern, M. Influence of Resistance Training Combined with Daily Consumption of an Egg-based or Bagel-based breakfast on risk factors for chronic diseases in healthy untrained Individuals. *J. Am. Coll. Nutr.* **2015**, *34*, 113–119. [CrossRef] [PubMed]

72. Andersen, C.J.; Blesso, C.N.; Lee, J.; Barona, J.; Shah, D.; Thomas, M.J.; Fernandez, M.L. Egg consumption modulates HDL lipid composition and increases the cholesterol-accepting Capacity of Serum in Metabolic Syndrome. *Lipids* **2013**, *48*, 557–567. [CrossRef] [PubMed]

73. Blesso, C.N.; Andersen, C.J.; Barona, J.; Volek, J.S.; Fernandez, M.L. Whole egg consumption improves lipoprotein profiles and insulin sensitivity to a greater extent than yolk-free egg substitute in individuals with metabolic syndrome. *Metab. Clin. Exp.* **2013**, *62*, 400–410. [CrossRef] [PubMed]

74. Blesso, C.N.; Andersen, C.J.; Barona, J.; Volk, B.; Volek, J.S.; Fernandez, M.L. Effects of carbohydrate restriction and dietary cholesterol provided by eggs on clinical risk factors in metabolic syndrome. *J. Clin. Lipidol.* **2013**, *7*, 463–471. [CrossRef] [PubMed]

75. Blesso, C.N.; Andersen, C.J.; Bolling, B.W.; Fernandez, M.L. Egg intake improves carotenoid status by increasing plasma HDL cholesterol in adults with metabolic syndrome. *Food Func.* **2013**, *4*, 213–221. [CrossRef] [PubMed]

76. Edington, J.; Geekie, M.; Carter, R.; Benfield, L.; Fisher, K.; Ball, M.; Mann, J. Effect Of Dietary Cholesterol on plasma cholesterol concentration in subjects following reduced fat, high fibre diet. *Br. Med. J.* **1987**, *294*, 333–336. [CrossRef]

77. Knopp, R.H.; Retzlaff, B.M.; Walden, C.E.; Dowdy, A.A.; Tsunehara, C.H.; Austin, M.A.; Nguyen, T. A double-blind, randomized, controlled trial of the effects of two eggs per day in moderately hypercholesterolemic and combined hyperlipidemic subjects taught the NCEP Step I diet. *J. Am. Coll. Nutr.* **1997**, *16*, 551–561. [PubMed]

78. Njike, V.; Faridi, Z.; Dutta, S.; Gonzalez-Simon, A.L.; Katz, D.L. Daily egg consumption in hyperlipidemic adults—Effects on endothelial function and cardiovascular risk. *Nutr. J.* **2010**, *9*, 28. [CrossRef] [PubMed]

79. Katz, D.L.; Gnanaraj, J.; Treu, J.A.; Ma, Y.; Kavak, Y.; Njike, V.Y. Effects of egg ingestion on endothelial function in adults with coronary artery disease: A randomized, controlled, crossover trial. *Am. Heart J.* **2015**, *169*, 162–169. [CrossRef] [PubMed]

80. Fuller, N.R.; Caterson, I.D.; Sainsbury, A.; Denyer, G.; Fong, M.; Gerofi, J.; Baqleh, K.; Williams, K.H.; Lau, N.S.; Markovic, T.P. The effect of a high-egg diet on cardiovascular risk factors in people with type 2 diabetes: The Diabetes and Egg (DIABEGG) study-a 3-mo randomized controlled trial. *Am. J. Clin. Nutr.* **2015**, *101*, 705–713. [CrossRef] [PubMed]

81. Pearce, K.L.; Clifton, P.M.; Noakes, M. Egg consumption as part of an energy-restricted high-protein diet improves blood lipid and blood glucose profiles in individuals with type 2 diabetes. *Br. J. Nutr.* **2011**, *105*, 584–592. [CrossRef] [PubMed]

82. Ballesteros, M.N.; Valenzuela, F.; Robles, A.E.; Artalejo, E.; Aguilar, D.; Andersen, C.J.; Valdez, H.; Fernandez, M.L. One Egg per Day improves inflammation when compared to an Oatmeal-Based Breakfast without increasing other cardiometabolic risk factors in diabetic patients. *Nutrients* **2015**, *7*, 3449–3463. [CrossRef] [PubMed]

83. Romano, G.; Tilly-Kiesi, M.K.; Patti, L.; Taskinen, M.R.; Pacioni, D.; Cassader, M.; Riccardi, G.; Rivellese, A.A. Effects of dietary cholesterol on plasma lipoproteins and their subclasses in IDDM patients. *Diabetologia* **1998**, *41*, 193–200. [CrossRef] [PubMed]

84. Chung, H.Y.; Rasmussen, H.M.; Johnson, E.J. Lutein bioavailability is higher from lutein-enriched eggs than from supplements and spinach in men. *J. Nutr.* **2004**, *134*, 1887–1893. [PubMed]

85. Preli, R.B.; Klein, K.P.; Herrington, D.M. Vascular effects of dietary L-arginine supplementation. *Atherosclerosis* **2002**, *162*, 1–15. [CrossRef]

86. Antoniades, C.; Antonopoulos, A.S.; Tousoulis, D.; Marinou, K.; Stefanadis, C. Homocysteine and coronary atherosclerosis: From folate fortification to the recent clinical trials. *Eur. Heart J.* **2009**, *30*, 6–15. [CrossRef] [PubMed]

87. Antonopoulos, A.S.; Shirodaria, C.; Antoniades, C. Vitamins and folate fortification in the context of cardiovascular disease prevention. In *B Vitamins and Folate: Chemistry, Analysis, Function and Effects*; Preedy, V.R., Ed.; Royal Society of Chemistry: Washington, DC, USA, 2013; pp. 35–54.

88. Pitkin, R.M. Folate and neural tube defects. *Am. J. Clin. Nutr.* **2007**, *85*, 285S–288S. [PubMed]

89. Bovet, P.; Faeh, D.; Madeleine, G.; Viswanathan, B.; Paccaud, F. Decrease in blood triglycerides associated with the consumption of eggs of hens fed with food supplemented with fish oil. *Nutr. Metab. Cardiovasc. Dis.* **2007**, *17*, 280–287. [CrossRef] [PubMed]

90. Jiang, Z.R.; Sim, J.S. Consumption of n-3 polyunsaturated fatty acid enriched eggs and changes in plasma lipids of human subjects. *Nutrition* **1993**, *9*, 513–518. [PubMed]

91. Din, J.N.; Newby, D.E.; Flapan, A.D. Science, medicine, and the future—Omega 3 fatty acids and cardiovascular disease—Fishing for a natural treatment. *Br. Med. J.* **2004**, *328*, 30–35. [CrossRef] [PubMed]

92. Harris, W.S. Fish oils and plasma lipid and lipoprotein metabolism in humans—A critical review. *J. Lipid Res.* **1989**, *30*, 785–807. [PubMed]

93. Sarter, M.; Parikh, V. Choline transporters, cholinergic transmission and cognition. *Nat. Rev. Neurosci.* **2005**, *6*, 48–56. [CrossRef] [PubMed]

94. Tang, W.H.W.; Wang, Z.; Levison, B.S.; Koeth, R.A.; Britt, E.B.; Fu, X.; Wu, Y.; Hazen, S.L. Intestinal microbial metabolism of phosphatidylcholine and cardiovascular Risk. *N. Engl. J. Med.* **2013**, *368*, 1575–1584. [CrossRef] [PubMed]

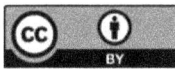

nutrients

MDPI

Review

Bioactive Egg Components and Inflammation

Catherine J. Andersen

Department of Biology, Fairfield University, Fairfield, CT 06824, USA; candersen@fairfield.edu;
Tel.: +1-203-254-4000 (ext. 2266); Fax: +1-203-254-4253

Received: 1 August 2015; Accepted: 9 September 2015; Published: 16 September 2015

Abstract: Inflammation is a normal acute response of the immune system to pathogens and tissue injury. However, chronic inflammation is known to play a significant role in the pathophysiology of numerous chronic diseases, such as cardiovascular disease, type 2 diabetes mellitus, and cancer. Thus, the impact of dietary factors on inflammation may provide key insight into mitigating chronic disease risk. Eggs are recognized as a functional food that contain a variety of bioactive compounds that can influence pro- and anti-inflammatory pathways. Interestingly, the effects of egg consumption on inflammation varies across different populations, including those that are classified as healthy, overweight, metabolic syndrome, and type 2 diabetic. The following review will discuss the pro- and anti-inflammatory properties of egg components, with a focus on egg phospholipids, cholesterol, the carotenoids lutein and zeaxanthin, and bioactive proteins. The effects of egg consumption of inflammation across human populations will additionally be presented. Together, these findings have implications for population-specific dietary recommendations and chronic disease risk.

Keywords: eggs; inflammation; phospholipids; cholesterol; lutein; bioactive proteins; healthy adults; metabolic syndrome; type 2 diabetes mellitus

1. Introduction

Inflammation is a normal, adaptive physiological response to pathogenic insult, including microbial infection and tissue injury; however the incidence of chronic low-grade, systemic inflammation underlying multiple highly prevalent chronic metabolic diseases has warranted the evaluation of inflammatory processes in disease pathogenesis [1,2]. Acute inflammatory responses mediated by immune system cells are considered beneficial if executed in a local, controlled manner, as they function to rapidly and effectively eliminate pathogenic stimuli and return the affected tissue to a normal, homeostatic state through coordinated activation and resolution of pro-inflammatory leukocyte activity [1]. However, failure of the body to appropriately execute and resolve acute inflammatory responses can lead to a detrimental chronic inflammatory tissue state, characterized by pathological tissue remodeling, fibrosis, and impaired functioning due to persistent inflammatory cell infiltration, activation, and leukocyte-mediated tissue damage [3,4]. These detrimental effects are observed in cases of inappropriate activation of the immune system, such as autoimmune conditions and allergic responses [5–7]. It has additionally been well established that similar adverse physiological adaptations occur in obesity-related disorders, where prolonged metabolic stress and tissue malfunction play a role in the development of chronic diseases, such as metabolic syndrome, cardiovascular disease (CVD), type 2 diabetes mellitus (T2DM), and cancer—all of which coincide with a chronic state of systemic, low-grade inflammation [8–11].

Given its significant role in the pathophysiology of many chronic diseases, inflammation has become a primary target for nutritional intervention. Various dietary patterns, functional foods, nutrients, and bioactive components have been shown to modulate inflammatory processes within the context of disease risk and progression [12–15]. Within this category, eggs are one of the most complex and controversial foods [16]. Eggs contain a variety of essential nutrients and bioactive components, but are most often recognized as a relatively rich source of high-quality protein and dietary cholesterol [17–19]. This had led to discrepancy in dietary recommendations across populations, where egg consumption has traditionally been considered more advisable to young, healthy populations and/or athletes (e.g., those with greater protein needs that can withstand a dietary cholesterol "challenge"), whereas egg intake by individuals at risk for CVD has been discouraged [20,21]. These recommendations have held, despite numerous epidemiological studies finding no association between egg intake and risk of coronary heart disease (CHD) mortality or stroke in the general U.S. population [22–25]. However, some studies have found eggs to be associated with an increased risk for T2DM [26,27], although these findings are not consistent across studies [28,29]. While the majority of egg nutrition studies have focused on parameters of lipid metabolism and markers of CVD risk, research has additionally revealed differential inflammatory responses across human populations. These findings indicate that healthy individuals often have greater pro-inflammatory responses to egg intake [30,31], whereas egg consumption by individuals who are overweight [32], classified with metabolic syndrome [33–37], or type 2 diabetic [38] is associated with a reduction in inflammatory markers. In this review, egg components known to modulate inflammatory pathways will be discussed, with a focus on their composition, bioavailability, and known mechanisms of action in cell, animal, and human models. The effects of egg consumption of inflammation across human populations will additionally be presented. Together, these findings have important implications for the role of eggs in modulating inflammation within the context of chronic diseases and immune defense.

2. Composition and Bioavailability of Egg Components

Eggs contain a wide variety of essential nutrients and bioactive compounds that can impact human health [17,39]. At only 72 kilocalories/large egg, eggs are a good source of high quality protein, fat-soluble and B vitamins, minerals, and choline, while providing relatively less saturated fat per gram compared to other animal protein sources [17,40]. This review will focus on primary components of eggs that are relatively abundant, bioavailable, and have pro- and anti-inflammatory properties: phospholipids, cholesterol, the carotenoids lutein and zeaxanthin, and egg white- and yolk-derived proteins.

2.1. Phospholipids

Eggs—particularly the yolk fractions—are one of the richest dietary sources of phospholipids [41, 42]. On average, one large egg contains approximately 1.3 g of phospholipids [43,44], which represent approximately 28%–30% of total lipids by weight [45]. The predominate phospholipid class found in eggs is the glycerophospholipid phosphatidylcholine, representing approximately ~72% of phospholipids. Additional phospholipid classes include phosphatidylethanolamine (~20%), lysophosphatidylcholine (3%), phosphatidylinositol (2%), and the sphingolipid sphingomyelin (3%) [46]. While the fatty acid composition of egg phospholipids varies across classes, the majority of phospholipids contain long-chain saturated and monounsaturated fatty acids—the distribution of which can be somewhat reflective of the hen's diet, age, and environmental conditions [44,47,48].

The majority of egg-derived phospholipids are highly bioavailable, with glycerophospholipid classes such as phosphatidylcholine being absorbed at >90% efficiency [49,50]. Tracer studies have demonstrated that dietary phospholipids are preferentially incorporated into plasma high-density lipoprotein (HDL) fractions over apoB-containing lipoproteins, red blood cells, or total blood fractions [50]. Similar findings were observed in subjects classified with metabolic syndrome, where consumption of 3 eggs per day for 12 weeks resulted in greater enrichment of HDL-phosphatidylethanolamine when compared to subjects consuming a yolk-free egg substitute. Further, subjects consuming whole eggs exhibited greater enrichment of egg-derived sphingomyelin species, indicative of the high bioavailability egg phospholipids and incorporation into HDL particles [46]. In general, phospholipids are known to influence plasma lipids and preferentially raise HDL-cholesterol [51,52], making them the likely egg component attributable to increases in HDL-cholesterol observed from egg intake [34,53].

2.2. Cholesterol

Eggs are one of the richest sources of dietary cholesterol, with an average large egg providing approximately 186 mg cholesterol [17]. Similar to the majority of phospholipids, cholesterol is localized to the yolk fraction; however, cholesterol only contributes ~5% of total yolk lipids by weight [45,54]. Although dietary recommendations for egg intake are often based on their cholesterol content, absorption efficiency of dietary cholesterol has been shown to be highly variable between individuals, ranging from 15% to 85% [55]. Efficiency of cholesterol absorption additionally seems to vary across human populations, with individuals who are insulin-resistant absorbing less cholesterol then insulin-sensitive counterparts [56,57], regardless of body weight status [58]. However, obese and insulin resistant subjects exhibit increased rates of endogenous cholesterol synthesis, contributing to hypercholesterolemia commonly observed in these populations [56–58]. Obesity is additionally associated with elevated secretion of biliary cholesterol, which may compete with dietary cholesterol for micellarization and absorption [59–61].

In addition to body weight and health status, cholesterol absorption efficiency is affected by food matrix composition [43,58,62,63]. The absorption of egg-derived cholesterol can be altered by interactions with phospholipids, potentially altering the mobilization of cholesterol from micelles in the intestine [41,43,63]. In Sprague-Dawley rats, egg-derived phosphatidylcholine and sphingomyelin lowered the intestinal absorption of cholesterol [43,63], whereas, the addition of lysophosphatidylcholine increased cholesterol absorption [64]. Given that phosphatidylcholine represents that vast majority of egg phospholipid species [46], intestinal cholesterol-phosphatidylcholine interactions likely limit egg-derived cholesterol absorption [43,64].

Cholesterol that is absorbed is packaged into chylomicrons and HDL by the enterocyte for ultimate release into the circulation and delivery to the liver and peripheral tissues [65,66]. Interestingly, in healthy young men (age 17–22 years), consumption of 3 whole eggs + labeled tracer led to a 52% slower fractional clearance rate of ^{14}C-cholesteryl ester in plasma, indicating an increased retention time in chylomicron remnants following egg consumption [67], potentially through downregulation of receptors involved in systemic cholesterol clearance [67,68]. Overall, while cholesterol intake is known to impact plasma lipid levels, it is difficult to attribute changes in plasma lipids solely to cholesterol provided in eggs, due to the similarity of effect on plasma lipids from providing whole eggs or isolated phospholipid [51–53].

2.3. Lutein and Zeaxanthin

In addition to phospholipids and cholesterol, egg yolks contain various antioxidant carotenoids [69]. Carotenoids are plant-derived pigments that confer yellow, orange, and red color to fruits and vegetables [70]. As such, the carotenoid composition of egg yolk is reflective of the hen's diet, with greater intake of carotenoid-rich grains resulting in greater yolk enrichment [71]. Lutein and zeaxanthin are the predominant carotenoid species found in egg yolk, although β-carotene, α-carotene, and β-cryptoxanthin are also present at lower levels [69].

Lutein and zeaxanthin are dipolar xanthophylls comprised of hydrophilic ionone ring structures with hydroxyl groups on each end, connected by a lipophilic central chain consisting of conjugated C = C bonds. Lutein and zeaxanthin structures are near identical, apart from a difference in the positioning of a double bond the ring structure [72,73]. The predominant isomers of carotenoids found in raw chicken eggs include all-E-lutein, all-E-zeaxanthin, 13′-Z-lutein, 13-Z-zeaxanthin [74,75].

Compared to plant sources, eggs contain a relatively low amount of lutein and zeaxanthin; however, egg-derived carotenoids have been shown to be significantly more bioavailable [76]. Factors affecting the bioavailability of egg-derived lutein and zeaxanthin include method of cooking and the food matrix [74,75,77]. Using an *in vitro* gastrointestinal model, Nimalaratne *et al.* [75] found that the primary egg carotenoids, all-E-lutein and all-E-zeaxanthin, were highly stable during digestion, yet the method of cooking impacted carotenoid bioaccessibility—the release of the carotenoids from the whole food matrix to allow for micellarization into an absorbable form [75,77]. Boiled eggs promoted the greatest bioaccessibility, whereas scrambling had the most deleterious effect [75]. Cooking methods have additionally been shown to differentially promote the formation of Z-isomers from all-E-lutein [74], which may impact downstream micellarization and absorption [78]. Carotenoid absorption can further be influenced by phospholipid interactions in the intestine [79–81].

Dietary consumption of egg-derived lutein and zeaxanthin often correlates with concentrations in plasma, where carotenoids are carried by lipoproteins [69]. In a crossover study conducted in healthy men, serum lutein concentrations were increased to the greatest extent following consumption of a lutein-enriched egg, as opposed to a lutein supplement, lutein ester supplement, or spinach [76]. Plasma lutein and zeaxanthin levels have also been shown to be increased in healthy adults following consumption of one lutein- or zeaxanthin-enriched egg per day for 90 days [82], as well as hypercholesterolemic adults who consumed 1.3 egg yolks per day for 4.5 weeks [83]. Increases in plasma lutein, zeaxanthin, and β-carotene were observed in subjects with metabolic syndrome who consumed 3 eggs per day for 3 weeks. These changes corresponded to enrichment of HDL (+20%, +57%) and low-density lipoproteins (LDL) (+9%, +46%) fractions with lutein and zeaxanthin, respectively [69].

Once in circulation, lutein is preferentially localized to the retina of the eye, which has been shown to increase macular pigment density and protect against age-related macular degeneration [72,84]. In older adults (60 years +), consumption or 2 or 4 eggs per day for 5 weeks increased serum lutein and zeaxanthin, in addition to increasing macular pigment optical density [85]. Serum zeaxanthin and macular pigment density was additionally increased in adult women (age 24–59) who consumed 6 eggs/week for 12 weeks [86]. In addition to accumulating in the eye, lutein supplementation increases lutein concentrations various other tissues, including skin [87], liver [84], and adipose [88, 89]. Interestingly, obesity is associated with increased carotenoid deposition in adipose and lower circulating levels of carotenoids, potentially making them less available for other tissues [90].

2.4. Egg Proteins

Eggs are a good source of high-quality protein that promote protein synthesis and maintenance of skeletal muscle mass [91–93]. On average, one large egg provides ~6.3 g protein that is rich in essential amino acids [17,94]. Eggs also contain a variety of bioactive proteins that possess antimicrobial and immunoprotective properties—that majority of which can be found in the egg white fraction [54,95–97]. The predominant egg white proteins that can impact inflammation include ovalbumin (54% of egg white protein by weight), ovotransferrin (12%), ovomucin (3.5%), lysozyme (3.4%), and avidin (0.5%) [54]. Egg white additionally contains ovoinhibitor, a serine proteinase inhibitor that can reduce enzymatic digestion by trypsin and chymotrypsin, and it has been demonstrated that certain egg proteins can be absorbed intact [98–100]. Lysozyme is absorbed intact via endocytic and paracellular transport in proximal intestine of rats [99], whereas ovalbumin is preferentially absorbed in the distal intestine via paracellular and receptor- and clatharin-mediated endocytic transport [100]. The absorption of intact egg proteins has been implicated in mediating allergic responses to egg proteins, whereas heating and digestion of egg proteins can lower allergenicity [99–101]. Methods of cooking and preparation of eggs may further impact overall egg protein bioavailability. Using tracer studies, cooked egg proteins have been found to be highly digestible (~91%) as compared to raw egg protein (~51%) [102].

3. Pro- and Anti-Inflammatory Properties of Egg Components: Mechanisms of Action

The components of eggs highlighted above each possess unique pro- and/or anti-inflammatory properties that likely contribute to the effects that egg intake has on inflammation in human populations [30–32,36,54,72,103]. The following section summarizes known mechanisms of action for each egg component as it relates to inflammation and human health.

3.1. Phospholipids

Egg-derived phospholipids have pro- and anti-inflammatory properties via both direct and indirect mechanisms. The majority of research investigating inflammatory properties of phospholipids has focused on phosphatidylcholine. In Caco-2 cells, phosphatidylcholine (200 μmol) has been shown to inhibit TNFα-induced alterations of plasma membrane architecture required for receptor-mediated signaling, activation of the pro-inflammatory mitogen-activated protein kinases (MAPKs), extracellular-signal-regulated kinase (ERK) and p38, nuclear factor κB (NF-κB) subunit translocation to the nucleus, and up-regulation of pro-inflammatory cytokines, such as tumor necrosis factor α (TNFα), interleukin (IL)-8, intercellular adhesion molecule (ICAM)-1, monocyte chemoattractant protein (MCP)-1, interferon γ-induced protein (IP)-10, and matrix metalloproteinase (MMP)-1 [104,105]. Individuals with ulcerative colitis have lower levels of phosphatidylcholine in the gastrointestinal mucus layer, and supplementation of phosphatidylcholine has positive clinical outcomes [106–108]. Phosphatidylcholine supplementation through diet enrichment has additionally been shown to reduce adverse leukocyte-endothelial interactions and inflammatory joint damage in a chronic murine model of rheumatoid arthritis [109]. In a rat model of neuroinflammation, oral administration of phosphatidylcholine reduced lipopolysaccharide (LPS)-induced plasma TNFα and mitigated disturbances in hippocampal neurogenesis [110].

Despite the evidence to suggest that phosphatidylcholine is anti-inflammatory, egg phospholipids have recently been implicated in the promotion of inflammation and atherosclerosis due formation of trimethylamine-*N*-oxide (TMAO) [31,111]. Production of TMAO is dependent upon intestinal microbiota-induced conversion of phosphatidylcholine to trimethylamine (TMA), followed by oxidation of TMA by hepatic flavin-containing monooxygenase 3 (FMO3). TMAO has been shown to promote atherosclerosis in animal models, whereas high levels of plasma TMAO has been associated with increased risk for major adverse cardiovascular events in a cohort of 4007 patients [31,112]. TMAO has additionally been shown to increase adipose tissue inflammation and impair glucose tolerance in mice [111]. Egg intake has also been shown to dose-dependently increase post-prandial TMAO concentrations in plasma, although large interindividual variability was observed [113]. Variation between individuals may be attributable to differences in FMO3 expression and/or intestinal microbiota composition [114]. However, intake of more than one egg per day has been associated with lower atherosclerotic burden, as determined by coronary angiography [115]. Given that numerous epidemiological studies have failed to find an association between egg intake and atherosclerosis, additional long-term studies are needed to determine whether egg-induced TMAO production has detrimental effects on inflammation and disease risk.

3.2. Cholesterol

Dietary cholesterol is known to be pro-atherogenic and pro-inflammatory in animal studies [116, 117]; however, these studies are often not representative of egg consumption, as cholesterol is provided in high doses as an isolated form, thus failing to take into account the phospholipid matrix, realistic dose provided by eggs, and the variability in cholesterol absorption across populations [17,43,55,57]. Nevertheless, cholesterol is known to possess pro-inflammatory properties by inducing cytotoxicity in its free, unesterified form, in addition to promoting the formation of lipid rafts in plasma membranes of leukocytes, resulting in greater hypersensitivity to activation by pro-inflammatory signaling pathways [118,119]. Increased lipid raft formation has been associated with increased pro-inflammatory responses in macrophages and T lymphocytes [119–122]. In mouse models, dietary cholesterol provided by standard atherogenic diets has additionally been shown to promote aortic inflammation and the formation of macrophage foam cells—the hallmark of atherosclerosis [123,124]. In guinea pigs fed a low-carbohydrate diet, the addition of high cholesterol (0.25/100 g) increased concentrations of total and free cholesterol in the aorta and adipose tissue, while also increasing pro-inflammatory cytokine levels in adipose [125]. In line with its atheroprotective properties, HDL and its related lipid transporter, ATP-binding cassette transport A 1 (ABCA1), have been shown to exert direct and indirect anti-inflammatory activity by reducing cellular cholesterol levels, lipid raft formation, and mitigating leukocyte inflammation [120,121,126–128]. This may have significant implications for egg consumption, which is known to favorably modulate HDL metabolism, as discussed in greater detail below [33,34,36,46].

3.3. Lutein and Zeaxanthin

Despite the relatively high bioavailability of both lutein and zeaxanthin from egg yolk [69,76], lutein has gained considerably more attention due to its protective effects against age-related macular degeneration [72,129]. Supplementation with lutein alone or in combination with zeaxanthin has been shown to have anti-inflammatory effects in a variety of experimental models. The anti-inflammatory properties of lutein are thought to be related to its antioxidant activity, conferred by its conjugated C = C double bonds that can readily quench singlet oxygen species, triplet states of photoreactive molecules, and scavenge free radicals [130,131]. Lutein has been shown to protect against cisplatin-induced DNA damage, chromosome instability, and oxidative stress in mice and HepG2 human liver cells [132–134]. In guinea pigs fed a hypercholesterolemic diet, lutein supplementation (0.01 g/100 g) has been shown to exert anti-inflammatory effects in the liver, aorta, and eye [84,131]. Following a 12-week period, lutein treatment lowered aortic pro-inflammatory cytokines, in addition to oxidized LDL (oxLDL) in plasma and aorta. Aortic morphology further indicated protective effects of lutein against atherosclerosis [131]. Similar anti-inflammatory effects were observed in the liver, as lutein supplementation lowered the NF-κB p65 DNA binding activity compared to control animals, in addition to lowering liver TNFα protein and hepatic free cholesterol by 43% [84]. Reductions in eye TNFα and IL-1β were additionally observed in the lutein-supplemented group [84]. In apoE$^{-/-}$ mice, combined supplementation of lutein and egg yolk reduced detrimental ultrastructural alterations of the retina, whereas egg yolk additionally reduced the degree of systemic lipid peroxidation [135].

Studies have further shown lutein to protect mice from LPS-induced lethality, while also inhibiting NF-κB-mediated pro-inflammatory gene expression induced by hydrogen peroxide [136]. Following LPS injection, dietary lutein supplementation (50 mg/kg of feed) dose-dependently reduced TNFα mRNA expression in the spleen of F-line turkeys, while increasing mRNA expression of anti-inflammatory IL-10 [137]. Interestingly, Meriwether *et al.* [138] found that the lutein status of laying hens impacted the inflammatory immune response in chick offspring, where depletion/deficiency of lutein during embryonic development and early life was associated with greater pro-inflammatory responses to LPS [138]. Lutein derivatives generated from UV-irradiation have additionally been shown to have anti-inflammatory effects via inhibition of serum TNFα and IL-6 in LPS-treated mice [139]. Lutein has additionally been shown to suppress T_h2 lymphocyte-mediated airway inflammation in a murine model of asthma [140]. However, in a study conducted in healthy adults by Graydon *et al.* [141], lutein (10 mg/day) and zeaxanthin (5 mg/day) supplementation for 8 weeks did not affect serum ICAM-1, VCAM-1 or CRP levels [141]. These results may be indicative of a lower bioavailability of lutein and zeaxanthin from supplements, or perhaps a lack of an anti-inflammatory effect in healthy individuals who do not exhibit physiological stress and tissue dysfunction [8,76].

3.4. Egg Proteins

As detailed above, eggs contain a variety of bioactive proteins in the white fraction, including ovalbumin, ovotransferrin, ovomucin, lysozyme, and avidin [54]. These proteins possess antibacterial and immunoprotective properties, yet are also capable of inducing unfavorable pro-inflammatory responses in individuals allergic to egg proteins [99–101]. Egg white-derived lysozyme naturally exerts antimicrobial activity against Gram-positive and Gram-negative bacteria through hydrolysis of structural peptidoglycans in the bacterial cell walls, in addition to giving rise to antibacterial peptides from within its complete protein structure through enzymatic hydrolysis [142,143]. In a porcine model of dextran sodium sulfate (DSS)-induced colitis, hen egg lysozyme supplementation reduced intestinal gene expression of pro-inflammatory cytokines (TNFα, IL-6, IFNγ, IL-8, IL-17) while increasing expression of anti-inflammatory IL-4 and transforming growth factor β (TGFβ). Further, lysozyme attenuated weight loss, colonic crypt distortion, muscle wall thickening, and gastric wall permeability observed in control DSS-treated animals [97]. Ovotransferrin, an iron-binding glycoprotein with antibacterial activity, has additionally been shown reduce inflammatory colitis pathology in a DSS-induced mouse model of colitis [95,144]. Oral administration of egg ovotransferrin reduced inflammatory cytokines, while additionally mitigating clinical markers of colitis, including weight loss and histological scores of the colon [95]. Egg yolk-derived phosvitin additionally has significant bactericidal activity against *E. coli*, which was shown to be attributable to its high metal-chelating properties, in addition to its high surface activity under thermal stress [145]. Ovokinin, a biologically active peptide derivative of ovalbumin, has been shown to lower blood pressure in spontaneously hypertensive rats when provided via oral administration [146]. This phenomenon was dependent upon the presence of egg yolk phospholipids during administration, provided as either the whole egg yolk, the yolk phospholipid fraction, or isolated egg phosphatidylcholine [146].

In addition to the bioactive proteins above, utilization of immunoglobulin Y (IgY) in medicine has additionally shown promising results in promoting passive immunity against a variety of pathogens in the treatment of conditions such as colitis, influenza, and infection of *Clostridium botulinum*, *Staphylococcus aureus*, *Candida albicans*, and *Helicobacter pylori* [96,147]. In cystic fibrosis patients, daily use of a mouthwash containing IgY antibody purified from eggs of hens immunized against *Pseudomonas aeruginosa* significantly decreased *Pseudomonas aeruginosa* colonization [148]. Together, these findings highlight a unique immunomodulatory and anti-inflammatory role of egg-derived proteins.

4. Effects of Egg Intake on Inflammation in Human Populations

As outlined above, eggs contain a variety of bioactive components that possess pro- and/or anti-inflammatory properties. Each of these components likely contribute to the overall response observed in human subjects following egg consumption; however, evidence suggests that the effects of egg intake on inflammatory markers differs across populations, based on body weight and health status [30–33,35,36]. The following section explores these findings, with a summary of the relationship between egg intake and inflammation presented in Table 2.

Table 1. Effects of egg intake on inflammation in different human populations.

Population, *n*	Intervention Conditions	Effect on Inflammation	Ref.
Healthy Adults			
n = 66	4 eggs/day for 4 weeks; AHA NCEP step 1 diet	↑ serum amyloid A, CRP	[30]
n = 40	2-egg meal	↑ postprandial TMAO	[31]
Young men, *n* = 24	1-, 2-, or 4-egg meal	↑ *ex vivo* J774 macrophage cell free cholesterol	[149]
Young men and women, n = 50	2 eggs/day for 4 weeks	↓ AST and ALT	[150]
Overweight			
Men, n = 28	3 eggs/day for 12 weeks, *ad libitum* carbohydrate-restricted diet	↓ CRP ↑ adiponectin	[32]

Table 2. Cont.

Population, *n*	Intervention Conditions	Effect on Inflammation	Ref.
Insulin resistant			
Lean, n = 76	4 eggs/day for 4 weeks; AHA NCEP step 1 diet	↔serum amyloid A, CRP	[30]
Obese, n = 59	4 eggs/day for 4 weeks; AHA NCEP step 1 diet	↔serum amyloid A, CRP	[30]
Metabolic syndrome			
Men and women, n = 37	3 eggs/day for 12 weeks, moderate carbohydrate-restricted diet	↓oxidized LDL	[34]
Men and women, n = 37	3 eggs/day for 12 weeks, moderate carbohydrate-restricted diet	↓TNFα, serum amyloid A	[35]
Men and women, n = 5	3 eggs/day for 12 weeks, moderate carbohydrate-restricted diet	↓LPS-induced TNFα and IL-1β production from PBMCs *ex vivo*	[36]
T2DM			
Men and women, n = 29	1 egg/day for 5 weeks	↓TNFα and AST ↔ CRP	[38]
Men and women, n = 65	2 eggs/day for 12 weeks	↔CRP and homocysteine	[151]

Abbreviations: ↑: increase; ↓: decrease; ↔: no change; AHA: American Heart Association; ALT: alanine aminotransferase; AST: aspartate aminotransferase; CRP: C-reactive protein; IL-1β: interleukin 1 β; NCEP: National Cholesterol Education Program; PBMC: peripheral blood mononuclear cells; T2DM: type 2 diabetes mellitus; TMAO: trimethylamine-N-oxide; TNFα: tumor necrosis factor α.

4.1. Healthy Populations

A number of intervention trials conducted in healthy adults have demonstrated a pro-inflammatory response to egg intake. Tannock *et al.* [30] investigated the effects of egg consumption in lean insulin sensitive, lean insulin resistant, and obese insulin resistant subjects on an American Heart Association (AHA)—National Cholesterol Education Program (NCEP) step 1 diet. Interestingly, after consuming 4 eggs per day for 4 weeks, CRP and serum amyloid A—both acute phase inflammatory proteins—were significantly increased in the lean insulin sensitive subjects, whereas no changes were observed in either lean or obese insulin resistant groups—despite their having higher baseline levels of inflammation [30]. This was associated with increased cholesterol absorption in the lean insulin sensitive subjects, whereas both lean and obese insulin resistant subjects exhibited greater cholesterol synthesis [58]. In a crossover study conducted in 13 subjects with LDL-C over 130 mg/dL (>3.36 mmol/L), addition of daily egg yolk to a diet of 30% fat (predominantly polyunsaturated and saturated fatty acids) for 32 days resulted in increased susceptibility of LDL to *in vitro* oxidation [152]. Increased susceptibility to plasma and LDL oxidation was additionally observed by Levy *et al.* [153] in subjects consuming 2 eggs per day for 3 weeks. These subjects additionally exhibited minor increases in plasma glucose [153], contributing to the controversial body of research regarding the effects of egg intake on T2DM risk [26,27]. Similarly, healthy subjects who consumed a 2-egg meal exhibited increased plasma levels of pro-inflammatory TMAO postprandially; however, these increases were dependent upon the presence of normal intestinal microbiota, as administration of an oral broad-spectrum antibiotic suppressed the egg-induced increase in TMAO [31]. In a study by Ginsberg *et al.* [149], the serum from healthy men following consumption of a meal containing 0, 1, 2, or 4 eggs was incubated with J774 murine macrophage cells for 18 h. Following incubation, cellular free cholesterol content of J774 cells was highest when incubated with serum post-egg consumption when compared to the 0-egg meal [149]. Although markers of inflammation were not assessed, elevated levels of leukocyte cholesterol is known to increase the pro-inflammatory potential of the cell [120,121]. Conversely, in a study in college-aged men and women participating a crossover study, liver enzymes aspartate aminotransferase (AST) and alanine aminotransferase (ALT) were lower following consumption of a 2-egg per day for 4 weeks *vs.* an oatmeal breakfast, whereas no changes were observed in CRP [150].

4.2. Overweight

It has been well established that excessive weight gain and obesity is associated with a chronic state of low-grade systemic inflammation and metabolic tissue dysfunction. This physiological milieu is thought to stem from dysfunctional adipose, which becomes stressed as it attempts to expand in order to accommodate an excess influx of nutrients [8]. In contrast to what is observed in most healthy populations, egg consumption in overweight populations shows beneficial anti-inflammatory effects. In a study by Ratliff *et al.* [32], overweight men consuming 3 eggs per day for 12 weeks while following an *ad libitum* carbohydrate-restricted diet showed reductions in plasma CRP, that were not observed in overweight men consuming a carbohydrate restriction diet with yolk-free egg substitute. However, men consuming the egg substitute showed significant decreases in pro-inflammatory MCP-1 [32]. Interestingly, men on both whole egg and egg substitute groups increased plasma levels of the anti-inflammatory adipokine adiponectin over 12 weeks, with greater increases observed in the whole egg group (+21% *vs.* +7%) [32]. Consumption of eggs for breakfast has additionally been shown to increased satiety in overweight/obese women [154] and healthy men [155] when compared to a bagel breakfast, while also promoting weight loss and reductions in daily caloric intake [155,156]. Increased satiety from egg consumption has also been observed in young adults [157]. Together, these findings suggest that egg consumption may improve inflammation in overweight/obese individuals undergoing weight loss—either through direct action of bioactive components or indirect action of promoting satiety, weight loss, and restoration of adipose tissue function.

4.3. Metabolic Syndrome

Metabolic syndrome is characterized by a clustering of cardiometabolic risk factors that increase an individual's risk of developing CVD and T2DM by 2- and 5-fold, respectively [20]. Individuals with metabolic syndrome commonly present with insulin resistance, endothelial dysfunction, adverse lipoprotein profiles, and a chronic state of low-grade inflammation [158]. However, similar to what has been observed in obesity, egg consumption has been shown to mitigate inflammation in metabolic syndrome. In men and women classified with metabolic syndrome following a moderate carbohydrate-restricted diet, consumption of either 3 eggs per day or the equivalent amount of yolk-free egg substitute for 12 weeks lowered oxLDL [34]. Interestingly, reductions in plasma TNFα and serum amyloid A were only observed in the group consuming whole eggs that included the yolk, whereas no changes in CRP, adiponectin, IL-6, or IL-10 were observed in either whole egg or egg substitute groups [35].

The effects of egg consumption during carbohydrate restriction in metabolic syndrome was further assessed in regard to peripheral blood mononuclear cell inflammation [33,36]. Despite increases in peripheral blood mononuclear cell (PBMC) toll-like receptor 4 (TLR4) mRNA expression, whole egg intake did not alter lipopolysaccharide-induced TNFα or IL-1β secretion by PBMCs. Surprisingly, lipopolysaccharide-induced TNFα or IL-1β secretion in PBMC was increased over the 12 week period in subjects consuming the yolk-free egg substitute. Interestingly, there was a trend toward a decrease in PBMC cholesterol content in the whole egg group, as changes in PBMC cholesterol content over the 12-week intervention positively correlated with lipid raft content [33,36]. These changes corresponded to increased PBMC mRNA expression of ABCA1, which is known to exert direct and indirect anti-inflammatory activity [120,121]. Egg consumption in metabolic syndrome has additionally been shown to increase HDL-phosphatidylethanolamine content and the *ex vivo* cholesterol-accepting capacity of serum from lipid-loaded macrophages [46]. While the anti-inflammatory properties of egg-induced, phosphatidylethanolamine-enriched HDL were not assessed, phosphatidylethanolamine may confer antithrombotic properties [159,160]. Thus, taken together with the reductions in serum amyloid A, which is predominantly associated with HDL in circulation, it is possible that some of these observations may be attributable to more anti-inflammatory and functional HDL [35,46,161].

4.4. T2DM

Of all populations, the recommendation of egg intake in T2DM is one of the most controversial, given the results of some epidemiological studies that found a positive association between egg intake and T2DM risk [26,27]. However, similar to what has been observed in obese and metabolic syndrome populations, egg intake in T2DM appears to reduce markers of inflammation. In a randomized, crossover study conducted in patients with well-controlled T2DM, intake of 1 whole egg per day breakfast for 5 weeks significantly reduced AST and TNFα when compared to an oatmeal-based breakfast [38]. Further, there were no differences in fasting glucose, glycosylated hemoglobin (HbA1c), CRP, or plasma lipids between the egg and oatmeal breakfast periods, suggesting that consumption of one egg per day may mitigate the inflammation characteristic of T2DM without negatively affecting traditional markers of glucose tolerance and CVD risk [38]. Similarly, in a study by Pearce *et al.* [151], T2DM patients fed a hypoenergetic high-protein, high-cholesterol diet (achieved by consuming 2 eggs/day) for 12 weeks exhibited no adverse changes in T2DM and CVD biomarkers. Conversely, egg consumption resulted in greater increases in serum HDL-cholesterol and plasma lutein when compared to T2DM patients consuming a low cholesterol hypoenergetic, high-protein diet that lacked eggs. However, no changes in serum CRP or plasma homocysteine were observed in either group [151]. Thus, it appears eggs may confer anti-inflammatory benefits in patients with well-controlled T2DM.

4.5. Acute Infection

The findings on egg intake and inflammation outlined above not only have implications for chronic metabolic diseases, but also for immune function in cases of acute infection, where inflammation is essential to clearing pathogenic factors. While research on egg intake in immunity is limited, one study by Pérez-Guzmán *et al.* [162] investigated the effects of a cholesterol-rich diet on the treatment of, and recovery from, pulmonary tuberculosis. Adult patients with newly diagnosed pulmonary tuberculosis were assigned to consume a cholesterol-rich diet (800 mg cholesterol/day, provided by egg yolk, butter, beef liver, and dairy products) or a control diet (250 mg cholesterol/day) for 8 weeks while remaining hospitalized and receiving anti-tubercular drug treatments. Interestingly, subjects following the cholesterol-rich diet exhibited faster reductions in sputum production and clearance of mycobacteria from sputum cultures [162]. Given these findings, and those highlighted above, the effects of egg intake in parameters of immunity across different populations warrants further investigation.

4.6. Implications from Human Studies

As presented above, the majority of research suggests that egg intake promotes a pro-inflammatory response in healthy adults [30,31], whereas the consumption of eggs in conditions of overweight [32], insulin resistance [30], metabolic syndrome [35,36], and T2DM [38,151] have either an anti-inflammatory or neutral effect. It is possible that this variation is attributable to differences in intestinal absorption of dietary cholesterol, which is known to be increased in healthy, non-insulin resistant individuals [30,56–58]; however, it is possible that other factors impact the dietary response to eggs, such as the composition of the microbiome or genetic variation [31,114]. It is additionally important to recognize potential confounding variables across studies, such as differences in the number of eggs consumed per day, concurrent dietary treatments/interventions, or medication regimens.

5. Conclusions

Bioactive egg components, including phospholipids, cholesterol, lutein, zeaxanthin, and proteins, possess a variety of pro- and/or anti-inflammatory properties, which may have important implications for the pathophysiology of numerous chronic diseases and immune responses to acute injury. The unique formulation of the egg food matrix significantly impacts the bioaccessibility and absorption of these components, allowing each bioactive component to likely contribute to the overall effects of egg intake on inflammatory processes. Thus, as opposed to solely basing dietary recommendations for egg intake on cholesterol content, it is likely more beneficial to consider the relationship between egg intake and inflammation in different populations. Moreover, given the essentiality of pro-inflammatory responses in normal immune defense against pathogens, further research into the role of egg intake on immunity is warranted. Together, the findings presented in this review have important implications for population-specific dietary recommendations that add complexity to current guidelines and standards of clinical practice.

Conflicts of Interest: The author declares no conflict of interest.

References

1. Medzhitov, R. Origin and physiological roles of inflammation. *Nature* **2008**, *454*, 428–435. [CrossRef] [PubMed]
2. Medzhitov, R. Recognition of microorganisms and activation of the immune response. *Nature* **2007**, *449*, 819–826. [CrossRef] [PubMed]
3. Huang, W.; Glass, C.K. Nuclear receptors and inflammation control: Molecular mechanisms and pathophysiological relevance. *Arterioscler. Thromb. Vasc. Biol.* **2010**, *30*, 1542–1549. [CrossRef] [PubMed]
4. Bannenberg, G.; Serhan, C.N. Specialized pro-resolving lipid mediators in the inflammatory response: An update. *Biochim. Biophys. Acta* **2010**, *1801*, 1260–1273. [CrossRef] [PubMed]
5. Amin, K. The role of mast cells in allergic inflammation. *Respir. Med.* **2012**, *106*, 9–14. [CrossRef] [PubMed]
6. Todd, D.J.; Lee, A.H.; Glimcher, L.H. The endoplasmic reticulum stress response in immunity and autoimmunity. *Nat. Rev. Immunol.* **2008**, *8*, 663–674. [CrossRef] [PubMed]
7. Rodriguez-Reyna, T.S.; Alarcon-Segovia, D. The different faces of shared autoimmunity. *Autoimmun. Rev.* **2006**, *5*, 86–88. [CrossRef] [PubMed]
8. Guilherme, A.; Virbasius, J.V.; Puri, V.; Czech, M.P. Adipocyte dysfunctions linking obesity to insulin resistance and type 2 diabetes. *Nat. Rev. Mol. Cell Biol.* **2008**, *9*, 367–377. [CrossRef] [PubMed]
9. Berg, A.H.; Scherer, P.E. Adipose tissue, inflammation, and cardiovascular disease. *Circ. Res.* **2005**, *96*, 939–949. [CrossRef] [PubMed]
10. Ndumele, C.E.; Nasir, K.; Conceicao, R.D.; Carvalho, J.A.; Blumenthal, R.S.; Santos, R.D. Hepatic steatosis, obesity, and the metabolic syndrome are independently and additively associated with increased systemic inflammation. *Arterioscler. Thromb. Vasc. Biol.* **2011**, *31*, 1927–1932. [CrossRef] [PubMed]
11. Elinav, E.; Nowarski, R.; Thaiss, C.A.; Hu, B.; Jin, C.; Flavell, R.A. Inflammation-induced cancer: Crosstalk between tumours, immune cells and microorganisms. *Nat. Rev. Cancer* **2013**, *13*, 759–771. [CrossRef] [PubMed]
12. Pan, M.H.; Lai, C.S.; Ho, C.T. Anti-inflammatory activity of natural dietary flavonoids. *Food Funct.* **2010**, *1*, 15–31. [CrossRef] [PubMed]
13. Siriwardhana, N.; Kalupahana, N.S.; Cekanova, M.; LeMieux, M.; Greer, B.; Moustaid-Moussa, N. Modulation of adipose tissue inflammation by bioactive food compounds. *J. Nutr. Biochem.* **2013**, *24*, 613–623. [CrossRef] [PubMed]
14. Zeng, C.; Zhong, P.; Zhao, Y.; Kanchana, K.; Zhang, Y.; Khan, Z.A.; Chakrabarti, S.; Wu, L.; Wang, J.; Liang, G. Curcumin protects hearts from FFA-induced injury by activating Nrf2 and inactivating NF-κB both *in vitro* and *in vivo*. *J. Mol. Cell Cardiol.* **2015**, *79*, 1–12. [CrossRef] [PubMed]
15. Figueras, M.; Olivan, M.; Busquets, S.; Lopez-Soriano, F.J.; Argiles, J.M. Effects of eicosapentaenoic acid (EPA) treatment on insulin sensitivity in an animal model of diabetes: Improvement of the inflammatory status. *Obesity (Silver Spring)* **2011**, *19*, 362–369. [CrossRef] [PubMed]
16. Herron, K.L.; Fernandez, M.L. Are the current dietary guidelines regarding egg consumption appropriate? *J. Nutr.* **2004**, *134*, 187–190. [PubMed]
17. *USDA National Nutrient Database for Standard Reference, Release 27 (Revised)*; May 2015 Version; US Department of Agriculture, Agricultural Research Service, Nutrient Data Laboratory: Beltsville, MD, USA.

18. Millward, D.J.; Layman, D.K.; Tome, D.; Schaafsma, G. Protein quality assessment: Impact of expanding understanding of protein and amino acid needs for optimal health. *Am. J. Clin. Nutr.* **2008**, *87*, 1576S–1581S. [PubMed]

19. Moore, D.R.; Robinson, M.J.; Fry, J.L.; Tang, J.E.; Glover, E.I.; Wilkinson, S.B.; Prior, T.; Tarnopolsky, M.A.; Phillips, S.M. Ingested protein dose response of muscle and albumin protein synthesis after resistance exercise in young men. *Am. J. Clin. Nutr.* **2009**, *89*, 161–168. [CrossRef] [PubMed]

20. Expert Panel on Detection, Evaluation, and Treatment of High Blood Cholesterol in Adults. Executive summary of the third report of the National Cholesterol Education Program (NCEP) Expert Panel on detection, evaluation, and treatment of high blood cholesterol in adults (Adult Treatment Panel III). *JAMA* **2001**, *285*, 2486–2497.

21. Krauss, R.M.; Deckelbaum, R.J.; Ernst, N.; Fisher, E.; Howard, B.V.; Knopp, R.H.; Kotchen, T.; Lichtenstein, A.H.; McGill, H.C.; Pearson, T.A.; *et al.* Dietary guidelines for healthy American adults. A statement for health professionals from the nutrition committee, American heart association. *Circulation* **1996**, *94*, 1795–1800. [CrossRef] [PubMed]

22. Scrafford, C.G.; Tran, N.L.; Barraj, L.M.; Mink, P.J. Egg consumption and chd and stroke mortality: A prospective study of US adults. *Public Health Nutr.* **2011**, *14*, 261–270. [CrossRef] [PubMed]

23. Hu, F.B.; Stampfer, M.J.; Rimm, E.B.; Manson, J.E.; Ascherio, A.; Colditz, G.A.; Rosner, B.A.; Spiegelman, D.; Speizer, F.E.; Sacks, F.M.; *et al.* A prospective study of egg consumption and risk of cardiovascular disease in men and women. *JAMA* **1999**, *281*, 1387–1394. [CrossRef] [PubMed]

24. Dawber, T.R.; Nickerson, R.J.; Brand, F.N.; Pool, J. Eggs, serum cholesterol, and coronary heart disease. *Am. J. Clin. Nutr.* **1982**, *36*, 617–625. [PubMed]

25. Barraj, L.; Tran, N.; Mink, P. A comparison of egg consumption with other modifiable coronary heart disease lifestyle risk factors: A relative risk apportionment study. *Risk Anal.* **2009**, *29*, 401–415. [CrossRef] [PubMed]

26. Djousse, L.; Gaziano, J.M.; Buring, J.E.; Lee, I.M. Egg consumption and risk of type 2 diabetes in men and women. *Diabetes Care* **2009**, *32*, 295–300. [CrossRef] [PubMed]

27. Radzeviciene, L.; Ostrauskas, R. Egg consumption and the risk of type 2 diabetes mellitus: A case-control study. *Public Health Nutr.* **2012**, *15*, 1437–1441. [CrossRef] [PubMed]

28. Zazpe, I.; Beunza, J.J.; Bes-Rastrollo, M.; Basterra-Gortari, F.J.; Mari-Sanchis, A.; Martinez-Gonzalez, M.A.; SUN Project Investigators. Egg consumption and risk of type 2 diabetes in a mediterranean cohort; the sun project. *Nutr. Hosp.* **2013**, *28*, 105–111. [PubMed]

29. Djousse, L.; Kamineni, A.; Nelson, T.L.; Carnethon, M.; Mozaffarian, D.; Siscovick, D.; Mukamal, K.J. Egg consumption and risk of type 2 diabetes in older adults. *Am. J. Clin. Nutr.* **2010**, *92*, 422–427. [CrossRef] [PubMed]

30. Tannock, L.R.; O'Brien, K.D.; Knopp, R.H.; Retzlaff, B.; Fish, B.; Wener, M.H.; Kahn, S.E.; Chait, A. Cholesterol feeding increases C-reactive protein and serum amyloid A levels in lean insulin-sensitive subjects. *Circulation* **2005**, *111*, 3058–3062. [CrossRef] [PubMed]

31. Tang, W.H.; Wang, Z.; Levison, B.S.; Koeth, R.A.; Britt, E.B.; Fu, X.; Wu, Y.; Hazen, S.L. Intestinal microbial metabolism of phosphatidylcholine and cardiovascular risk. *N. Engl. J. Med.* **2013**, *368*, 1575–1584. [CrossRef] [PubMed]

32. Ratliff, J.C.; Mutungi, G.; Puglisi, M.J.; Volek, J.S.; Fernandez, M.L. Eggs modulate the inflammatory response to carbohydrate restricted diets in overweight men. *Nutr. Metab. (Lond.)* **2008**, *5*. [CrossRef] [PubMed]

33. Andersen, C.J.; Blesso, C.N.; Lee, J.; Fernandez, M.L. Egg intake increases peripheral blood mononuclear cell expression of ATP-binding cassette transporter A1 in parallel with Toll-like receptor 4 as a potential mechanism to reduce cellular inflammation in metabolic syndrome. *FASEB* **2013**, *27*, 846.7.

34. Blesso, C.N.; Andersen, C.J.; Barona, J.; Volek, J.S.; Fernandez, M.L. Whole egg consumption improves lipoprotein profiles and insulin sensitivity to a greater extent than yolk-free egg substitute in individuals with metabolic syndrome. *Metabolism* **2013**, *62*, 400–410. [CrossRef] [PubMed]

35. Blesso, C.N.; Andersen, C.J.; Barona, J.; Volk, B.; Volek, J.S.; Fernandez, M.L. Effects of carbohydrate restriction and dietary cholesterol provided by eggs on clinical risk factors in metabolic syndrome. *J. Clin. Lipidol.* **2013**, *7*, 463–471. [CrossRef] [PubMed]

36. Andersen, C.J.; Lee, J.Y.; Blesso, C.N.; Carr, T.P.; Fernandez, M.L. Egg intake during carbohydrate restriction alters peripheral blood mononuclear cell inflammation and cholesterol homeostasis in metabolic syndrome. *Nutrients* **2014**, *6*, 2650–2667. [CrossRef] [PubMed]

37. Jones, J.L.; Ackermann, D.; Barona, J.; Calle, M.; Andersen, C.; Kim, J.E.; Volek, J.S.; McIntosh, M.; Najm, W.; Lerman, R.H.; *et al.* A mediterranean low-glycemic-load diet alone or in combination with a medical food improves insulin sensitivity and reduces inflammation in women with metabolic syndrome. *Br. J. Med. Med. Res.* **2011**, *1*, 356–370. [CrossRef] [PubMed]

38. Ballesteros, M.N.; Valenzuela, F.; Robles, A.E.; Artalejo, E.; Aguilar, D.; Andersen, C.J.; Valdez, H.; Fernandez, M.L. One egg per day improves inflammation when compared to an oatmeal-based breakfast without increasing other cardiometabolic risk factors in diabetic patients. *Nutrients* **2015**, *7*, 3449–3463. [CrossRef] [PubMed]

39. Miranda, J.M.; Anton, X.; Redondo-Valbuena, C.; Roca-Saavedra, P.; Rodriguez, J.A.; Lamas, A.; Franco, C.M.; Cepeda, A. Egg and egg-derived foods: Effects on human health and use as functional foods. *Nutrients* **2015**, *7*, 706–729. [CrossRef] [PubMed]

40. Naviglio, D.; Gallo, M.; le Grottaglie, L.; Scala, C.; Ferrara, L.; Santini, A. Determination of cholesterol in Italian chicken eggs. *Food Chem.* **2012**, *132*, 701–708. [CrossRef]

41. Cohn, J.S.; Kamili, A.; Wat, E.; Chung, R.W.; Tandy, S. Dietary phospholipids and intestinal cholesterol absorption. *Nutrients* **2010**, *2*, 116–127. [CrossRef] [PubMed]

42. Weihrauch, J.; Son, Y.S. The phospholipid content of foods. *J. Am. Oil. Chem. Soc.* **1983**, *60*, 1971–1978. [CrossRef]

43. Jiang, Y.; Noh, S.K.; Koo, S.I. Egg phosphatidylcholine decreases the lymphatic absorption of cholesterol in rats. *J. Nutr.* **2001**, *131*, 2358–2363. [PubMed]

44. An, B.K.; Nishiyama, H.; Tanaka, K.; Ohtani, S.; Iwata, T.; Tsutsumi, K.; Kasai, M. Dietary safflower phospholipid reduces liver lipids in laying hens. *Poult. Sci.* **1997**, *76*, 689–695. [CrossRef] [PubMed]

45. Tsiagbe, V.K.; Cook, M.E.; Harper, A.E.; Sunde, M.L. Alterations in phospholipid composition of egg yolks from laying hens fed choline and methionine-supplemented diets. *Poult. Sci.* **1988**, *67*, 1717–1724. [CrossRef] [PubMed]

46. Andersen, C.J.; Blesso, C.N.; Lee, J.; Barona, J.; Shah, D.; Thomas, M.J.; Fernandez, M.L. Egg consumption modulates HDL lipid composition and increases the cholesterol-accepting capacity of serum in metabolic syndrome. *Lipids* **2013**, *48*, 557–567. [CrossRef] [PubMed]

47. Beynen, A.C. Fatty acid composition of eggs produced by hens fed diets containing groundnut, soya bean or linseed. *NJAS Wagening. J. Life Sci.* **2004**, *52*, 3–10. [CrossRef]

48. Schreiner, M.; Hulan, H.W.; Razzazi-Fazeli, E.; Bohm, J.; Iben, C. Feeding laying hens seal blubber oil: Effects on egg yolk incorporation, stereospecific distribution of omega-3 fatty acids, and sensory aspects. *Poult. Sci.* **2004**, *83*, 462–473. [CrossRef] [PubMed]

49. Kullenberg, D.; Taylor, L.A.; Schneider, M.; Massing, U. Health effects of dietary phospholipids. *Lipids. Health. Dis.* **2012**, *11*, 3. [CrossRef] [PubMed]

50. Zierenberg, O.; Grundy, S.M. Intestinal absorption of polyenephosphatidylcholine in man. *J. Lipid. Res.* **1982**, *23*, 1136–1142. [PubMed]

51. Klimov, A.N.; Konstantinov, V.O.; Lipovetsky, B.M.; Kuznetsov, A.S.; Lozovsky, V.T.; Trufanov, V.F.; Plavinsky, S.L.; Gundermann, K.J.; Schumacher, R. "Essential" phospholipids *versus* nicotinic acid in the treatment of patients with type IIb hyperlipoproteinemia and ischemic heart disease. *Cardiovasc. Drugs. Ther.* **1995**, *9*, 779–784. [CrossRef] [PubMed]

52. Bunea, R.; el Farrah, K.; Deutsch, L. Evaluation of the effects of neptune krill oil on the clinical course of hyperlipidemia. *Altern. Med. Rev.* **2004**, *9*, 420–428. [PubMed]

53. Mutungi, G.; Ratliff, J.; Puglisi, M.; Torres-Gonzalez, M.; Vaishnav, U.; Leite, J.O.; Quann, E.; Volek, J.S.; Fernandez, M.L. Dietary cholesterol from eggs increases plasma HDL cholesterol in overweight men consuming a carbohydrate-restricted diet. *J. Nutr.* **2008**, *138*, 272–276. [PubMed]

54. Kovacs-Nolan, J.; Phillips, M.; Mine, Y. Advances in the value of eggs and egg components for human health. *J. Agric. Food Chem.* **2005**, *53*, 8421–8431. [CrossRef] [PubMed]

55. Miettinen, T.A.; Gylling, H. Cholesterol absorption efficiency and sterol metabolism in obesity. *Atherosclerosis* **2000**, *153*, 241–248. [CrossRef]

56. Pihlajamaki, J.; Gylling, H.; Miettinen, T.A.; Laakso, M. Insulin resistance is associated with increased cholesterol synthesis and decreased cholesterol absorption in normoglycemic men. *J. Lipid. Res.* **2004**, *45*, 507–512. [CrossRef] [PubMed]

57. Simonen, P.P.; Gylling, H.K.; Miettinen, T.A. Diabetes contributes to cholesterol metabolism regardless of obesity. *Diabetes Care* **2002**, *25*, 1511–1515. [CrossRef] [PubMed]
58. Paramsothy, P.; Knopp, R.H.; Kahn, S.E.; Retzlaff, B.M.; Fish, B.; Ma, L.; Ostlund, R.E., Jr. Plasma sterol evidence for decreased absorption and increased synthesis of cholesterol in insulin resistance and obesity. *Am. J. Clin. Nutr.* **2011**, *94*, 1182–1188. [CrossRef] [PubMed]
59. Bennion, L.J.; Grundy, S.M. Effects of obesity and caloric intake on biliary lipid metabolism in man. *J. Clin. Investig.* **1975**, *56*, 996–1011. [CrossRef] [PubMed]
60. Shaffer, E.A.; Small, D.M. Biliary lipid secretion in cholesterol gallstone disease. The effect of cholecystectomy and obesity. *J. Clin. Investig.* **1977**, *59*, 828–840. [CrossRef] [PubMed]
61. Ros, E. Intestinal absorption of triglyceride and cholesterol. Dietary and pharmacological inhibition to reduce cardiovascular risk. *Atherosclerosis* **2000**, *151*, 357–379. [CrossRef]
62. Noh, S.K.; Koo, S.I. Milk sphingomyelin is more effective than egg sphingomyelin in inhibiting intestinal absorption of cholesterol and fat in rats. *J. Nutr.* **2004**, *134*, 2611–2616. [PubMed]
63. Noh, S.K.; Koo, S.I. Egg sphingomyelin lowers the lymphatic absorption of cholesterol and alpha-tocopherol in rats. *J. Nutr.* **2003**, *133*, 3571–3576. [PubMed]
64. Koo, S.I.; Noh, S.K. Phosphatidylcholine inhibits and lysophosphatidylcholine enhances the lymphatic absorption of α-tocopherol in adult rats. *J. Nutr.* **2001**, *131*, 717–722. [PubMed]
65. Brunham, L.R.; Singaraja, R.R.; Duong, M.; Timmins, J.M.; Fievet, C.; Bissada, N.; Kang, M.H.; Samra, A.; Fruchart, J.C.; McManus, B.; *et al.* Tissue-specific roles of abca1 influence susceptibility to atherosclerosis. *Arterioscler. Thromb. Vasc. Biol.* **2009**, *29*, 548–554. [CrossRef] [PubMed]
66. Van Greevenbroek, M.M.; de Bruin, T.W. Chylomicron synthesis by intestinal cells *in vitro* and *in vitro*. *Atherosclerosis* **1998**, *141*, S9–S16. [CrossRef]
67. Cesar, T.B.; Oliveira, M.R.; Mesquita, C.H.; Maranhao, R.C. High cholesterol intake modifies chylomicron metabolism in normolipidemic young men. *J. Nutr.* **2006**, *136*, 971–976. [PubMed]
68. Nervi, F.O.; Dietschy, J.M. Ability of six different lipoprotein fractions to regulate the rate of hepatic cholesterogenesis *in vivo*. *J. Biol. Chem.* **1975**, *250*, 8704–8711. [PubMed]
69. Blesso, C.N.; Andersen, C.J.; Bolling, B.W.; Fernandez, M.L. Egg intake improves carotenoid status by increasing plasma HDL cholesterol in adults with metabolic syndrome. *Food Funct.* **2013**, *4*, 213–221. [CrossRef] [PubMed]
70. Johnson, E.J. The role of carotenoids in human health. *Nutr. Clin. Care* **2002**, *5*, 56–65. [CrossRef] [PubMed]
71. Karadas, F.; Pappas, A.C.; Surai, P.F.; Speake, B.K. Embryonic development within carotenoid-enriched eggs influences the post-hatch carotenoid status of the chicken. *Comp. Biochem. Physiol. B. Biochem. Mol. Biol.* **2005**, *141*, 244–251. [CrossRef] [PubMed]
72. Abdel-Aal el, S.M.; Akhtar, H.; Zaheer, K.; Ali, R. Dietary sources of lutein and zeaxanthin carotenoids and their role in eye health. *Nutrients* **2013**, *5*, 1169–1185. [CrossRef] [PubMed]
73. Kotake-Nara, E.; Nagao, A. Absorption and metabolism of xanthophylls. *Mar. Drugs* **2011**, *9*, 1024–1037. [CrossRef] [PubMed]
74. Nimalaratne, C.; Lopes-Lutz, D.; Schieber, A.; Wu, J. Effect of domestic cooking methods on egg yolk xanthophylls. *J. Agric. Food Chem.* **2012**, *60*, 12547–12552. [CrossRef] [PubMed]
75. Nimalaratne, C.; Savard, P.; Gauthier, S.F.; Schieber, A.; Wu, J. Bioaccessibility and digestive stability of carotenoids in cooked eggs studied using a dynamic *in vitro* gastrointestinal model. *J. Agric. Food Chem.* **2015**, *63*, 2956–2962. [CrossRef] [PubMed]
76. Chung, H.Y.; Rasmussen, H.M.; Johnson, E.J. Lutein bioavailability is higher from lutein-enriched eggs than from supplements and spinach in men. *J. Nutr.* **2004**, *134*, 1887–1893. [PubMed]
77. Faulks, R.M.; Southon, S. Challenges to understanding and measuring carotenoid bioavailability. *Biochim. Biophys. Acta* **2005**, *1740*, 95–100. [CrossRef] [PubMed]
78. Ryan, L.; O'Connell, O.; O'Sullivan, L.; Aherne, S.A.; O'Brien, N.M. Micellarisation of carotenoids from raw and cooked vegetables. *Plant Foods. Hum. Nutr.* **2008**, *63*, 127–133. [CrossRef] [PubMed]
79. Baskaran, V.; Sugawara, T.; Nagao, A. Phospholipids affect the intestinal absorption of carotenoids in mice. *Lipids* **2003**, *38*, 705–711. [CrossRef] [PubMed]
80. Lakshminarayana, R.; Raju, M.; Krishnakantha, T.P.; Baskaran, V. Enhanced lutein bioavailability by lyso-phosphatidylcholine in rats. *Mol. Cell Biochem.* **2006**, *281*, 103–110. [CrossRef] [PubMed]

81. Kotake-Nara, E.; Yonekura, L.; Nagao, A. Effect of glycerophospholipid class on the beta-carotene uptake by human intestinal Caco-2 cells. *Biosci. Biotechnol. Biochem.* **2010**, *74*, 209–211. [CrossRef] [PubMed]

82. Kelly, E.R.; Plat, J.; Haenen, G.R.; Kijlstra, A.; Berendschot, T.T. The effect of modified eggs and an egg-yolk based beverage on serum lutein and zeaxanthin concentrations and macular pigment optical density: Results from a randomized trial. *PLoS ONE* **2014**, *9*, e92659. [CrossRef] [PubMed]

83. Handelman, G.J.; Nightingale, Z.D.; Lichtenstein, A.H.; Schaefer, E.J.; Blumberg, J.B. Lutein and zeaxanthin concentrations in plasma after dietary supplementation with egg yolk. *Am. J. Clin. Nutr.* **1999**, *70*, 247–251. [PubMed]

84. Kim, J.E.; Clark, R.M.; Park, Y.; Lee, J.; Fernandez, M.L. Lutein decreases oxidative stress and inflammation in liver and eyes of guinea pigs fed a hypercholesterolemic diet. *Nutr. Res. Pract.* **2012**, *6*, 113–119. [CrossRef] [PubMed]

85. Vishwanathan, R.; Goodrow-Kotyla, E.F.; Wooten, B.R.; Wilson, T.A.; Nicolosi, R.J. Consumption of 2 and 4 egg yolks/d for 5 wk increases macular pigment concentrations in older adults with low macular pigment taking cholesterol-lowering statins. *Am. J. Clin. Nutr.* **2009**, *90*, 1272–1279. [CrossRef] [PubMed]

86. Wenzel, A.J.; Gerweck, C.; Barbato, D.; Nicolosi, R.J.; Handelman, G.J.; Curran-Celentano, J. A 12-wk egg intervention increases serum zeaxanthin and macular pigment optical density in women. *J. Nutr.* **2006**, *136*, 2568–2573. [PubMed]

87. Lee, E.H.; Faulhaber, D.; Hanson, K.M.; Ding, W.; Peters, S.; Kodali, S.; Granstein, R.D. Dietary lutein reduces ultraviolet radiation-induced inflammation and immunosuppression. *J. Investig. Dermatol.* **2004**, *122*, 510–517. [CrossRef] [PubMed]

88. Johnson, E.J.; Hammond, B.R.; Yeum, K.J.; Qin, J.; Wang, X.D.; Castaneda, C.; Snodderly, D.M.; Russell, R.M. Relation among serum and tissue concentrations of lutein and zeaxanthin and macular pigment density. *Am. J. Clin. Nutr.* **2000**, *71*, 1555–1562. [PubMed]

89. Chung, H.Y.; Ferreira, A.L.; Epstein, S.; Paiva, S.A.; Castaneda-Sceppa, C.; Johnson, E.J. Site-specific concentrations of carotenoids in adipose tissue: Relations with dietary and serum carotenoid concentrations in healthy adults. *Am. J. Clin. Nutr.* **2009**, *90*, 533–539. [CrossRef] [PubMed]

90. Bovier, E.R.; Lewis, R.D.; Hammond, B.R., Jr. The relationship between lutein and zeaxanthin status and body fat. *Nutrients* **2013**, *5*, 750–757. [CrossRef] [PubMed]

91. Hoffman, J.R.; Falvo, M.J. Protein—Which is best? *J. Sports. Sci. Med.* **2004**, *3*, 118–130. [PubMed]

92. Borsheim, E.; Tipton, K.D.; Wolf, S.E.; Wolfe, R.R. Essential amino acids and muscle protein recovery from resistance exercise. *Am. J. Physiol. Endocrinol. Metable* **2002**, *283*, E648–E657. [CrossRef] [PubMed]

93. Paddon-Jones, D.; Sheffield-Moore, M.; Urban, R.J.; Sanford, A.P.; Aarsland, A.; Wolfe, R.R.; Ferrando, A.A. Essential amino acid and carbohydrate supplementation ameliorates muscle protein loss in humans during 28 days bedrest. *J. Clin. Endocrinol. Metable* **2004**, *89*, 4351–4358. [CrossRef] [PubMed]

94. Lewis, J.C.; Snell, N.S.; Hirschmann, D.J.; Fraenkel-Conrat, H. Amino acid composition of egg proteins. *J. Biol. Chem.* **1950**, *186*, 23–35. [PubMed]

95. Kobayashi, Y.; Rupa, P.; Kovacs-Nolan, J.; Turner, P.V.; Matsui, T.; Mine, Y. Oral administration of hen egg white ovotransferrin attenuates the development of colitis induced by dextran sodium sulfate in mice. *J. Agric. Food Chem.* **2015**, *63*, 1532–1539. [CrossRef] [PubMed]

96. Kovacs-Nolan, J.; Mine, Y. Egg yolk antibodies for passive immunity. *Annu. Rev. Food. Sci. Technol.* **2012**, *3*, 163–182. [CrossRef] [PubMed]

97. Lee, M.; Kovacs-Nolan, J.; Yang, C.; Archbold, T.; Fan, M.Z.; Mine, Y. Hen egg lysozyme attenuates inflammation and modulates local gene expression in a porcine model of dextran sodium sulfate (DSS)-induced colitis. *J. Agric. Food Chem.* **2009**, *57*, 2233–2240. [CrossRef] [PubMed]

98. Jahan-Mihan, A.; Luhovyy, B.L.; el Khoury, D.; Anderson, G.H. Dietary proteins as determinants of metabolic and physiologic functions of the gastrointestinal tract. *Nutrients* **2011**, *3*, 574–603. [CrossRef] [PubMed]

99. Yokooji, T.; Hamura, K.; Matsuo, H. Intestinal absorption of lysozyme, an egg-white allergen, in rats: Kinetics and effect of nsaids. *Biochem. Biophys. Res. Commun.* **2013**, *438*, 61–65. [CrossRef] [PubMed]

100. Yokooji, T.; Nouma, H.; Matsuo, H. Characterization of ovalbumin absorption pathways in the rat intestine, including the effects of aspirin. *Biol. Pharm. Bull.* **2014**, *37*, 1359–1365. [CrossRef] [PubMed]

101. Kovacs-Nolan, J.; Zhang, J.W.; Hayakawa, S.; Mine, Y. Immunochemical and structural analysis of pepsin-digested egg white ovomucoid. *J. Agric. Food Chem.* **2000**, *48*, 6261–6266. [CrossRef] [PubMed]

102. Evenepoel, P.; Geypens, B.; Luypaerts, A.; Hiele, M.; Ghoos, Y.; Rutgeerts, P. Digestibility of cooked and raw egg protein in humans as assessed by stable isotope techniques. *J. Nutr.* **1998**, *128*, 1716–1722. [PubMed]

103. Tall, A.R.; Yvan-Charvet, L. Cholesterol, inflammation and innate immunity. *Nat. Rev. Immunol.* **2015**, *15*, 104–116. [CrossRef] [PubMed]

104. Treede, I.; Braun, A.; Sparla, R.; Kuhnel, M.; Giese, T.; Turner, J.R.; Anes, E.; Kulaksiz, H.; Fullekrug, J.; Stremmel, W.; *et al.* Anti-inflammatory effects of phosphatidylcholine. *J. Biol. Chem.* **2007**, *282*, 27155–27164. [CrossRef] [PubMed]

105. Treede, I.; Braun, A.; Jeliaskova, P.; Giese, T.; Fullekrug, J.; Griffiths, G.; Stremmel, W.; Ehehalt, R. Tnf-alpha-induced up-regulation of pro-inflammatory cytokines is reduced by phosphatidylcholine in intestinal epithelial cells. *BMC Gastroenterol.* **2009**, *9*, 53. [CrossRef] [PubMed]

106. Ehehalt, R.; Wagenblast, J.; Erben, G.; Lehmann, W.D.; Hinz, U.; Merle, U.; Stremmel, W. Phosphatidylcholine and lysophosphatidylcholine in intestinal mucus of ulcerative colitis patients. A quantitative approach by nanoelectrospray-tandem mass spectrometry. *Scand. J. Gastroenterol.* **2004**, *39*, 737–742. [CrossRef] [PubMed]

107. Stremmel, W.; Ehehalt, R.; Autschbach, F.; Karner, M. Phosphatidylcholine for steroid-refractory chronic ulcerative colitis: A randomized trial. *Ann. Intern. Med.* **2007**, *147*, 603–610. [CrossRef] [PubMed]

108. Stremmel, W.; Merle, U.; Zahn, A.; Autschbach, F.; Hinz, U.; Ehehalt, R. Retarded release phosphatidylcholine benefits patients with chronic active ulcerative colitis. *Gut* **2005**, *54*, 966–971. [CrossRef] [PubMed]

109. Eros, G.; Ibrahim, S.; Siebert, N.; Boros, M.; Vollmar, B. Oral phosphatidylcholine pretreatment alleviates the signs of experimental rheumatoid arthritis. *Arthritis Res. Ther.* **2009**, *11*, R43. [CrossRef] [PubMed]

110. Tokes, T.; Eros, G.; Bebes, A.; Hartmann, P.; Varszegi, S.; Varga, G.; Kaszaki, J.; Gulya, K.; Ghyczy, M.; Boros, M. Protective effects of a phosphatidylcholine-enriched diet in lipopolysaccharide-induced experimental neuroinflammation in the rat. *Shock* **2011**, *36*, 458–465. [CrossRef] [PubMed]

111. Gao, X.; Liu, X.; Xu, J.; Xue, C.; Xue, Y.; Wang, Y. Dietary trimethylamine *N*-oxide exacerbates impaired glucose tolerance in mice fed a high fat diet. *J. Biosci. Bioeng.* **2014**, *118*, 476–481. [CrossRef] [PubMed]

112. Wang, Z.; Klipfell, E.; Bennett, B.J.; Koeth, R.; Levison, B.S.; Dugar, B.; Feldstein, A.E.; Britt, E.B.; Fu, X.; Chung, Y.M.; *et al.* Gut flora metabolism of phosphatidylcholine promotes cardiovascular disease. *Nature* **2011**, *472*, 57–63. [CrossRef] [PubMed]

113. Miller, C.A.; Corbin, K.D.; da Costa, K.A.; Zhang, S.; Zhao, X.; Galanko, J.A.; Blevins, T.; Bennett, B.J.; O'Connor, A.; Zeisel, S.H. Effect of egg ingestion on trimethylamine-*N*-oxide production in humans: A randomized, controlled, dose-response study. *Am. J. Clin. Nutr.* **2014**, *100*, 778–786. [CrossRef] [PubMed]

114. Tang, W.H.; Hazen, S.L. The contributory role of gut microbiota in cardiovascular disease. *J. Clin. Investig.* **2014**, *124*, 4204–4211. [CrossRef] [PubMed]

115. Chagas, P.; Caramori, P.; Galdino, T.P.; Barcellos Cda, S.; Gomes, I.; Schwanke, C.H. Egg consumption and coronary atherosclerotic burden. *Atherosclerosis* **2013**, *229*, 381–384. [CrossRef] [PubMed]

116. Wouters, K.; van Gorp, P.J.; Bieghs, V.; Gijbels, M.J.; Duimel, H.; Lutjohann, D.; Kerksiek, A.; van Kruchten, R.; Maeda, N.; Staels, B.; *et al.* Dietary cholesterol, rather than liver steatosis, leads to hepatic inflammation in hyperlipidemic mouse models of nonalcoholic steatohepatitis. *Hepatology* **2008**, *48*, 474–486. [CrossRef] [PubMed]

117. Kleemann, R.; Verschuren, L.; van Erk, M.J.; Nikolsky, Y.; Cnubben, N.H.; Verheij, E.R.; Smilde, A.K.; Hendriks, H.F.; Zadelaar, S.; Smith, G.J.; *et al.* Atherosclerosis and liver inflammation induced by increased dietary cholesterol intake: A combined transcriptomics and metabolomics analysis. *Genome. Biol.* **2007**, *8*, R200. [CrossRef] [PubMed]

118. Kellner-Weibel, G.; Luke, S.J.; Rothblat, G.H. Cytotoxic cellular cholesterol is selectively removed by ApoA-I via ABCA1. *Atherosclerosis* **2003**, *171*, 235–243. [CrossRef] [PubMed]

119. Surls, J.; Nazarov-Stoica, C.; Kehl, M.; Olsen, C.; Casares, S.; Brumeanu, T.D. Increased membrane cholesterol in lymphocytes diverts T-cells toward an inflammatory response. *PLoS ONE* **2012**, *7*, e38733. [CrossRef] [PubMed]

120. Zhu, X.; Owen, J.S.; Wilson, M.D.; Li, H.; Griffiths, G.L.; Thomas, M.J.; Hiltbold, E.M.; Fessler, M.B.; Parks, J.S. Macrophage ABCA1 reduces MyD88-dependent toll-like receptor trafficking to lipid rafts by reduction of lipid raft cholesterol. *J. Lipid. Res.* **2010**, *51*, 3196–3206. [CrossRef] [PubMed]

121. Zhu, X.; Lee, J.Y.; Timmins, J.M.; Brown, J.M.; Boudyguina, E.; Mulya, A.; Gebre, A.K.; Willingham, M.C.; Hiltbold, E.M.; Mishra, N.; *et al.* Increased cellular free cholesterol in macrophage-specific ABCA1 knock-out

mice enhances pro-inflammatory response of macrophages. *J. Biol. Chem.* **2008**, *283*, 22930–22941. [CrossRef] [PubMed]

122. Bensinger, S.J.; Bradley, M.N.; Joseph, S.B.; Zelcer, N.; Janssen, E.M.; Hausner, M.A.; Shih, R.; Parks, J.S.; Edwards, P.A.; Jamieson, B.D.; *et al.* LXR signaling couples sterol metabolism to proliferation in the acquired immune response. *Cell* **2008**, *134*, 97–111. [CrossRef] [PubMed]

123. Wang, S.; Wu, D.; Matthan, N.R.; Lamon-Fava, S.; Lecker, J.L.; Lichtenstein, A.H. Enhanced aortic macrophage lipid accumulation and inflammatory response in LDL receptor null mice fed an atherogenic diet. *Lipids* **2010**, *45*, 701–711. [CrossRef] [PubMed]

124. Aviram, M. Macrophage foam cell formation during early atherogenesis is determined by the balance between pro-oxidants and anti-oxidants in arterial cells and blood lipoproteins. *Antioxid. Redox. Signal.* **1999**, *1*, 585–594. [CrossRef] [PubMed]

125. Aguilar, D.; deOgburn, R.C.; Volek, J.S.; Fernandez, M.L. Cholesterol-induced inflammation and macrophage accumulation in adipose tissue is reduced by a low carbohydrate diet in guinea pigs. *Nutr. Res. Pract.* **2014**, *8*, 625–631. [CrossRef] [PubMed]

126. Yvan-Charvet, L.; Pagler, T.; Gautier, E.L.; Avagyan, S.; Siry, R.L.; Han, S.; Welch, C.L.; Wang, N.; Randolph, G.J.; Snoeck, H.W.; *et al.* ATP-binding cassette transporters and HDL suppress hematopoietic stem cell proliferation. *Science* **2010**, *328*, 1689–1693. [CrossRef] [PubMed]

127. Zhu, X.; Parks, J.S. New roles of HDL in inflammation and hematopoiesis. *Annu. Rev. Nutr.* **2012**, *32*, 161–182. [CrossRef] [PubMed]

128. Zhu, X.; Westcott, M.M.; Bi, X.; Liu, M.; Gowdy, K.M.; Seo, J.; Cao, Q.; Gebre, A.K.; Fessler, M.B.; Hiltbold, E.M.; *et al.* Myeloid cell-specific ABCA1 deletion protects mice from bacterial infection. *Circ. Res.* **2012**, *111*, 1398–1409. [CrossRef] [PubMed]

129. Murthy, R.K.; Ravi, K.; Balaiya, S.; Brar, V.S.; Chalam, K.V. Lutein protects retinal pigment epithelium from cytotoxic oxidative stress. *Cutan. Ocul. Toxicol.* **2014**, *33*, 132–137. [CrossRef] [PubMed]

130. Krinsky, N.I.; Landrum, J.T.; Bone, R.A. Biologic mechanisms of the protective role of lutein and zeaxanthin in the eye. *Annu. Rev. Nutr.* **2003**, *23*, 171–201. [CrossRef] [PubMed]

131. Kim, J.E.; Leite, J.O.; DeOgburn, R.; Smyth, J.A.; Clark, R.M.; Fernandez, M.L. A lutein-enriched diet prevents cholesterol accumulation and decreases oxidized LDL and inflammatory cytokines in the aorta of guinea pigs. *J. Nutr.* **2011**, *141*, 1458–1463. [CrossRef] [PubMed]

132. Serpeloni, J.M.; Barcelos, G.R.; Friedmann Angeli, J.P.; Mercadante, A.Z.; Lourdes Pires Bianchi, M.; Antunes, L.M. Dietary carotenoid lutein protects against DNA damage and alterations of the redox status induced by cisplatin in human derived HepG2 cells. *Toxicol. Vitro* **2012**, *26*, 288–294. [CrossRef] [PubMed]

133. Serpeloni, J.M.; Colus, I.M.; de Oliveira, F.S.; Aissa, A.F.; Mercadante, A.Z.; Bianchi, M.L.; Antunes, L.M. Diet carotenoid lutein modulates the expression of genes related to oxygen transporters and decreases DNA damage and oxidative stress in mice. *Food Chem. Toxicol.* **2014**, *70C*, 205–213. [CrossRef] [PubMed]

134. Serpeloni, J.M.; Grotto, D.; Mercadante, A.Z.; de Lourdes Pires Bianchi, M.; Antunes, L.M. Lutein improves antioxidant defense *in vivo* and protects against DNA damage and chromosome instability induced by cisplatin. *Arch. Toxicol.* **2010**, *84*, 811–822. [CrossRef] [PubMed]

135. Fernandez-Robredo, P.; Rodriguez, J.A.; Sadaba, L.M.; Recalde, S.; Garcia-Layana, A. Egg yolk improves lipid profile, lipid peroxidation and retinal abnormalities in a murine model of genetic hypercholesterolemia. *J. Nutr. Biochem.* **2008**, *19*, 40–48. [CrossRef] [PubMed]

136. Kim, J.H.; Na, H.J.; Kim, C.K.; Kim, J.Y.; Ha, K.S.; Lee, H.; Chung, H.T.; Kwon, H.J.; Kwon, Y.G.; Kim, Y.M. The non-provitamin a carotenoid, lutein, inhibits NF-κB-dependent gene expression through redox-based regulation of the phosphatidylinositol 3-kinase/pten/akt and nf-kappab-inducing kinase pathways: Role of H_2O_2 in NF-κB activation. *Free. Radic. Biol. Med.* **2008**, *45*, 885–896. [CrossRef] [PubMed]

137. Shanmugasundaram, R.; Selvaraj, R.K. Lutein supplementation alters inflammatory cytokine production and antioxidant status in F-line turkeys. *Poult. Sci.* **2011**, *90*, 971–976. [CrossRef] [PubMed]

138. Meriwether, L.S.; Humphrey, B.D.; Peterson, D.G.; Klasing, K.C.; Koutsos, E.A. Lutein exposure, in ovo or in the diet, reduces parameters of inflammation in the liver and spleen laying-type chicks (*gallus gallus domesticus*). *J. Anim. Physiol. Anim. Nutr. (Berl.)* **2010**, *94*, e115–e122. [CrossRef] [PubMed]

139. Nidhi, B.; Sharavana, G.; Ramaprasad, T.R.; Vallikannan, B. Lutein derived fragments exhibit higher antioxidant and anti-inflammatory properties than lutein in lipopolysaccharide induced inflammation in rats. *Food Funct.* **2015**, *6*, 450–460. [CrossRef] [PubMed]

140. Song, J.Y.; Lee, C.M.; Lee, M.K. Lutein modulates Th2 immune response in ovalbumin-induced airway inflammation. *J. Life Sci.* **2012**, *22*, 298–305. [CrossRef]

141. Graydon, R.; Hogg, R.E.; Chakravarthy, U.; Young, I.S.; Woodside, J.V. The effect of lutein- and zeaxanthin-rich foods v. Supplements on macular pigment level and serological markers of endothelial activation, inflammation and oxidation: Pilot studies in healthy volunteers. *Br. J. Nutr.* **2012**, *108*, 334–342. [CrossRef] [PubMed]

142. Ibrahim, H.R.; Aoki, T.; Pellegrini, A. Strategies for new antimicrobial proteins and peptides: Lysozyme and aprotinin as model molecules. *Curr. Pharm. Des.* **2002**, *8*, 671–693. [CrossRef] [PubMed]

143. Pellegrini, A.; Thomas, U.; Bramaz, N.; Klauser, S.; Hunziker, P.; von Fellenberg, R. Identification and isolation of a bactericidal domain in chicken egg white lysozyme. *J. Appl. Microbiol.* **1997**, *82*, 372–378. [CrossRef] [PubMed]

144. Giansanti, F.; Leboffe, L.; Pitari, G.; Ippoliti, R.; Antonini, G. Physiological roles of ovotransferrin. *Biochim. Biophys. Acta* **2012**, *1820*, 218–225. [CrossRef] [PubMed]

145. Sattar Khan, M.A.; Nakamura, S.; Ogawa, M.; Akita, E.; Azakami, H.; Kato, A. Bactericidal action of egg yolk phosvitin against *Escherichia coli* under thermal stress. *J. Agric. Food Chem.* **2000**, *48*, 1503–1506. [CrossRef] [PubMed]

146. Fujita, H.; Sasaki, R.; Yoshikawa, M. Potentiation of the antihypertensive activity of orally administered ovokinin, a vasorelaxing peptide derived from ovalbumin, by emulsification in egg phosphatidylcholine. *Biosci. Biotechnol. Biochem.* **1995**, *59*, 2344–2345. [CrossRef] [PubMed]

147. Horie, K.; Horie, N.; Abdou, A.M.; Yang, J.O.; Yun, S.S.; Chun, H.N.; Park, C.K.; Kim, M.; Hatta, H. Suppressive effect of functional drinking yogurt containing specific egg yolk immunoglobulin on *Helicobacter pylori* in humans. *J. Dairy Sci.* **2004**, *87*, 4073–4079. [CrossRef]

148. Kollberg, H.; Carlander, D.; Olesen, H.; Wejaker, P.E.; Johannesson, M.; Larsson, A. Oral administration of specific yolk antibodies (IgY) may prevent pseudomonas aeruginosa infections in patients with cystic fibrosis: A phase I feasibility study. *Pediatr. Pulmonol.* **2003**, *35*, 433–440. [CrossRef] [PubMed]

149. Ginsberg, H.N.; Karmally, W.; Siddiqui, M.; Holleran, S.; Tall, A.R.; Rumsey, S.C.; Deckelbaum, R.J.; Blaner, W.S.; Ramakrishnan, R. A dose-response study of the effects of dietary cholesterol on fasting and postprandial lipid and lipoprotein metabolism in healthy young men. *Arterioscler. Thromb.* **1994**, *14*, 576–586. [CrossRef] [PubMed]

150. Missimer, A.; DiMarco, D.; Murillo, G.; Creighton, B.; Andersen, C.J.; Ketzmer, R.; Fernandez, M.L. Intake of 2 eggs or oatmeal for breakfast does not increase biomarkers for heart disease while eggs improve liver enzymes and raise HDL cholesterol in young healthy individuals. *FASEB* **2015**, *29*, 274.2.

151. Pearce, K.L.; Clifton, P.M.; Noakes, M. Egg consumption as part of an energy-restricted high-protein diet improves blood lipid and blood glucose profiles in individuals with type 2 diabetes. *Br. J. Nutr.* **2011**, *105*, 584–592. [CrossRef] [PubMed]

152. Schwab, U.S.; Ausman, L.M.; Vogel, S.; Li, Z.; Lammi-Keefe, C.J.; Goldin, B.R.; Ordovas, J.M.; Schaefer, E.J.; Lichtenstein, A.H. Dietary cholesterol increases the susceptibility of low density lipoprotein to oxidative modification. *Atherosclerosis* **2000**, *149*, 83–90. [CrossRef]

153. Levy, Y.; Maor, I.; Presser, D.; Aviram, M. Consumption of eggs with meals increases the susceptibility of human plasma and low-density lipoprotein to lipid peroxidation. *Ann. Nutr. Metable* **1996**, *40*, 243–251. [CrossRef]

154. Vander Wal, J.S.; Marth, J.M.; Khosla, P.; Jen, K.L.; Dhurandhar, N.V. Short-term effect of eggs on satiety in overweight and obese subjects. *J. Am. Coll. Nutr.* **2005**, *24*, 510–515. [CrossRef] [PubMed]

155. Ratliff, J.; Leite, J.O.; de Ogburn, R.; Puglisi, M.J.; VanHeest, J.; Fernandez, M.L. Consuming eggs for breakfast influences plasma glucose and ghrelin, while reducing energy intake during the next 24 h in adult men. *Nutr. Res.* **2010**, *30*, 96–103. [CrossRef] [PubMed]

156. Vander Wal, J.S.; Gupta, A.; Khosla, P.; Dhurandhar, N.V. Egg breakfast enhances weight loss. *Int. J. Obes. (Lond.)* **2008**, *32*, 1545–1551.

157. Rueda, J.M.; Khosla, P. Impact of breakfasts (with or without eggs) on body weight regulation and blood lipids in university students over a 14-week semester. *Nutrients* **2013**, *5*, 5097–5113. [CrossRef] [PubMed]

158. Huang, P.L. A comprehensive definition for metabolic syndrome. *Dis. Model. Mech.* **2009**, *2*, 231–237. [CrossRef] [PubMed]

159. Smirnov, M.D.; Esmon, C.T. Phosphatidylethanolamine incorporation into vesicles selectively enhances factor Va inactivation by activated protein C. *J. Biol. Chem.* **1994**, *269*, 816–819. [PubMed]
160. Griffin, J.H.; Kojima, K.; Banka, C.L.; Curtiss, L.K.; Fernandez, J.A. High-density lipoprotein enhancement of anticoagulant activities of plasma protein S and activated protein C. *J. Clin. Investig.* **1999**, *103*, 219–227. [CrossRef] [PubMed]
161. Andersen, C.J.; Fernandez, M.L. Dietary approaches to improving atheroprotective HDL functions. *Food Funct.* **2013**, *4*, 1304–1313. [CrossRef] [PubMed]
162. Perez-Guzman, C.; Vargas, M.H.; Quinonez, F.; Bazavilvazo, N.; Aguilar, A. A cholesterol-rich diet accelerates bacteriologic sterilization in pulmonary tuberculosis. *Chest* **2005**, *127*, 643–651. [CrossRef] [PubMed]

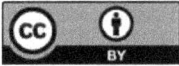

nutrients

MDPI

Review

Hen Egg as an Antioxidant Food Commodity: A Review

Chamila Nimalaratne and Jianping Wu *

Department of Agricultural, Food and Nutritional Science (AFNS), 4-10 Agriculture/Forestry Centre, University of Alberta, Edmonton, AB T6G 2P5, Canada; nimalara@ualberta.ca
* Correspondence: jwu3@ualberta.ca; Tel.: +780-492-6885; Fax: +780-492-4265

Received: 22 July 2015; Accepted: 18 September 2015; Published: 24 September 2015

Abstract: Intake of antioxidants through diet is known to be important in reducing oxidative damage in cells and improving human health. Although eggs are known for their exceptional, nutritional quality, they are not generally considered as antioxidant foods. This review aims to establish the importance of eggs as an antioxidant food by summarizing the current knowledge on egg-derived antioxidants. Eggs have various natural occurring compounds including the proteins ovalbumin, ovotransferrin and lysozyme in egg white, as well as phosvitin, carotenoids and free aromatic amino acids in egg yolk. Some lipophilic antioxidants such as vitamin E, carotenoids, selenium, iodine and others can be transferred from feed into egg yolk to produce antioxidant-enriched eggs. The bioactivity of egg antioxidants can be affected by food processing, storage and gastrointestinal digestion. Generally thermal processing methods can promote loss of antioxidant properties in eggs due to oxidation and degradation, whereas gastrointestinal digestion enhances the antioxidant properties, due to the formation of new antioxidants (free amino acids and peptides). In summary, in addition to its well-known nutritional contribution to our diet, this review emphasizes the role of eggs as an important antioxidant food.

Keywords: hen eggs; naturally-occurring antioxidants; antioxidant-enriched eggs; processing; gastrointestinal digestion

1. Antioxidants in Human

An antioxidant can be defined as "any substance that delays, prevents or removes oxidative damage to a target molecule" [1] or "any substance that directly scavenges reactive oxygen species (ROS) or indirectly acts to up-regulate antioxidant defenses or inhibit ROS production" [2]. The human body produces many enzymatic and nonenzymatic endogenous antioxidants in order to provide the primary defense against superoxide and hydrogen peroxides. The major antioxidant enzymes are superoxide dismutase (SOD), catalase (CAT), glutathione peroxidase (GPx), glutathione reductase (GRx) and peroxiredoxins [3]. Nonenzymatic endogenous antioxidants include coenzyme Q10, vitamin A, glutathione, uric acid, lipoic acid, bilirubin, L-carnitine, *etc.* [3,4]. There are many different mechanisms by which antioxidants exert protective effects against oxidative damage. They can scavenge free radicals and other reactive species by stopping initiation or propagation of free radicals chain reactions in the system, scavenging singlet oxygen, sequestering transition metal ions to prevent generation of free radicals, reducing localized oxygen concentration, and inhibiting pro-oxidative enzymes such as lipoxygenases [3,5,6]. Antioxidants can work synergistically with each other against different types of free radicals and reactive species. The most efficient enzymatic antioxidants are glutathione peroxidase (GSH-Px), catalase, and SOD [7]. GSH-Px and SOD (in two forms: CuZnSOD and MnSOD) are found in mitochondria and cytosol, whereas catalases are located in peroxisomes [8]. SOD converts superoxide into H_2O_2 and oxygen, while GSH-Px and catalase react with H_2O_2 to produce water and oxygen [8]. Although the gene expression and activity of these enzymes in the cell are well regulated to maintain redox homeostasis, internal and external factors such as aging, inflammation, smoking and toxins can influence the balance [7].

Glutathione (GSH) is a water soluble tripeptide (L-γ-glutamyl-L-cysteinylglycine) that can react with ROS using its thiol group and oxidized to form glutathione disulfide (GSSG) which can then convert back to GSH by combined action of NADPH (reduced nicotinamide-adenine di-nucleotide phosphate) cofactor and GRx [3,4]. GSH is also involved in regeneration of ascorbate [3]. Coenzyme Q10, present in all cells and membranes, is the only endogenously synthesized liposoluble antioxidant. It is an effective antioxidant which prevents lipid peroxidation during the initiation step and is involved in regenerating vitamin E [9]. Uric acid is a metabolic product of purine nucleotide, and can be absorbed back into the body during kidney filtration into the plasma [3]. A potent singlet oxygen and hydroxyl radical scavenger, uric acid prevents lysis of red blood cells by peroxidation [10].

2. Dietary Antioxidants

Intake of antioxidants through diet is thought to be important in reducing oxidative damage [11–14]. These antioxidants play a critical role in protecting cellular components from potentially damaging ROS and thereby maintaining homeostasis and optimal cellular functions. Synthetic antioxidants such as butylated hydroxyanisole (BHA), butylated hydroxytoluene (BHT), tert-butylhydroquinone (TBHQ) and propyl gallate (PG) have been used in both food and pharmacological applications [15]. However, because of the possible toxic and carcinogenic effects associated with BHT and BHA, their use is legally restricted [16,17]. As a result, there is a growing interest in using natural antioxidants for food and therapeutic applications which prompt the scientific community to explore new sources of natural and dietary antioxidants [3,15,18,19]. The most known groups of natural antioxidants are vitamin C, vitamin E, carotenoids and flavonoids and more recently, peptides with antioxidant properties derived from various plant and animal sources [15,19].

Most of the plant derived antioxidant compounds are phytochemicals including phenolics, flavonoids and carotenoids whereas the prominent animal-derived antioxidants are amino-derived compounds such as amino acids, peptides and proteins [20].

Vitamin E, a well-known chain breaking antioxidant, prevents propagation of lipid peroxidation reactions by donating its phenolic hydrogen to the lipid peroxyl radical [15]. Vitamin E will become a radical itself (tocopheroxyl radical), but is more stable due to delocalization of the solitary electron over the aromatic ring structure [15,21]. Lipid soluble vitamin E is considered the most important antioxidant in preventing lipid peroxidation. Carotenoids are another class of lipid soluble compounds with antioxidant properties. The main mechanisms are singlet oxygen quenching, reacting with free radicals and delocalizing the unpaired electrons with the aid of unsaturation and resonant stabilization [22,23]. Singlet oxygen scavenging ability of lutein and zeaxanthin is suggested as the main protective mechanism of eye macular against blue light-induced oxidative damage [24,25]. Carotenoids can also prevent lipid peroxidation and play a protective role in carcinogenesis [26]. Although beneficial at moderate concentration, high doses of supplementation of β-carotenoids in high concentration can act as a pro-oxidant [22,27].

Vitamin C or ascorbic acid, a water soluble vitamin, has been shown to be effective against the superoxide radical anion, H_2O_2, the hydroxyl radical and singlet oxygen [15,28]. It also acts synergistically with vitamin E by reacting with tocopheroxyl radical to regenerate its antioxidant ability [29]. Flavonoids represent a class of phytochemicals which are known to have antioxidant properties depending on structural features such as the number and position of the hydroxyl groups and number of phenolic rings, *etc.* [27,30]. They have been reported to scavenge peroxyl radicals, inhibit lipid peroxidation, and chelate metal ions [27,31].

Fruits, vegetables, oil seeds, nuts, cereals, spices, herbs, and grains are important sources of antioxidants such as phenolics, flavonoids and carotenoids. A great deal of research has been conducted on their antioxidant properties *in vivo, in vitro* as well as on extraction and purification methods, applications in food products, bioavailability, and anti-nutritional aspects [32–36]. Among many plant sources, berries and fruits are known for their high phenolic content including phenolic acids, and anthocyanins and their high antioxidant capacity [37]. Most vegetables including tomatoes, red pepper, *Brassica* vegetables, onion, garlic and red beet are found to have high antioxidant capacity mainly attributed to their flavonoid, carotenoid, vitamin C contents [38–41]. Although cereal grains are not considered rich sources of antioxidants compared to fruits and vegetables, grains and grain products are staple food components in the human diet and therefore their contribution is still significant [42–44]. The major phenolic compounds are phenolic acids such as ferulic acid, the dominating phenolic acid in wheat, caffeic acid, *p*-coumaric acid, *p*-hydroxybenzoic acid, vanillic acid and protocatechuic acid, *etc.* [44]. In addition, they contain other compounds which may exert antioxidant effects, for example, vitamin E, folates, minerals (iron, zinc) and trace elements (selenium, copper and manganese), carotenoids, *etc.* It has been suggested that antioxidant capacity of cereals is usually underestimated because of the bound phenolic compounds which do not contribute during *in vitro* assays, but can be released in the gut to exert the antioxidant activity [45,46].

Compared to antioxidants from plant sources, the available research on animal-derived antioxidants is limited. Proteins and peptides have been known to inhibit lipid oxidation through inactivation of ROS, scavenging free radicals, chelation of prooxidative transition metals, reduction of hydroperoxides, and alteration of the physical properties of food systems [47]. The most abundant antioxidant dipeptides in skeletal muscles are histidine-containing dipeptides, such as carnosine and anserine [48]. The peptide concentration varies from about 500 mg per kg of chicken thigh to 2700 mg per kg of pork shoulder depending on the type of muscle [47]. Their antioxidant properties are believed to arise through radical scavenging and metal chelation abilities [48]. The presence of thiol groups and aromatic side chains (tryptophan, tyrosine and phenyl alanine) and imidazole ring in histidine [49,50] are recognized as important structural features for their antioxidant properties. Casein derived peptides from milk proteins have been reported to inhibit enzymatic as well as non-enzymatic oxidation of lipids [51,52]. Generation of antioxidative peptides from milk proteins has been studied in detail [53]. Antioxidant peptides from egg proteins have also been reported [54,55]. Apart from proteins, other antioxidant compounds in animal tissues such as vitamin E and ascorbic acid are well-known for their antioxidant properties [56]. Some aquatic animals including salmon and shrimp contain high amounts of carotenoids with strong antioxidant properties. Astaxanthin, a carotenoid found in high concentrations in fish and shrimp, showed strong singlet oxygen and radical scavenging ability, which was 100 times greater than α-tocopherol activity [57]. The activity was mainly attributable to the presence of hydroxyl and keto endings on each ionone ring in the structure of astaxanthin [58].

3. Egg as an Antioxidant Food Commodity

3.1. Chemical and Nutritional Composition of Eggs

Egg is composed of three parts: egg shell with membranes, egg white albumen, and yolk, accounting for approximately 9.5%, 63% and 27.5% of the whole shell egg [59]. The edible portion of the egg consists of water (74%), proteins (12%), lipids (12%), carbohydrate (<1%) as well as vitamins and minerals [60]. The chemical and nutrient composition of egg is well documented [60–63]. The protein fraction is distributed in both egg white (ovalbumin, ovotransferrin, ovomucoid, ovomucin, *etc.*) and yolk (high density lipoproteins, low density lipoproteins and livetins). Eggs proteins are high quality proteins and are used as a golden standard for measuring the quality of other food proteins [61]. Almost all egg lipids are located in yolk and approximately 65% of yolk lipids are triglycerides, while phospholipids, cholesterol and carotenoids make 30%, 4%, <1%, respectively [64]. The fatty acid composition of egg yolk can be manipulated through feed formulation to produce eggs enriched with polyunsaturated fatty acids with benefits beyond basic nutrition [65]. Based on the standardized poultry feed, about 30%–35% from the total fatty acids are saturated fatty acids (SFA), 40%–45% are monounsaturated fatty acids (MUFA), and 20%–25% are polyunsaturated fatty acids (PUFA) [66]. Egg yolk lipids have been used as a source of long-chain polyunsaturated fatty acids, Docosahexaenoic acid (DHA) and phospholipids to incorporate into infant formula [67,68]. Eggs are also considered a good source of micronutrients such as vitamins and minerals. Eggs contain ~16%, 29%, 9% and 9% of the recommended daily intake (RDI) of phosphorus, selenium, iron, and zinc, and 10% of the RDI of vitamin A, D, E, K, B2, B12, biotin and pantothenic acid [61]. It has been shown that some minerals like selenium, and iodine can be enriched through fortification of feed [69,70]. In the same way as minerals, vitamin contents of egg can be manipulated through hen's feed formulation [71].

In addition to the nutritional value, egg components have various biological activities which may render important health benefits [72]. Egg is a complete biological system designed to nourish and protect the growing embryo from various pathogen invasions. As a result, egg shell with membranes and egg white proteins possess physical and biological defense mechanisms such as viscosity, pH, antimicrobial properties, *etc.* For a list of egg compounds with various bioactivities please refer to [62,73].

3.2. Antioxidant Compounds in Eggs

Numerous compounds in both egg white and yolk exhibit antioxidant properties (Table 1). Many egg proteins such as ovalbumin, ovotransferrin, phosvitin, egg lipids such as phospholipids, as well as certain micronutrients such as vitamin E, vitamin A, selenium, and carotenoids, are reported to have antioxidant properties. In addition, eggs can be further enriched with antioxidants (*i.e.*, carotenoids, vitamin E, selenium and iodine) through manipulation of poultry feed [58–61].

Table 1. Antioxidants in Egg.

Name of Compound	Amount in Egg	Mechanisms of Action
Egg white	(% of egg white proteins)	
Ovalbumin	54	Free thiol (SH) groups in ovalbumin regulate the redox status and bind metal ions, thereby exert antioxidant properties [74]; Increased antioxidant activity when conjugated with saccharides [74,75]
Ovotransferrin	12	Possess SOD-like superoxide scavenging activity due to its metal chelating ability [76]
Ovomucin	3.5	Inhibit H_2O_2-induced oxidative stress in human embryonic kidney [77]
Lysozyme	3.4	Suppress reactive oxygen species (ROS) and oxidative stress genes [78]
Cystatin	0.05	Modulate the synthesis and release of NO• production and thereby play a role in cellular antioxidant pathways [79,80]
Egg yolk	(% of yolk dry matter)	
Phosvitin	4	Antioxidant activity based on metal chelating ability; chelates iron and protects against Fe-induced oxidative damage [81,82]
Phospholipids	10	Hydrolyl amines in the side chains of phospholipids play a role in radical scavenging and exert antioxidant properties [83]
Carotenoids	<1	Unsaturated backbone and aromatic rings of carotenoids aid in neutralizing singlet oxygen and free radicals and protect against oxidative damage [22,25,26]

Table 1. *Cont.*

Name of Compound	Amount in Egg	Mechanisms of Action
Vitamin E	<1	Vitamin E can donate its phenolic hydrogen to scavenge free radicals [15]; protect membrane fatty acids and plasma Low density lipoproteins (LDL), High density lipoproteins (HDL) against lipid oxidation [84]
Aromatic amino acids	<1	Aromatic nature of tryptophan and tyrosine contribute to the total antioxidant capacity [85]

3.2.1. Antioxidants Naturally Occurring in Eggs

Ovalbumin

Ovalbumin is a glycoprotein made of 385 amino acids and constitutes approximately 54% (w/w) of the total egg white protein [60,86]. It contains six cysteine residues with a single disulfide bond and is the only egg white protein with free SH (thiol) groups [60]. The presence of thiol groups enable its ability to play a role in redox regulation and binding metal ions therefore exert antioxidant properties [87–89]. In 1971, Goto and Shibasaki observed the protective effects of ovalbumin against lipid oxidation in a linolenic model system [90]. When covalently attached with polysaccharides, the radical scavenging activity of ovalbumin was significantly increased [74]. It was speculated that free SH groups are responsible for the antioxidant activity of ovalbumin, which were effectively exposed upon the conjugation with polysaccharides [74]. Further studies on glycated ovalbumin showed that the activity is dependent on the type of sugars used and also the configuration of hydroxyl groups in the sugar molecule [75,91].

Ovotransferrin

Ovotransferrin (also known as conalbumin), representing 12%–13% of the total egg white protein, is a member of the transferrin family, a group of ion-binding proteins with an *in vivo* preference for iron [60,92]. Ovotransferrin consists of two lobes, each capable of binding one atom of Fe^{3+} and carbonate anion [60]. Among the two, the *N*-lobe is found to be more important for its antioxidant properties [76].

Ovotransferrin was reported to possess SOD-like activity against superoxide anion promoted by metal binding. The scavenging activity was dose-dependent and considerably higher than known for antioxidants such as ascorbate or serum albumin [76]. Additionally, the iron-binding ability of ovotransferrin has an indirect role in preventing iron-induced lipid peroxidation [60].

Lysozyme

Lysozyme is an enzyme present in almost all organisms. One egg contains approximately 0.3–0.4 g of lysozyme [93]. Lysozyme is a defensin, a member of the family of native, highly conserved host-defense proteins [78]. It contains an 18-amino acid domain that binds agents such as advanced glycation end products (AGE), which contribute to the production of ROS and increased oxidative stress (ROS). Liu *et al.*, showed that lysozyme protects transgenic mice against acute and chronic oxidative injury [78]. They also showed that hepatocytes incubated with lysozyme suppress cellular ROS levels and oxidative response genes. In another study, the survival rate following acute or chronic oxidative injury in lysozyme deficient transgenic mice was found to be significantly lower compared to the control, indicating its protective role as an antioxidant [94].

Cystatin

Egg white cystatin is the first identified member of the cystatin family [95]. It is a small protein of approximately 13 kDa molecular weight which makes up 0.05% of the total egg white proteins and contains two disulfide bonds [60]. Cystatin is an inhibitor of cysteine proteinases, thereby exerting antibacterial properties [96,97]. It is also reported that chicken cystatin exerts immunomodulatory activities by modulating the synthesis and release of NO$^\bullet$ production in interferon γ-activated murine macrophages [78–80,98,99]. Optimum levels of NO$^\bullet$ is essential for regulation of certain cellular antioxidant pathways [100]. Moreover, cystatin B, the group which chicken cystatin belongs to, has recently found to involve in protecting cerebellar granule neurons from oxidative stress by playing a role in oxidative stress-responsive signaling pathway [79]. Taken together, the role of cystatin in modulating the NO$^\bullet$ synthesis and protecting brain neurons from oxidative damage, provide us with evidence of its potential activity as an antioxidant.

Ovoinhibitor

Ovoinhibitor, which makes approximately 1.5% of egg white proteins, inhibits serine proteinases such as trypsin and chymotrypsin and also bacterial and fungal proteinases [93]. It was shown that chymotrypsin proteinase inhibitors including ovoinhibtor are capable of inhibiting the formation of ROS in activated human polymorphonuclear leukocytes during the inflammatory response [100]. They demonstrated that about 29% of formation of H_2O_2 was inhibited by ovoinhibitor at a concentration of 20 μM [100].

Phosvitin

Phosvitin is the most phosphorylated protein containing nearly 80% of yolk protein phosphorous and represents ~11% of yolk proteins [101]. More than half of its amino acid composition is serine, which exists as phosphoserine. It has a strong metal-binding ability and approximately 95% of yolk iron is bound to phosvitin. This high metal-binding capacity makes phosvitin a potential antioxidant, particularly against iron induced oxidative damage [82]. Iron is essential for life; under normal physiological conditions, the level is controlled by iron binding proteins ferritin and transferrin. However, if the balance is disturbed causing iron overload in cells, the effects could be lethal as humans have a very limited capacity to excrete excess iron. The excess iron in the form of Fe^{2+} can participate in Fenton reaction to produce toxic OH$^\bullet$ by reacting with H_2O_2.

Moreover, the circulating free iron can oxidize heart-muscle membranes, causing arrhythmia and heart failure. The iron-chelating ability of phosvitin indicates its possible role in protecting iron-induced oxidative damage. Phosvitin accelerates Fe^{2+} autoxidation, thereby reducing the availability of Fe^{2+} and inhibiting Fe^{2+}-catalyzed OH$^\bullet$ generation through Fenton reaction [102]. Additionally, phosvitin is also proven to be effective against UV-induced lipid peroxidation in the presence of excess iron [103].

Phospholipids

Egg yolk phospholipids consist of 84% phosphatidylcholine (PC), 12% phosphatidylethanolamine (PE), 2% sphingomyelin and 2% lysophosphatidylcholine and other minor compounds [64]. King, Boyd, and Sheldon (1992) reported that egg yolk phospholipids exhibit antioxidant activity in a refined salmon oil model system, and also demonstrated that the presence of nitrogen improved the antioxidant activity of phospholipids [104]. The antioxidant activity was positively associated with the degree of fatty acid unsaturation [81]. Hydroxy amines in the side chains of choline and ethanolamines showed strong inhibition of lipid peroxidation, indicating the importance of side-chain amino acids with hydroxyl groups in the antioxidant activity [105].

Carotenoids

Carotenoids are lipid soluble compounds responsible for the orange-yellow color of the egg yolk. The health promoting properties of carotenoids are well documented [106,107]. More than 600 carotenoids have been identified to date and it is suggested than around 50 of them might occur in our diet and 14 in human blood [107,108]. Human body do not synthesize carotenoids and must be obtained through the diet. Therefore, it is important to consider the type and bioavailability of dietary carotenoids. Bioavailability of egg carotenoids is superior to those from green leafy vegetables [109,110] due to the solubilization of yolk lipids, which makes eggs a unique and important carrier of bioactive carotenoids. The profile of egg carotenoids is largely depend on hen's feed composition, therefore it can vary among different types of eggs [111,112]. Certain carotenoids are allowed to use as poultry feed additives to improve color of the egg yolk, however, the amount and types of carotenoid can be varied as per the country's feed regulation [113]. In general, lutein, zeaxanthin, canthaxanthin, β-apo-8'-carotenal, capsanthin, β-apo-8'-carotenoic acid ethyl ester, β-cryptoxanthin, and citranaxanthin can be present in egg yolk [114].

Human plasma contains several carotenoids including β-carotene, α-carotene, β-cryptoxanthin, lutein and zeaxanthin and their isomers [115]. Lutein, zeaxanthin and *meso*-zeaxanthin are the main components of the eye macular pigment [116]. Lutein and zeaxanthin are well known for their role in protecting the eye from age-related macular degeneration (AMD) [117]. The singlet oxygen and radical scavenging activity of lutein and zeaxanthin is considered one of the two major mechanisms for their beneficial effects against light-induced oxidative damage in eye macular, in particular, against AMD [117–119]. The other major mechanism is their ability to absorb blue light, particularly before it damages the photoreceptor cells, which is also considered a passive antioxidant action [117]. A recent study demonstrated that pre-incubation of human lens epithelial cells (HLEC) with lutein, zeaxanthin and α-tocopherol, dramatically reduced the levels of H_2O_2-induced protein carbonyl, MDA, and DNA damage [120]. Further, lutein, zeaxanthin and α-tocopherol supplementation increased GSH levels and GSH: GSSG ratio, particularly in response to oxidative stress [120]. Dietary supplementation with lutein reduced plasma lipid hydroperoxides and the size of aortic lesions in mice [121] and reduced the plasma levels of oxidized-LDL in guinea pigs [122], indicating a protective role in ROS induced early atherosclerosis. The ability of lutein and zeaxanthin to scavenge hydroxyl and superoxide radicals is attributed to the presence of double bonds which makes a bond with the free radical to produce a highly resonance-stabilized C-centered radical [123]. Lutein, zeaxanthin and β-cryptoxanthin have also been shown to scavenge peroxynitrite which may play a role in LDL protection against oxidative damage [124].

Vitamins and Minerals

On average egg contains around 1.1 mg of vitamin E [61] which is equivalent to 8.5% of RDA. Vitamin E, especially α-tocopherol as the most active form, is a well-known lipophilic chain-breaking antioxidant known to protect long-chain polyunsaturated fatty acids in the membranes of cells and thus maintain their bioactivity [125,126]. In plasma, vitamin E exists with LDL and HDL, providing protection against oxidation [84,127]. Supplementing with vitamin E increased resistance to LDL-oxidation and is associated with a lower risk of coronary diseases in both men [128] and women [129]. Eggs can be enriched with vitamin E to provide up to 150% RDA without formation of off flavour [130], not only providing the aforementioned benefits, but also protecting against oxidation of long chain fatty acids in yolk [130].

Certain minerals present in egg yolk including selenium and iodine also contribute to the antioxidant properties. Selenium is an essential mineral present in antioxidant selenoproteins such as GPx, thioredoxin reductases (TrxR) and selenoprotein P (Sepp1) [131]. Iodine has a potential role as an antioxidant in human systems including the eye, thyroid and the breast [132]. Iodine deficiency can increase the stimulation of thyroid gland by TSH resulting in excessive H_2O_2 [132].

Egg-Derived Antioxidative Peptides

Antioxidant activity was reported from egg white and egg yolk proteins. Recently, many studies have reported antioxidant properties of egg white proteins hydrolyzed using different enzymes and some have even purified the potential antioxidant peptides [133–136]. For example, Liu *et al.*, used alcalase to produce and purified three novel peptides with antioxidant properties, DHTKE (Asp-His-Thr-Lys-Glu), FFGFN (Phe-Phe-Glu-Phe-His) and MPDAHL

(Met-Pro-Asp-Ala-His-Leu) [137]. Similarly, our recent studies showed that "protease P" hydrolysed egg white produce twopotent antioxidant peptides, AEERYP (Ala-Glu-Glu-Arg-Tyr-Pro) and DEDTQAMP (Asp-Glu-Asp-Thr-Gln-Ala-Met-Pro) [138]. Trypsin hydrolysate prepared from egg white protein precipitate, obtained as a by-product in cystatin and lysozyme isolation, showed a considerably better radical scavenging activity than those prepared from chymotrypsin and elastase [139,140]. Adult male spontaneously hypertensive rats fed with peptic digested egg white for 17 weeks showed increased radical-scavenging capacity of the plasma and lowered MDA concentration in the aorta, and exerted a beneficial effect on the lipid profile, lowering triglycerides and total cholesterol without changing HDL levels [141]. Two peptides derived from lecithin-free egg yolk exhibit protection against lipid peroxidation in intoxicated normal human liver cells [142]. Both peptides contained a leucine residue at their *N*-terminal positions which were thought to contribute to their antioxidant properties [142]. Another study showed that egg yolk protein hydrolysate exhibited superoxide and hydroxyl radical scavenging activity, effectively inhibiting thiobarbituric acid reactive substances (TBARS) formation from ground beef and tuna homogenates, indicating its potential as a natural antioxidant [143].

The peptide, Tyr-Ala-Glu-Glu-Arg-Tyr-Pro-Ile-Leu, derived from pepsin hydrolyzed ovalbumin, which was previously reported to possess angiotensin converting enzyme (ACE)-inhibitory activity, also exhibited a strong radical scavenging activity and delayed the LDL-oxidation induced by Cu^{2+} [54]. Peptic digests of ovalbumin inhibited the action of $OH^\bullet$ and $O_2^{\bullet-}$ and also prevented the oxidation of linoleic acid in linoleic acid autoxidation system [144]. *In-vivo* studies showed that supplementation with these peptic digests of ovalbumin significantly decreased the production of oxidants and oxidative damage in serum and liver of aged mice [144].

Enzymatic hydrolysis of ovotransferrin was shown to lead to enhanced overall antioxidant activity. Two tetrapeptides (Trp-Asn-Ile-Pro and Gly-Trp-Asn-Ile) were characterized from thermolytic hydrolysate of ovotransferrin [145]. Trp-Asn-Ile was suggested as the responsible peptide motif for the high activity of the above tetrapeptides [146]. A tripeptide Ile-Arg-Trp, derived from ovotransferrin showed strong radical scavenging activity which was attributed to tryptophan and the peptide bond between Trp and Arg [146]. It is known that Trp can exert radical scavenging properties mainly due to the presence of the indole ring [147,148]. A recent study demonstrated that grafting a catechin moiety significantly increased the antioxidant activity of ovotransferrin implicating its potential as neutraceutical and functional food [149]. Peptides derived from lysozyme are reported to possess antioxidant properties [150–152].

Egg white ovomucin, a sulfated glycoprotein accounting for 3.5%–4% of egg white proteins, is responsible for the jelly-like structure of egg white [60,153]. Recently, ovomucin derived pentapeptide Trp-Asn-Trp-Ala-Asp was reported to reduce H_2O_2-induced oxidative stress in human embryonic kidney (HEK-293) cells by inhibiting intracellular ROS accumulation and blocking the ROS activated mitochondria-mediated cell apoptosis pathway [154]. Others also reported on antioxidant properties of peptides derived from ovomucin [75,134].

Phosvitin phosphopeptides (PPP) obtained from tryptic digestion of egg yolk phosvitin showed protective effects against H_2O_2-induced oxidative stress in human intestinal epithelial cells [155,156]. The antioxidative activity of PPP was similar to that of glutathione and positively related to the phosphorous content. PPPs are also assumed to be involved with up-regulating glutathione and associated antioxidative enzymes such as glutathione reductase, glutathione *S*-transferase, and catalase and thus reducing the oxidative stress [157]. Furthermore, the antioxidative activity of PPPs on H_2O_2-induced oxidative stress retained after gastrointestinal digestion [81].

3.2.2. Antioxidant Enriched Eggs

Owing to its high lipid content, many lipid-soluble antioxidant compounds such as lutein/zeaxanthin, vitamin E, selenium, iodine lycopene can be incorporated into egg yolk [158]. The most studied are omega-3 fatty acids, which are incorporated into eggs by feeding fish oil, flax seed, algae, or other ingredients to laying hens [159]. High contents of omega-3 fatty acids might increase susceptibility to fatty acid oxidation therefore simultaneously enrichment of eggs with antioxidants such as vitamin E and carotenoids was suggested to decrease fatty acid oxidation and provide a good source of dietary antioxidant [158].

Carotenoids are naturally occurring in egg yolk in varied amounts depending on hen's feed. Feed fortification with natural sources such as marigold (*Tagetes erecta*) or alfalfa (*Medicago sativa*) extracts are sources of lutein, while other sources such as corn (*Zea mays*) and red pepper (*Capsicum annuum*) provide zeaxanthin and capsanthin respectively [113,160]. Canthaxanthin, β-apo-8′-carotenal and β-apo-8′-carotenoic acid ethyl ester are chemically synthesized and incorporated into the feed [114]. Lutein and zeaxanthin are two major egg carotenoids that can be found in human serum, skin and eye macular and involved in the protective roles against oxidative stress [161,162]. Lutein content of enriched eggs can be increased up to 15-fold compared to the control group, for example enriched egg contains around 1.9 mg of lutein [130]. Lutein enriched eggs show a higher lutein bioavailability compared to lutein, lutein ester supplements, and spinach [110]. Lycopene is a hydrocarbon carotenoid reported to have strong antioxidant properties effective in reducing the risk of prostate carcinoma [163,164]. Although lycopene is not usually found in eggs, lycopene enrichment can be achieved via feed fortification with tomato powder and lycopene could reduce yolk lipid peroxidation [165].

Vitamin E is the major lipophilic antioxidant compound in our body that may provide the primary protection against free radical induced lipid peroxidation [125]. The daily requirement is approximately 15 mg α-tocopherol equivalents per day [166]. Since vitamin E is needed to protect membrane lipids from being peroxidized, this amount can be increased with higher intake of polyunsaturated fatty acids [167,168]. Egg can be enriched to provide around 20 mg of vitamin E per egg, which is more than the daily requirement, and also provide protection against unsaturated fatty acid peroxidation [158]. Folate, a water soluble B-group vitamin is shown to reduce the incidence of neural tube defects in newborns [169]. Egg yolk can be enriched with highly bioavailable folate through fortification of feed with folic acid to provide up to 12.5% of the recommended daily intake of folate [170,171]. Almost all the folate in egg exists in the form of 5-methyltetrahydrofolate (5-MTHF), and showed high stability during cooking [172]. Folates are reported to have antioxidant properties and among different forms, 5-MTHF was reported to have the most prominent antioxidant activity, which was attributed to the electron donating effect of the 5-amino group [173]. *In vivo* and *ex vivo* studies with human vessels showed that 5-MTHF improves NO-mediated endothelial function, decreases superoxide production, scavenge peroxynitrite and also reversed endothelial nitric oxide synthase (eNOS) uncoupling, thereby exerts antioxidant effects [174,175].

Both selenium and iodine, which are known to have antioxidant properties, can be effectively transferred into the egg yolk. Eggs can be supplemented to provide up to 50% and 150% of the daily requirements of selenium and iodine respectively [158,176]. Collectively, these antioxidant enriched eggs provide multiple advantages by serving as a dietary source of several nutrients including omega 3, vitamin E, vitamin D, selenium, iodine and also as an important source of antioxidants such as lutein.

3.3. Effect of Processing, Storage Conditions and Gastrointestinal Digestion on Egg Antioxidants

Foods are subjected to various processing and storage conditions before consumption, which may influence the antioxidant capacity of food components. The effect of food processing and storage conditions on the overall antioxidant activity of a particular food is a result of several different events occurring consecutively or simultaneously. According to Nicoli *et al.*, there are three possible effects of food processing on the overall antioxidant capacity [177]:

1. The total antioxidant capacity is not affected: as a result of no changes in natural antioxidant compounds or loss of naturally occurring antioxidants balanced by formation of compounds with novel or improved antioxidant properties,

2. The total antioxidant capacity is increased: as a result of improvement of antioxidant properties of naturally occurring compounds or formation of new antioxidant,
3. The total antioxidant capacity is decreased: loss of naturally occurring antioxidants or formation of new compounds with pro-oxidant activity.

Most thermal processing methods can create environments that can lead to oxidation, thermal degradation, and leaching of vitamin C and phenolic compounds, which would reduce the antioxidant activity [178]. With regard to carotenoids, processing can lead to the dissociation of compounds from plant matrix resulting in increased carotenoid antioxidants, and improved digestive absorption [179–181]. Most of the fruits and vegetables contain phenolic compounds, carotenoids and vitamin C, which are differently affected by processing conditions. Consequently, the total antioxidant capacity can be increased [182–184] or decreased [184–187]. In animal-derived foods, the antioxidant capacity depends mainly on amino compounds (proteins, peptides and amino acids) and vitamin E.

Heat modification of egg white proteins, ovalbumin, lysozyme and ovomucoid via Maillard reaction resulted in protein-sugar conjugates, leading to increased radical scavenging properties [188]. Chen, Chi, and Xu showed that there are no significant differences in terms of DPPH (1,1-diphenyl-2-picrylhydrazyl) radical-scavenging activity, reducing power, and lipid peroxidation inhibitory activity of spray dried and freeze-dried egg white protein hydrolysates compared to the undried sample [135]. Antioxidant properties of egg yolk phosvitin is due to its iron binding abilities; heating phosvitin at 110 °C for 40 min did not change the iron binding ability of phosvitin [189].

Carotenoids and vitamin E in egg yolk are reported to be influenced by thermal processing. In the presence of heat, light, oxygen, *etc.*, carotenoids can undergo *trans-cis* isomerization, or they can be degraded resulting in altered or loss of bioactivity [190]. Boiling of eggs resulted in a 10%–20% carotenoid loss [112], whereas pasteurizarion did not change the carotenoid content [191]. Storage conditions such as temperature can also affect the antioxidant properties of eggs. Storage at refrigeration temperature for two weeks reduced significantly the total carotenoid content in raw eggs enriched with omega-3 and carophyll (canthaxanthin preparation), while at room temperature, the losses were observed after 7 days of storage [192]. The vitamin E content of eggs was also significantly reduced by thermal processing accompanied with increased lipid oxidation products [193,194].

Pretreatments with ultrasound, high-intensity pulsed electric field (PEF) or high pressure can affect the antioxidant activity of egg proteins/peptides. Pretreatment with PEF significantly increased the antioxidant activity of egg white protein hydrolysate which was attributed to the release of free amino acids and small peptides with antioxidant properties [134]. Also, high pressure processing and sonication or ultrasound pretreatments are shown to improve the degree of hydrolysis of egg white proteins which result increased antioxidant properties [195,196].

Gastrointestinal digestion involves extreme pH conditions and various enzymes which might cause degradation of antioxidant componds or generation of novel antioxidant compounds. Many recent research activities have evaluated the changes in antioxidant capacity of different food products after gastrointestinal digestion using diverse model systems. After gastrointestinal digestion, the antioxidant activity of wheat [197], gooseberries [198], grapes [199], soymilk [200], saithe and shrimp [201] and loach protein hydrolysate [202] increased several times, attributed mainly to increased free amino acid content and short chain peptides generated during digestion. However, the antioxidant activity of some foods such as apples [203] and *Feijoada* whole meal (a traditional Brazilian dish containing vegetables) [204] was significantly reduced.

Many studies have reported the formation of antioxidant peptides after simulated gastrointestinal digestion of egg components [81,134,150]. A recent study showed that different types of domestic cooking methods such as boiling and frying decreased the antioxidant activity [134]. Nevertheless, simulated gastrointestinal digestion of cooked egg with pepsin and pancreatin significantly increased the antioxidant activity, which was attributed to the release of amino acids and antioxidant peptides [134]. Our recent studies on effect of simulated gastrointestinal digestion of egg yolk antioxidant using highly sophisticated intestinal model TIM-1 showed that, lutein and zeaxanthin, the main egg carotenoids, remain stable during the gastrointestinal digestion and also highly bioaccessible possibly due to the association with yolk fat [205], it is likely that they retain their antioxidant activity. Moreover, gastrointestinal digestion significantly increased the total antioxiant activity of cooked egg yolk (about 5–8 fold), which is presumed to be a result of increased free amino acid content and release of antioxidant peptides

4. Summary

Oxidative stress is hypothesized to be responsible for the onset and development of various diseases and ageing. Dietary antioxidants are thought to impart potential benefits in reducing the risk of some chronic diseases by maintaining redox homeostasis. There is extensive research on the presence and characterization of antioxidants from fruits, vegetables, cereals and herbs; however, there is only limited research with regard to antioxidants from animal products. Eggs are an important part of our breakfast and an excellent source of high quality proteins, lipids, vitamins and minerals. Many egg proteins such as ovalbumin, ovotransferrin, phosvitin, and egg lipids such as phospholipids, as well as certain micronutrients such as vitamin E, vitamin A, selenium, and carotenoids, are reported to have antioxidant properties. Furthermore, eggs can be enriched with antioxidants (*i.e.*, carotenoids, vitamin E, selenium and iodine) through manipulation of poultry feed. Domestic cooking tended to reduce the antioxidant activity of egg, while gastrointestinal digestion of cooked eggs increased the antioxidant due to the release of amino acid and peptides.

Acknowledgments: This review was funded by grants from Egg Farmers of Canada (EFC), Alberta Egg Producers (AEP), the Agriculture and Food Council, which is responsible for delivering Agriculture and Agri-Food Canada's Advancing Canadian Agriculture and Agri-Food (ACAAF) Program in Alberta, Food for Health Initiative (Vitamin Fund) of the Faculty of Agricultural, Life and Environmental Science of the University of Alberta, Burnbrae Farms Limited, Poultry Industry Council and Natural Sciences and Engineering Research Council (NSERC) of Canada to Jianping Wu.

Author Contributions: Jianping Wu and Chamila Nimalaratne generated the concept of review. Chamila Nimalaratne drafted the manuscript and Jianping Wu reviewed and edited the manuscript.

Conflicts of Interest: The authors declare no conflict of interest.

References

1. Halliwell, B. Biochemistry of oxidative stress. *Biochem. Soc. Trans.* **2007**, *35*, 1147–1150. [PubMed]
2. Khlebnikov, A.I.; Schepetkin, I.A.; Domina, N.G.; Kirpotina, L.N.; Quinn, M.T. Improved quantitative structure-activity relationship models to predict antioxidant activity of flavonoids in chemical, enzymatic, and cellular systems. *Bioorganic Med. Chem.* **2007**, *15*, 1749–1770.
3. Carocho, M.; Ferreira, I.C.F.R. A review on antioxidants, prooxidants and related controversy: Natural and synthetic compounds, screening and analysis methodologies and future perspectives. *Food Chem. Toxicol.* **2013**, *51*, 15–25. [CrossRef] [PubMed]
4. Rizzo, A.M.; Berselli, P.; Zava, S.; Montorfano, G.; Negroni, M.; Corsetto, P.; Berra, B. Endogenous antioxidants and radical scavengers. *Adv. Exp. Med. Biol.* **2010**, *698*, 52–67. [PubMed]
5. Lobo, V.; Patil, A.; Phatak, A.; Chandra, N. Free radicals, antioxidants and functional foods: Impact on human health. *Pharmacogn. Rev.* **2010**, *4*, 118–126. [CrossRef] [PubMed]
6. Brewer, M.S. Natural antioxidants: Sources, compounds, mechanisms of action, and potential applications. *Compr. Rev. Food Sci. Food Saf.* **2011**, *10*, 221–247. [CrossRef]
7. Matés, J.M.; Pérez-Gómez, C.; de Castro, I.N. Antioxidant enzymes and human diseases. *Clin. Biochem.* **1999**, *32*, 595–603. [CrossRef]
8. Rodriguez, C.; Mayo, J.C.; Sainz, R.M.; Antolin, I.; Herrera, F.; Martin, V.; Reiter, R.J. Regulation of antioxidant enzymes: A significant role for melatonin. *J. Pineal Res.* **2004**, *36*, 1–9. [PubMed]
9. Littarru, G.P.; Tiano, L. Bioenergetic and antioxidant properties of coenzyme q10: Recent developments. *Mol. Biotechnol.* **2007**, *37*, 31–37. [CrossRef] [PubMed]

10. Ames, B.N.; Cathcart, R.; Schwiers, E.; Hochstein, P. Uric acid provides an antioxidant defense in humans against oxidant- and radical-caused aging and cancer: A hypothesis. *Proc. Natl. Acad. Sci. USA* **1981**, *78*, 6858–6862. [CrossRef] [PubMed]
11. Halliwell, B. Antioxidants in human health and disease. *Annu. Rev. Nutr.* **1996**, *16*, 33–50. [CrossRef] [PubMed]
12. Halliwell, B. Free radicals and antioxidants: Updating a personal view. *Nutr. Rev.* **2012**, *70*, 257–265. [CrossRef] [PubMed]
13. Sies, H. Oxidative stress: Oxidants and antioxidants. *Exp. Physiol.* **1997**, *82*, 291–295. [CrossRef] [PubMed]
14. Valko, M.; Leibfritz, D.; Moncol, J.; Cronin, M.T.D.; Mazur, M.; Telser, J. Free radicals and antioxidants in normal physiological functions and human disease. *Int. J. Biochem. Cell Biol.* **2007**, *39*, 44–84. [CrossRef] [PubMed]
15. Gülçin, İ. Antioxidant activity of food constituents: An overview. *Arch. Toxicol.* **2012**, *86*, 345–391. [CrossRef] [PubMed]
16. Vandghanooni, S.; Forouharmehr, A.; Eskandani, M.; Barzegari, A.; Kafil, V.; Kashanian, S.; Dolatabadi, J.E.N. Cytotoxicity and DNA fragmentation properties of butylated hydroxyanisole. *DNA Cell Biol.* **2013**, *32*, 98–103. [CrossRef] [PubMed]
17. Williams, G.; Iatropoulos, M.; Whysner, J. Safety Assessment of butylated hydroxyanisole and butylated hydroxytoluene as antioxidant food additives. *Food Chem. Toxicol.* **1999**, *37*, 1027–1038. [CrossRef]
18. Halliwell, B.; Murcia, M.A.; Chirico, S.; Aruoma, O.I. Free radicals and antioxidants in food and *in vivo*: What they do and how they work. *Crit. Rev. Food Sci. Nutr.* **1995**, *35*, 7–20. [PubMed]
19. Samaranayaka, A.G.P.; Li-Chan, E.C.Y. Food-derived peptidic antioxidants: A review of their production, assessment, and potential applications. *J. Funct. Foods* **2011**, *3*, 229–254. [CrossRef]
20. Sikora, E.; Cieślik, E.; Topolska, K. The sources of natural antioxidants. *Acta Sci. Pol. Technol. Aliment.* **2008**, *7*, 5–17.
21. Niki, E. Role of vitamin E as a lipid-soluble peroxyl radical scavenger: *In vitro* and *in vivo* evidence. *Free Radic. Biol. Med.* **2014**, *66*, 3–12. [CrossRef] [PubMed]
22. Stahl, W.; Sies, H. Antioxidant activity of carotenoids. *Mol Aspect Med.* **2003**, *24*, 345–351. [CrossRef]
23. Tang, G. Lycopenes and related 351.compounds. In *Encyclopedia of Human Nutrition*, 3rd ed.; Caballero, B., Ed.; Academic Press: Waltham, MA, USA, 2013; pp. 124–130.
24. Alves-Rodrigues, A.; Shao, A. The science behind lutein. *Toxicol. Lett.* **2004**, *150*, 57–83. [CrossRef] [PubMed]
25. Ma, L.; Lin, X.-M. Effects of lutein and zeaxanthin on aspects of eye health. *J. Sci. Food Agric.* **2010**, *90*, 2–12. [CrossRef] [PubMed]
26. Zhang, L.-X.; Cooney, R.V.; Bertram, J.S. Carotenoids enhance gap junctional communication and inhibit lipid peroxidation in C3H/10T1/2 cells: Relationship to their cancer chemopreventive action. *Carcinogenesis* **1991**, *12*, 2109–2114. [CrossRef] [PubMed]
27. Procházková, D.; Boušová, I.; Wilhelmová, N. Antioxidant and prooxidant properties of flavonoids. *Fitoterapia* **2011**, *82*, 513–523. [CrossRef] [PubMed]
28. Benzie, I.F.F.; Choi, S.-W. Chapter One—Antioxidants in food: Content, measurement, significance, action, cautions, caveats, and research needs. *Adv. Food Nutr. Res.* **2014**, *71*, 1–53. [PubMed]
29. Fang, Y.-Z.; Yang, S.; Wu, G. Free radicals, antioxidants, and nutrition. *Nutrition* **2002**, *18*, 872–879. [CrossRef]
30. Rice-Evans, C.; Miller, N.; Paganga, G. Structure-antioxidant activity relationships of flavonoids and phenolic acids. *Free Radic. Biol. Med.* **1996**, *20*, 933–956. [CrossRef]
31. Brunetti, C.; di Ferdinando, M.; Fini, A.; Pollastri, S.; Tattini, M. Flavonoids as antioxidants and developmental regulators: Relative significance in plants and humans. *Int. J. Mol. Sci.* **2013**, *14*, 3540–3555.
32. Duthie, G.; Crozier, A. Plant-derived phenolic antioxidants. *Curr. Opin. Lipidol.* **2000**, *11*, 43–47. [CrossRef] [PubMed]
33. Abourashed, E. Bioavailability of plant-derived antioxidants. *Antioxidants* **2013**, *2*, 309–325. [CrossRef]
34. Re, R.; Pellegrini, N.; Proteggente, A.; Pannala, A.; Yang, M.; Rice-Evans, C. Antioxidant activity applying an improved ABTS radical cation decolorization assay. *Free Radic. Biol. Med.* **1999**, *26*, 1231–1237. [CrossRef]
35. Rice-evans, C.A.; Miller, N.J.; Bolwell, P.G.; Bramley, P.M.; Pridham, J.B. The relative antioxidant activities of plant-derived polyphenolic flavonoids. *Free Radic. Res.* **2009**, *22*, 375–383. [CrossRef]
36. Pokorný, J. Natural antioxidants for food use. *Trends Food Sci. Technol.* **1991**, *2*, 223–227. [CrossRef]

37. Kahkonen, M.P.; Hopia, A.I.; Vuorela, H.J.; Rauha, J.P.; Pihlaja, K.; Kujala, T.S.; Heinonen, M. Antioxidant activity of plant extracts containing phenolic compounds. *J. Agric. Food Chem.* **1999**, *47*, 3954–3962. [CrossRef] [PubMed]

38. Podsędek, A. Natural antioxidants and antioxidant capacity of Brassica vegetables: A review. *LWT Food Sci. Technol.* **2007**, *40*, 1–11. [CrossRef]

39. Cao, G.; Sofic, E.; Prior, R.L. Antioxidant Capacity of Tea and Common Vegetables. *J. Agric. Food Chem.* **1996**, *44*, 3426–3431. [CrossRef]

40. Velioglu, Y.S.; Mazza, G.; Gao, L.; Oomah, B.D. Antioxidant activity and total phenolics in selected fruits, vegetables, and grain products. *J. Agric. Food Chem.* **1998**, *46*, 4113–4117. [CrossRef]

41. Chu, Y.; Sun, J.; Wu, X.; Liu, R. Antioxidant and antiproliferative activities of common vegetables. *J. Agric. Food Chem.* **2002**, *50*, 6910–6916. [CrossRef] [PubMed]

42. Dykes, L.; Rooney, L.W. Phenolic compounds in cereal grains and their health benefits. *Cereal Food World* **2007**, *52*, 105–111. [CrossRef]

43. Adom, K.K.; Liu, R.H. Antioxidant activity of grains. *J. Agric. Food Chem.* **2002**, *50*, 6182–6187. [CrossRef] [PubMed]

44. Van Hung, P. Phenolic compounds of cereals and their antioxidant capacity. *Crit. Rev. Food Sci. Nutr.* **2014**. [CrossRef]

45. Fardet, A.; Rock, E.; Rémésy, C. Is the *in vitro* antioxidant potential of whole-grain cereals and cereal products well reflected *in vivo*? *J. Cereal Sci.* **2008**, *48*, 258–276. [CrossRef]

46. Pérez-Jiménez, J.; Saura-Calixto, F. Literature data may underestimate the actual antioxidant capacity of cereals. *J. Agric. Food Chem.* **2005**, *53*, 5036–5040. [CrossRef] [PubMed]

47. Elias, R.J.; Kellerby, S.S.; Decker, E.A. Antioxidant activity of proteins and peptides. *Crit. Rev. Food Sci. Nutr.* **2008**, *48*, 430–441. [CrossRef] [PubMed]

48. Chan, K.M.; Decker, E.A. Endogenous skeletal muscle antioxidants. *Crit. Rev. Food Sci. Nutr.* **1994**, *34*, 403–426. [CrossRef] [PubMed]

49. Stadtman, E.R.; Levine, R.L. Free radical-mediated oxidation of free amino acids and amino acid residues in proteins. *Amino Acids* **2003**, *25*, 207–218. [CrossRef] [PubMed]

50. Atmaca, G. Antioxidant effects of sulfur-containing amino acids. *Yonsei Med. J.* **2004**, *45*, 776–788. [CrossRef] [PubMed]

51. Suetsuna, K.; Ukeda, H.; Ochi, H. Isolation and characterization of free radical scavenging activities peptides derived from casein. *J. Nutr. Biochem.* **2000**, *11*, 128–131. [CrossRef]

52. Sakanaka, S.; Tachibana, Y.; Ishihara, N.; Juneja, L.R. Antioxidant properties of casein calcium peptides and their effects on lipid oxidation in beef homogenates. *J. Agric. Food Chem.* **2005**, *53*, 464–468. [CrossRef] [PubMed]

53. Power, O.; Jakeman, P.; FitzGerald, R.J. Antioxidative peptides: Enzymatic production, *in vitro* and *in vivo* antioxidant activity and potential applications of milk-derived antioxidative peptides. *Amino Acids* **2013**, *44*, 797–820. [CrossRef] [PubMed]

54. Dávalos, A.; Miguel, M.; Bartolomé, B.; López-Fandiño, R. Antioxidant activity of peptides derived from egg white proteins by enzymatic hydrolysis. *J. Food Prot.* **2004**, *67*, 1939–1944. [PubMed]

55. Huang, W.-Y.; Majumder, K.; Wu, J. Oxygen radical absorbance capacity of peptides from egg white protein ovotransferrin and their interaction with phytochemicals. *Food Chem.* **2010**, *123*, 635–641. [CrossRef]

56. Sies, H.; Stahl, W. Vitamins E and C, β-carotene, and other carotenoids as antioxidants. *Am. J. Clin. Nutr.* **1995**, *62*, 1315S–1321S. [PubMed]

57. Miki, W. Biological functions and activities of animal carotenoids. *Pure Appl. Chem.* **1991**, *63*, 141–146. [CrossRef]

58. Ngo, D.; Wijesekara, I.; Vo, T. Marine food-derived functional ingredients as potential antioxidants in the food industry: An overview. *Food Res. Int.* **2011**, *44*, 523–529. [CrossRef]

59. Cotterill, O.J.; Geiger, G.S. Egg product yield trends from shell eggs. *Poult. Sci.* **1977**, *56*, 1027–1031. [CrossRef]

60. Li-Chan, E.C.Y.; Kim, H.O. Structure and chemical composition of eggs. In *Egg Bioscience and Biotechnology*; Mine, Y., Ed.; John Wiley & Sons, Ltd: Hoboken, NJ, USA, 2008; pp. 1–95.

61. Seuss-baum, I. Nutritional evaluation of egg compounds. In *Bioactive Egg Compounds*; Huopalahti, R., Lopez-Fandino, R., Anton, M., Schade, R., Eds.; Springer-Verlag: Heidelbert, Germany; Berlin, Germany, 2007; pp. 117–144.

62. Kovacs-Nolan, J.; Phillips, M.; Mine, Y. Advances in the value of eggs and egg components for human health. *J. Agric. Food Chem.* **2005**, *53*, 8421–8431. [CrossRef] [PubMed]

63. United States Department of Agriculture. United States Department of Agriculture: National Nutrient Database for standard reference Release 27. Available online: http://ndb.nal.usda.gov/ndb/ (accessed on 25 September 2014).

64. Hatta, H.; Kapoor, M.; Juneja, L. Bioactive components in egg yolk. In *Egg Bioscience and Biotechnology*; Mine, Y., Ed.; John Wiley & Sons, Ltd.: Hoboken, NJ, USA, 2008; pp. 185–237.

65. Surai, P.F. Effect of selenium and vitamin E content of the maternal diet on the antioxidant system of the yolk and the developing chick. *Br. Poult. Sci.* **2000**, *41*, 235–243. [CrossRef] [PubMed]

66. Anton, M. Composition and structure of hen egg yolk. In *Bioactive Egg Compounds*; Huopalahti, R., Lopez-Fandino, R., Eds.; Springer-Verlag: Heidelbert, Germany, 2007; pp. 17–24.

67. Carlson, S.; Montalto, M.; Ponder, D. Lower incidence of necrotizing enterocolitis in infants fed a preterm formula with egg phospholipids. *Pediatr. Res.* **1998**, *44*, 491–498. [CrossRef] [PubMed]

68. Hoffman, D.R.; Theuer, R.C.; Castaneda, Y.S.; Wheaton, D.H.; Bosworth, R.G.; O'Connor, A.R.; Morale, S.E.; Wiedemann, L.E.; Birch, E.E. Maturation of visual acuity is accelerated in breast-fed term infants fed baby food containing DHA-enriched egg yolk. *J. Nutr.* **2004**, *134*, 2307–2313. [PubMed]

69. Charoensiriwatana, W.; Srijantr, P.; Teeyapant, P.; Wongvilairattana, J. Consuming iodine enriched eggs to solve the iodine deficiency endemic for remote areas in Thailand. *Nutr. J.* **2010**, *9*, 68. [CrossRef] [PubMed]

70. Bourre, J.M.; Galea, F. An important source of omega-3 fatty acids, vitamins D and E, carotenoids, iodine and selenium: A new natural multi-enriched egg. *J. Nutr. Health Aging* **2006**, *10*, 371–376. [PubMed]

71. Naber, E.C. Modifying Vitamin Composition of Eggs: A Review. *J. Appl. Poult. Res.* **1993**, *2*, 385–393. [CrossRef]

72. Miranda, J.M.; Anton, X.; Redondo-Valbuena, C.; Roca-Saavedra, P.; Rodriguez, J.A.; Lamas, A.; Franco, C.M.; Cepeda, A. Egg and egg-derived foods: Effects on human health and use as functional foods. *Nutrients* **2015**, *7*, 706–729. [CrossRef] [PubMed]

73. Mine, Y.; D'Silva, I. Bioactive Components in Egg White. In *Egg Bioscience and Biotechnology*; Mine, Y., Ed.; John Wiley & Sons, Inc.: Hoboken, NJ, USA, 2007; pp. 141–184.

74. Nakamura, S.; Kato, A.; Kobayashi, K. Enhanced antioxidative effect of ovalbumin due to covalent binding of polysaccharides. *J. Agric. Food Chem.* **1992**, *40*, 2033–2037. [CrossRef]

75. Huang, X.; Tu, Z.; Xiao, H.; Wang, H.; Zhang, L. Characteristics and antioxidant activities of ovalbumin glycated with different saccharides under heat moisture treatment. *Food Res. Int.* **2012**, *48*, 866–872. [CrossRef]

76. Ibrahim, H.; Hoq, M.; Aoki, T. Ovotransferrin possesses SOD-like superoxide anion scavenging activity that is promoted by copper and manganese binding. *Int. J. Biol. Macromol.* **2007**, *41*, 631–640. [CrossRef] [PubMed]

77. Chang, O.; Ha, G.; Han, G. Novel antioxidant peptide derived from the ultrafiltrate of ovomucin hydrolysate. *J. Agric. Food Chem.* **2013**, *61*, 7294–7300. [CrossRef] [PubMed]

78. Liu, H.; Zheng, F.; Cao, Q.; Ren, B.; Zhu, L.; Striker, G.; Vlassara, H. Amelioration of oxidant stress by the defensin lysozyme. *Am. J. Physiol. Endocrinol. Metab.* **2006**, *290*, E824–E832. [CrossRef] [PubMed]

79. Lehtinen, M.K.; Tegelberg, S.; Schipper, H.; Su, H.; Zukor, H.; Manninen, O.; Kopra, O.; Joensuu, T.; Hakala, P.; Bonni, A.; *et al.* Cystatin B deficiency sensitizes neurons to oxidative stress in progressive myoclonus epilepsy, EPM1. *J. Neurosci.* **2009**, *29*, 5910–5915. [CrossRef] [PubMed]

80. Verdot, L.; Lalmanach, G.; Vercruysse, V.; Hartmann, S.; Lucius, R.; Hoebeke, J.; Gauthier, F.; Vray, B. Cystatins up-regulate nitric oxide release from interferon-gamma-activated mouse peritoneal macrophages. *J. Biol. Chem.* **1996**, *271*, 28077–28081. [CrossRef] [PubMed]

81. Young, D.; Nau, F.; Pasco, M.; Mine, Y. Identification of hen egg yolk-derived phosvitin phosphopeptides and their effects on gene expression profiling against oxidative stress-induced Caco-2 cells. *J. Agric. Food Chem.* **2011**, *59*, 9207–9218. [CrossRef] [PubMed]

82. Lu, C.-L.; Baker, R.C. Characteristics of egg yolk phosvitin as an antioxidant for inhibiting metal-catalyzed phospholipid oxidations. *Poult. Sci.* **1986**, *65*, 2065–2070. [CrossRef] [PubMed]

83. Sugino, H.; Ishikawa, M.; Nitoda, T.; Koketsu, M.; Juneja, L.R.; Kim, M.; Yamamoto, T. Antioxidative activity of egg yolk phospholipids. *J. Agric. Food Chem.* **1997**, *45*, 551–554. [CrossRef]

84. Ricciarelli, R.; Zingg, J.M.; Azzi, A. Vitamin E reduces the uptake of oxidized LDL by inhibiting cd36 scavenger receptor expression in cultured aortic smooth muscle cells. *Circulation* **2000**, *102*, 82–87. [CrossRef] [PubMed]

85. Nimalaratne, C.; Lopes-Lutz, D.; Schieber, A.; Wu, J. Free aromatic amino acids in egg yolk show antioxidant properties. *Food Chem.* **2011**, *129*, 155–161. [CrossRef]

86. Lechevalier, V.; Croguennec, T. Ovalbumin and gene-related proteins. In *Bioactive Egg Compounds*; Springer-Verlag: Berlin, Germany, 2007.

87. Deneke, S. Thiol-based antioxidants. *Curr. Top. Cell. Regul.* **2001**, *36*, 151–181.

88. Thomas, J.A.; Poland, B.; Honzatko, R. Protein sulfhydryls and their role in the antioxidant function of protein *S*-thiolation. *Arch. Biochem. Biophys.* **1995**, *319*, 1–9. [CrossRef] [PubMed]

89. Roos, G.; Messens, J. Protein sulfenic acid formation: From cellular damage to redox regulation. *Free Radic. Biol. Med.* **2011**, *51*, 314–326. [CrossRef]

90. Goto, M.; Shibasaki, K. Effect of oxidation of oils on deterioration of foods. II. Effect of food components on the oxidation of linoleic acid. *Nihon Shokuhin Kogyo Gakkai-Shi* **1971**, *18*, 277–283. [CrossRef]

91. Sun, Y.; Hayakawa, S. Antioxidant effects of Maillard reaction products obtained from ovalbumin and different *D*-aldohexoses. *Biosci. Biotechnol. Biochem.* **2006**, *70*, 598–605. [CrossRef] [PubMed]

92. Superti, F.; Ammendolia, M. Ovotransferrin. In *Bioactive Egg Compounds*; Huopalahti, R., Lopez-Fandino, R., Anton, M., Eds.; Springer-Verlag: Heidelbert, Germany; Berlin, Germany, 2007; pp. 43–50.

93. Mine, Y.; Kovacs-Nolan, J. Biologically Active Hen Egg Components in Human Health and Disease. *J. Poult. Sci.* **2004**, *41*, 1–29. [CrossRef]

94. Fritz, J.; Ikegami, M. Lysozyme ameliorates oxidant-induced lung injury. *Am. J. Respir. Crit. Care Med.* **2009**, *179*, A4005.

95. Fossum, K.; Whitaker, J.R. Ficin and papain inhibitor from chicken egg white. *Arch. Biochem. Biophys.* **1968**, *125*, 367–375. [CrossRef]

96. Wesierska, E.; Saleh, Y.; Trziszka, T.; Kopec, W.; Siewinski, M.; Korzekwa, K. Antimicrobial activity of chicken egg white cystatin. *World J. Microbiol. Biotechnol.* **2005**, *21*, 59–64. [CrossRef]

97. Nicklin, M.; Barrett, A. Inhibition of cysteine proteinases and dipeptidyl peptidase I by egg-white cystatin. *Biochem. J.* **1984**, *223*, 245–253. [CrossRef] [PubMed]

98. Vray, B.; Hartmann, S.; Hoebeke, J. Immunomodulatory properties of cystatins. *Cell. Mol. Life Sci.* **2002**, *59*, 1503–1512. [CrossRef] [PubMed]

99. Abbas, K.; Breton, J.; Planson, A.G.; Bouton, C.; Bignon, J.; Seguin, C.; Riquier, S.; Toledano, M.B.; Drapier, J.C. Nitric oxide activates an Nrf2/sulfiredoxin antioxidant pathway in macrophages. *Free Radic. Biol. Med.* **2011**, *51*, 107–114. [CrossRef] [PubMed]

100. Frenkel, K.; Chrzan, K.; Ryan, C.A.; Wiesner, R.; Troll, W. Chymotrypsin-specific protease inhibitors decrease H_2O_2 formation by activated human polymorphonuclear leukocytes. *Carcinogenesis* **1987**, *8*, 1207–1212. [CrossRef] [PubMed]

101. Joubert, F.J.; Cook, W.H. Preparation and characterization of phosvitin from hen egg yolk. *Can. J. Biochem. Physiol.* **2011**, *36*, 399–408. [CrossRef]

102. Ishikawa, S.I.; Yano, Y.; Arihara, K.; Itoh, M. Egg yolk phosvitin inhibits hydroxyl radical formation from the fenton reaction. *Biosci. Biotechnol. Biochem.* **2004**, *68*, 1324–1331. [CrossRef] [PubMed]

103. Ishikawa, S.; Ohtsuki, S.; Tomita, K.; Arihara, K.; Itoh, M. Protective effect of egg yolk phosvitin against ultraviolet- light-induced lipid peroxidation in the presence of iron ions. *Biol. Trace Element Res.* **2005**, *105*, 249–256. [CrossRef]

104. King, M.F.; Boyd, L.C.; Sheldon, B.W. Antioxidant properties of individual phospholipids in a salmon oil model system. *J. Am. Oil Chem. Soc.* **1992**, *69*, 545–551. [CrossRef]

105. Saito, H.; Ishihara, K. Antioxidant activity and active sites of phospholipids as antioxidants. *J. Am. Oil Chem. Soc.* **1997**, *74*, 1531–1536. [CrossRef]

106. Rao, A.V.; Rao, L.G. Carotenoids and human health. *Nutr. Pharmacol.* **2007**, *55*, 207–216. [CrossRef] [PubMed]

107. Fiedor, J.; Burda, K. Potential role of carotenoids as antioxidants in human health and disease. *Nutrients* **2014**, *6*, 466–488. [CrossRef] [PubMed]

108. Voutilainen, S.; Nurmi, T.; Mursu, J.; Rissanen, T.H. Carotenoids and cardiovascular health. *Am. J. Clin. Nutr.* **2006**, *83*, 1265–1271. [PubMed]

109. Handelman, G.J.; Nightingale, Z.D.; Lichtenstein, A.H.; Schaefer, E.J.; Blumberg, J.B. Lutein and zeaxanthin concentrations in plasma after dietary supplementation with egg yolk. *Am. J. Clin. Nutr.* **1999**, *70*, 247–251. [PubMed]

110. Chung, H.-Y.; Rasmussen, H.M.; Johnson, E.J. Lutein bioavailability is higher from lutein-enriched eggs than from supplements and spinach in men. *J. Nutr.* **2004**, *134*, 1887–1893. [PubMed]

111. Karadas, F.; Grammenidis, E.; Surai, P.F.; Acamovic, T.; Sparks, N.H. Effects of carotenoids from lucerne, marigold and tomato on egg yolk pigmentation and carotenoid composition. *Br. Poult. Sci.* **2006**, *47*, 561–566. [CrossRef] [PubMed]

112. Schlatterer, J.; Breithaupt, D.E. Xanthophylls in commercial egg yolks: Quantification and identification by HPLC and LC-(APCI)MS using a C_{30} phase. *J. Agric. Food Chem.* **2006**, *54*, 2267–2273. [CrossRef] [PubMed]

113. Breithaupt, D.E. Modern application of xanthophylls in animal feeding—A review. *Trends Food Sci. Technol.* **2007**, *18*, 501–506. [CrossRef]

114. Breithaupt, D.R. Xanthophylls in Poultry Feeding. In *Carotenoids*; Pfander, H., Ed.; Birkhauser: Basel, Switzerland, 2008; Volume 4, pp. 255–264.

115. Krinsky, N.; Russett, M. Structural and geometrical isomers of carotenoids in human plasma. *J. Nutr.* **1990**, *120*, 1654–1662. [PubMed]

116. Landrum, J.T.; Bone, R.A. Lutein, zeaxanthin, and the macular pigment. *Arch. Biochem. Biophys.* **2001**, *385*, 28–40. [CrossRef] [PubMed]

117. Krinsky, N.; Landrum, J.; Bone, R. Biologic mechanisms of the protective role of lutein and zeaxanthin in the eye. *Annu. Rev. Nutr.* **2003**, *23*, 171–201. [CrossRef] [PubMed]

118. Li, B.; Ahmed, F.; Bernstein, P.S. Studies on the singlet oxygen scavenging mechanism of human macular pigment. *Arch. Biochem. Biophys.* **2010**, *504*, 56–60. [PubMed]

119. Böhm, F.; Edge, R.; Truscott, G. Interactions of dietary carotenoids with activated (singlet) oxygen and free radicals: Potential effects for human health. *Mol. Nutr. Food Res.* **2012**, *56*, 205–216. [PubMed]

120. Gao, S.; Qin, T.; Liu, Z.; Caceres, M.A.; Ronchi, C.F.; Chen, C.Y.O.; Yeum, K.J.; Taylor, A.; Blumberg, J.B.; Liu, Y.; *et al.* Lutein and zeaxanthin supplementation reduces H_2O_2-induced oxidative damage in human lens epithelial cells. *Mol. Vis.* **2011**, *17*, 3180–3190. [PubMed]

121. Dwyer, J.H.; Navab, M.; Dwyer, K.M.; Hassan, K.; Sun, P.; Shircore, A.; Hama-Levy, S.; Hough, G.; Wang, X.; Drake, T.; *et al.* Oxygenated Carotenoid Lutein and Progression of Early Atherosclerosis: The Los Angeles Atherosclerosis Study. *Circulation* **2001**, *103*, 2922–2927. [CrossRef] [PubMed]

122. Kim, J.E.; Leite, J.O.; DeOgburn, R.; Smyth, J.A.; Clark, R.M.; Fernandez, M.L. A lutein-enriched diet prevents cholesterol accumulation and decreases oxidized LDL and inflammatory cytokines in the aorta of guinea pigs. *J. Nutr.* **2011**, *141*, 1458–1463. [CrossRef] [PubMed]

123. Trevithick-Sutton, C.C.; Foote, C.S.; Collins, M.; Trevithick, J.R. The retinal carotenoids zeaxanthin and lutein scavenge superoxide and hydroxyl radicals: A chemiluminescence and ESR study. *Mol. Vis.* **2006**, *12*, 1127–1135. [PubMed]

124. Panasenko, O.M.; Sharov, V.S.; Briviba, K.; Sies, H. Interaction of peroxynitrite with carotenoids in human low density lipoproteins. *Arch. Biochem. Biophys.* **2000**, *373*, 302–305. [CrossRef] [PubMed]

125. Traber, M.G.; Atkinson, J. Vitamin E, antioxidant and nothing more. *Free Radic. Biol. Med.* **2007**, *43*, 4–15. [CrossRef] [PubMed]

126. Burton, G.W.; Traber, M.G. Vitamin E: Antioxidant activity, biokinetics, and bioavailability. *Annu. Rev. Nutr.* **1990**, *10*, 357–382. [CrossRef] [PubMed]

127. Esterbauer, H.; Puhl, H.; Dieber-Rotheneder, M.; Waeg, G.; Rabl, H. Effect of antioxidants on oxidative modification of LDL. *Ann. Med.* **1991**, *23*, 573–581. [CrossRef] [PubMed]

128. Rimm, E.B.; Stampfer, M.J.; Ascherio, A.; Giovannucci, E.; Colditz, G.A.; Willett, W.C. Vitamin E consumption and the risk of coronary heart disease in men. *N. Engl. J. Med.* **1993**, *328*, 1450–1456. [CrossRef] [PubMed]

129. Stampfer, M.J.; Hennekens, C.H.; Manson, J.E.; Colditz, G.A.; Rosner, B.; Willett, W.C. Vitamin E consumption and the risk of coronary disease in women. *N. Engl. J. Med.* **1993**, *328*, 1444–1449. [CrossRef]

130. Surai, P.F.; MacPherson, A.; Speake, B.K.; Sparks, N.H.C. Designer egg evaluation in a controlled trial. *Eur. J. Clin. Nutr.* **2000**, *54*, 298–305. [CrossRef] [PubMed]

131. Tapiero, H.; Townsend, D.; Tew, K. The antioxidant role of selenium and seleno-compounds. *Biomed. Pharmacother.* **2003**, *57*, 134–144. [CrossRef]

132. Smyth, P.P.A. Role of iodine in antioxidant defence in thyroid and breast disease. *BioFactors* **2003**, *19*, 121–130. [CrossRef] [PubMed]

133. Chen, C.; Chi, Y.-J.; Zhao, M.-Y.; Lv, L. Purification and identification of antioxidant peptides from egg white protein hydrolysate. *Amino Acids* **2012**, *43*, 457–466. [CrossRef] [PubMed]

134. Remanan, M.K.; Wu, J. Antioxidant activity in cooked and simulated digested eggs. *Food Funct.* **2014**, *5*, 1464–1474. [PubMed]

135. Chen, C.; Chi, Y.; Xu, W. Comparisons on the functional properties and antioxidant activity of spray-dried and freeze-dried egg white protein hydrolysate. *Food Bioprocess Technol.* **2012**, *5*, 2342–2352. [CrossRef]

136. Lin, S.; Jin, Y.; Liu, M.; Yang, Y.; Zhang, M.; Guo, Y. Research on the preparation of antioxidant peptides derived from egg white with assisting of high-intensity pulsed electric field. *Food Chem.* **2013**, *139*, 300–306. [CrossRef] [PubMed]

137. Liu, J.; Jin, Y.; Lin, S.; Jones, G.S.; Chen, F. Purification and identification of novel antioxidant peptides from egg white protein and their antioxidant activities. *Food Chem.* **2015**, *175*, 258–266. [CrossRef] [PubMed]

138. Nimalaratne, C.; Bandara, N.; Wu, J. Purification and characterization of antioxidant peptides from enzymatically hydrolyzed chicken egg white. *Food Chem.* **2015**, *188*, 467–472. [CrossRef] [PubMed]

139. Graszkiewicz, A.; Zelazko, M. Antioxidative capacity of hydrolysates of hen egg proteins. *Pol. J. Food Nutr. Sci.* **2007**, *57*, 195–199.

140. Graszkiewicz, A.; Zelazko, M.; Trziszka, T. Application of pancreatic enzymes in hydrolysis of egg-white proteins. *Pol. J. Food Nutr. Sci.* **2010**, *60*, 57–61.

141. Manso, M.; Miguel, M.; Even, J.; Hernandez, R.; Aleixandre, A.; Lopezfandino, R. Effect of the long-term intake of an egg white hydrolysate on the oxidative status and blood lipid profile of spontaneously hypertensive rats. *Food Chem.* **2008**, *109*, 361–367. [CrossRef]

142. Park, P.-J.; Jung, W.-K.; Nam, K.-S.; Shahidi, F.; Kim, S.-K. Purification and characterization of antioxidative peptides from protein hydrolysate of lecithin-free egg yolk. *J. Am. Oil Chem. Soc.* **2001**, *78*, 651–656. [CrossRef]

143. Sakanaka, S.; Tachibana, Y. Active oxygen scavenging activity of egg-yolk protein hydrolysates and their effects on lipid oxidation in beef and tuna homogenates. *Food Chem.* **2006**, *95*, 243–249. [CrossRef]

144. Xu, M.; Shangguan, X.; Wang, W.; Chen, J. Antioxidative activity of hen egg ovalbumin hydrolysates. *Asia Pac. J. Clin. Nutr.* **2007**, *16*, 178–182. [PubMed]

145. Shen, S.; Chahal, B.; Majumder, K. Identification of novel antioxidative peptides derived from a thermolytic hydrolysate of ovotransferrin by LC-MS/MS. *J. Agric. Food Chem.* **2010**, *58*, 7664–7672. [CrossRef] [PubMed]

146. Huang, W.; Shen, S.; Nimalaratne, C.; Li, S.; Majumder, K.; Wu, J. Effects of addition of egg ovotransferrin-derived peptides on the oxygen radical absorbance capacity of different teas. *Food Chem.* **2012**, *135*, 1600–1607. [CrossRef] [PubMed]

147. Galisteo, J.; Herraiz, T. Endogenous and Dietary Indoles: A Class of Antioxidants and Radical Scavengers in the ABTS Assay. *Free Radic. Res.* **2004**, *38*, 323–331.

148. Christen, S.; Peterhans, E.; Stocker, R. Antioxidant activities of some tryptophan metabolites: Possible implication for inflammatory diseases. *Proc. Natl. Acad. Sci. USA* **1990**, *87*, 2506–2510. [CrossRef] [PubMed]

149. You, J.; Luo, Y.; Wu, J. Conjugation of Ovotransferrin with Catechin Shows Improved Antioxidant Activity. *J. Agric. Food Chem.* **2014**, *62*, 2581–2587. [CrossRef] [PubMed]

150. Rao, S.; Sun, J.; Liu, Y.; Zeng, H.; Su, Y.; Yang, Y. ACE inhibitory peptides and antioxidant peptides derived from *in vitro* digestion hydrolysate of hen egg white lysozyme. *Food Chem.* **2012**, *135*, 1245–1252. [CrossRef] [PubMed]

151. You, S.-J.; Udenigwe, C.C.; Aluko, R.E.; Wu, J. Multifunctional peptides from egg white lysozyme. *Food Res. Int.* **2010**, *43*, 848–855. [CrossRef]

152. Memarpoor-Yazdi, M. A novel antioxidant and antimicrobial peptide from hen egg white lysozyme hydrolysates. *J. Funct. Foods* **2012**, *4*, 278–286. [CrossRef]

153. Omana, D.A.; Wang, J.; Wu, J. Ovomucin—A glycoprotein with promising potential. *Trends Food Sci. Technol.* **2010**, *21*, 455–463. [CrossRef]

154. Liu, J.; Chen, Z.; He, J.; Zhang, Y.; Zhang, T.; Jiang, Y. Anti-oxidative and anti-apoptosis effects of egg white peptide, Trp-Asn-Trp-Ala-Asp, against H_2O_2-induced oxidative stress in human embryonic kidney 293 cells. *Food Funct.* **2014**, *5*, 3179–3188. [CrossRef] [PubMed]

155. Katayama, S.; Xu, X.; Fan, M.Z.; Mine, Y. Antioxidative stress activity of oligophosphopeptides derived from hen egg yolk phosvitin in Caco-2 cells. *J. Agric. Food Chem.* **2006**, *54*, 773–778. [PubMed]

156. Xu, X.; Katayama, S.; Mine, Y. Antioxidant activity of tryptic digests of hen egg yolk phosvitin. *J. Sci. Food Agric.* **2007**, *87*, 2604–2608. [CrossRef] [PubMed]

157. Katayama, S.; Mine, Y. Antioxidative activity of amino acids on tissue oxidative stress in human intestinal epithelial cell model. *J. Agric. Food Chem.* **2007**, *55*, 8458–8464. [CrossRef] [PubMed]

158. Surai, P.F.; Simons, P.C.M.; Dvorska, J.E.; Aradas, F.; Sparks, N.H.C. Antioxidant-enriched eggs: Opportunities and limitations. In *The Amazing Egg: Nature's Perfect Functional Food for Health Promotion*; Sim, J.S., Sunwoo, H.H., Eds.; University of Alberta: Edmonton, AB, Canada, 2006; pp. 68–93.

159. Fraeye, I.; Bruneel, C.; Lemahieu, C.; Buyse, J.; Muylaert, K.; Foubert, I. Dietary enrichment of eggs with omega-3 fatty acids: A review. *Food Res. Int.* **2012**, *48*, 961–969. [CrossRef]

160. Leeson, S. Lutein-Enriched eggs: Transfer of lutein into eggs and health benefits. In *The Amazing Egg: Nature's Perfect Functional Food for Health Promotion*; Sim, J.S., Sunwoo, H.H., Eds.; Department of Agricultural, Food and Nutritional Science, University of Alberta: Edmonton, AB, Canada, 2006; pp. 171–179.

161. Serpeloni, J.M.; Grotto, D.; Mercadante, A.Z.; de Lourdes Pires Bianchi, M.; Antunes, L.M.G. Lutein improves antioxidant defense *in vivo* and protects against DNA damage and chromosome instability induced by cisplatin. *Arch. Toxicol.* **2010**, *84*, 811–822. [CrossRef] [PubMed]

162. Roberts, R.L.; Green, J.; Lewis, B. Lutein and zeaxanthin in eye and skin health. *Clin. Dermatol.* **2009**, *27*, 195–201. [CrossRef] [PubMed]

163. Wertz, K.; Siler, U.; Goralczyk, R. Lycopene: Modes of action to promote prostate health. *Arch. Biochem. Biophys.* **2004**, *430*, 127–134. [CrossRef] [PubMed]

164. Olson, J.B.; Ward, N.E.; Koutsos, E.A. Lycopene Incorporation into Egg Yolk and Effects on Laying Hen Immune Function. *Poult. Sci.* **2008**, *87*, 2573–2580. [CrossRef] [PubMed]

165. Akdemir, F.; Orhan, C.; Sahin, N.; Sahin, K.; Hayirli, A. Tomato powder in laying hen diets: Effects on concentrations of yolk carotenoids and lipid peroxidation. *Br. Poult. Sci.* **2012**, *53*, 675–680. [CrossRef]

166. Péter, S.; Moser, U. The challenge of setting appropriate intake recommendations for vitamin E: Considerations on status and functionality to define nutrient requirements. *Int. J. Vitam. Nutr. Res.* **2013**, *83*, 129–136. [CrossRef] [PubMed]

167. Sanders, T.A.B.; Hinds, A. The influence of a fish oil high in docosahexaenoic acid on plasma lipoprotein and vitamin E concentrations and haemostatic function in healthy male volunteers. *Br. J. Nutr.* **2007**, *68*, 163–173. [CrossRef]

168. Valk, E.; Hornstra, G. Relationship between vitamin E requirement and polyunsaturated fatty acid intake in man: A review. *Int. J. Vitam. Nutr. Res.* **2000**, *70*, 31–42. [CrossRef] [PubMed]

169. Honein, M.A. Impact of folic acid fortification of the US food supply on the occurrence of neural tube defects. *JAMA* **2001**, *285*, 2981–2986. [CrossRef] [PubMed]

170. House, J.D.; Braun, K.; Ballance, D.; O'Connor, C.; Guenter, W. The enrichment of eggs with folic acid through supplementation of the laying hen diet. *Poult. Sci.* **2002**, *81*, 1332–1337. [CrossRef] [PubMed]

171. House, J.D.; O'Connor, C.; Guenter, W. Plasma homocysteine and glycine are sensitive indices of folate status in a rodent model of folate depletion and repletion. *J. Agric. Food Chem.* **2003**, *51*, 4461–4467. [CrossRef] [PubMed]

172. Seyoum, E.; Selhub, J. Properties of Food Folates Determined by Stability and Susceptibility to Intestinal Pteroylpolyglutamate Hydrolase Action. *J. Nutr.* **1998**, *128*, 1956–1960. [PubMed]

173. Rezk, B.M.; Haenen, G.R.M.; van der Vijgh, W.J.; Bast, A. Tetrahydrofolate and 5-methyltetrahydrofolate are folates with high antioxidant activity. Identification of the antioxidant pharmacophore. *FEBS Lett.* **2003**, *555*, 601–605. [CrossRef]

174. Antoniades, C.; Shirodaria, C.; Warrick, N.; Cai, S.; de Bono, J.; Lee, J.; Leeson, P.; Neubauer, S.; Ratnatunga, C.; Pillai, R.; *et al.* 5-methyltetrahydrofolate rapidly improves endothelial function and decreases superoxide production in human vessels: Effects on vascular tetrahydrobiopterin availability and endothelial nitric oxide synthase coupling. *Circulation* **2006**, *114*, 1193–1201. [CrossRef] [PubMed]

175. Verhaar, M.C.; Wever, R.M.F.; Kastelein, J.J.P.; van Dam, T.; Koomans, H.A.; Rabelink, T.J. 5-Methyltetrahydrofolate, the Active Form of Folic Acid, Restores Endothelial Function in Familial Hypercholesterolemia. *Circulation* **1998**, *97*, 237–241. [CrossRef] [PubMed]

176. Dobrzanski, Z.; Gorecka, H.; Strzelbicka, G.; Szczypel, J.; Trziszka, T. Study on enrichment of hen eggs with selenium and iodine. *Electron. J. Pol. Agric. Univ. Ser. Anim. Husb.* **2001**, *4*. Available online: http://www.ejpau.media.pl/volume4/issue2/animal/art-01.html (accessed on 25 September 2014).

177. Nicoli, M.; Anese, M.; Parpinel, M. Influence of processing on the antioxidant properties of fruit and vegetables. *Trends Food Sci. Technol.* **1999**, *10*, 94–100. [CrossRef]

178. Kalt, W. Effects of production and processing factors on major fruit and vegetable antioxidants. *J. Food Sci.* **2005**, *70*, R11–R19. [CrossRef]

179. Shi, J.; le Maguer, M. Lycopene in tomatoes: Chemical and physical properties affected by food processing. *Crit. Rev. Food Sci. Nutr.* **2000**, *40*, 1–42. [CrossRef] [PubMed]

180. Dewanto, V.; Wu, X.; Adom, K.K.; Liu, R.H. Thermal processing enhances the nutritional value of tomatoes by increasing total antioxidant activity. *J. Agric. Food Chem.* **2002**, *50*, 3010–3014. [CrossRef] [PubMed]

181. Dewanto, V.; Wu, X.; Liu, R.H. Processed sweet corn has higher antioxidant activity. *J. Agric. Food Chem.* **2002**, *50*, 4959–4964. [CrossRef] [PubMed]

182. Adefegha, S.; Oboh, G. Cooking enhances the antioxidant properties of some tropical green leafy vegetables. *Afr. J. Biotechnol.* **2013**, *10*, 632–639.

183. Turkmen, N.; Sari, F.; Velioglu, Y.S. The effect of cooking methods on total phenolics and antioxidant activity of selected green vegetables. *Food Chem.* **2005**, *93*, 713–718. [CrossRef]

184. Ravichandran, K.; Saw, N.M.M.T.; Mohdaly, A.A.A.; Gabr, A.M.M.; Kastell, A.; Riedel, H.; Cai, Z.; Knorr, D.; Smetanska, I. Impact of processing of red beet on betalain content and antioxidant activity. *Food Res. Int.* **2013**, *50*, 670–675. [CrossRef]

185. Ismail, A.; Marjan, Z.M.; Foong, C.W. Total antioxidant activity and phenolic content in selected vegetables. *Food Chem.* **2004**, *87*, 581–586. [CrossRef]

186. Natella, F.; Belelli, F.; Ramberti, A.; Scaccini, C. Microwave and traditional cooking methods: Effect of cooking on antioxidant. *J. Food Biochem.* **2010**, *34*, 796–810.

187. Zhang, D.; Hamauzu, Y. Phenolics, ascorbic acid, carotenoids and antioxidant activity of broccoli and their changes during conventional and microwave cooking. *Food Chem.* **2004**, *88*, 503–509. [CrossRef]

188. Jing, H.; Yap, M.; Wong, P.Y.Y.; Kitts, D.D. Comparison of physicochemical and antioxidant properties of egg-white proteins and fructose and inulin maillard reaction products. *Food Bioprocess Technol.* **2009**, *4*, 1489–1496. [CrossRef]

189. Albright, K.; Gordon, D.; Cotterill, O. Release of iron from phosvitin by heat and food additives. *J. Food Sci.* **1984**, *49*, 78–81. [CrossRef]

190. Schieber, A.; Carle, R. Occurrence of carotenoid *cis*-isomers in food: Technological, analytical, and nutritional implications. *Pigment. Food* **2005**, *16*, 416–422. [CrossRef]

191. Wenzel, M.; Seuss-Baum, I.; Schlich, E. Influence of pasteurization, spray- and freeze-drying, and storage on the carotenoid content in egg yolk. *J. Agric. Food Chem.* **2010**, *58*, 1726–1731. [CrossRef] [PubMed]

192. Barbosa, V.C.; Gaspar, A.; Calixto, L.F.L.; Agostinho, T.S.P. Stability of the pigmentation of egg yolks enriched with omega-3 and carophyll stored at room temperature and under refrigeration. *Rev. Bras. Zootec.* **2011**, *40*, 1540–1544.

193. Galobart, J.; Barroeta, A. α-Tocopherol transfer efficiency and lipid oxidation in fresh and spray-dried eggs enriched with omega-3-polyunsaturated fatty acids. *Poult. Sci.* **2001**, *80*, 1496–1505. [CrossRef] [PubMed]

194. Caboni, M.; Boselli, E.; Messia, M. Effect of processing and storage on the chemical quality markers of spray-dried whole egg. *Food Chem.* **2005**, *92*, 293–303. [CrossRef]

195. Stefanović, A.B.; Jovanović, J.R.; Grbavčić, S.Ž.; Šekuljica, N.Ž.; Manojlović, V.B.; Bugarski, B.M.; Knežević-Jugović, Z.D. Impact of ultrasound on egg white proteins as a pretreatment for functional hydrolysates production. *Eur. Food Res. Technol.* **2014**, *239*, 979–993. [CrossRef]

196. Van der Plancken, I.; Van Loey, A.; Hendrickx, M.E. Combined effect of high pressure and temperature on selected properties of egg white proteins. *Innov. Food Sci. Emerg. Technol.* **2005**, *6*, 11–20. [CrossRef]

197. Mateo Anson, N.; Havenaar, R.; Bast, A.; Haenen, G.R.M.M. Antioxidant and anti-inflammatory capacity of bioaccessible compounds from wheat fractions after gastrointestinal digestion. *J. Cereal Sci.* **2010**, *51*, 110–114. [CrossRef]

198. Chiang, C.-J.; Kadouh, H.; Zhou, K. Phenolic compounds and antioxidant properties of gooseberry as affected by *in vitro* digestion. *LWT Food Sci. Technol.* **2013**, *51*, 417–422. [CrossRef]

199. Tagliazucchi, D.; Verzelloni, E.; Bertolini, D.; Conte, A. *In vitro* bio-accessibility and antioxidant activity of grape polyphenols. *Food Chem.* **2010**, *120*, 599–606. [CrossRef]

200. Rodríguez-Roque, M.J.; Rojas-Graü, M.A.; Elez-Martínez, P.; Martín-Belloso, O. Soymilk phenolic compounds, isoflavones and antioxidant activity as affected by *in vitro* gastrointestinal digestion. *Food Chem.* **2013**, *136*, 206–212. [CrossRef] [PubMed]

201. Jensen, I.-J.; Abrahamsen, H.; Maehre, H.K.; Elvevoll, E.O. Changes in antioxidative capacity of saithe (*Pollachius virens*) and shrimp (*Pandalus borealis*) during *in vitro* digestion. *J. Agric. Food Chem.* **2009**, *57*, 10928–10932. [CrossRef] [PubMed]

202. You, L.; Zhao, M.; Regenstein, J.M.; Ren, J. Changes in the antioxidant activity of loach (*Misgurnus anguillicaudatus*) protein hydrolysates during a simulated gastrointestinal digestion. *Food Chem.* **2010**, *120*, 810–816. [CrossRef]

203. Bouayed, J.; Hoffmann, L.; Bohn, T. Total phenolics, flavonoids, anthocyanins and antioxidant activity following simulated gastro-intestinal digestion and dialysis of apple varieties: Bioaccessibility and potential uptake. *Food Chem.* **2011**, *128*, 14–21. [CrossRef] [PubMed]

204. Faller, A.L.K.; Fialho, E.; Liu, R.H. Cellular antioxidant activity of feijoada whole meal coupled with an *in vitro* digestion. *J. Agric. Food Chem.* **2012**, *60*, 4826–4832. [PubMed]

205. Nimalaratne, C.; Savard, P.; Gauthier, S.F.; Schieber, A.; Wu, J. Bioaccessibility and digestive stability of carotenoids in cooked eggs studied using a dynamic *in vitro* gastrointestinal model. *J. Agric. Food Chem.* **2015**, *63*, 2956–2962. [CrossRef] [PubMed]

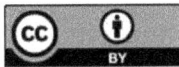

nutrients

MDPI

Article

Egg Intake and Dietary Quality among Overweight and Obese Mexican-American Postpartum Women

Sonia Vega-López [1,2,*], Giselle A. P. Pignotti [3], Michael Todd [4] and Colleen Keller [2,4]

[1] School of Nutrition and Health Promotion, Arizona State University, 500 North 3rd Street, Phoenix, AZ 85004, USA

[2] Southwestern Interdisciplinary Research Center, Arizona State University, 411 North Central Avenue, Suite #720, Phoenix, AZ 85004, USA; colleen.keller@asu.edu

[3] Department of Nutrition, Food Science and Packaging, San Jose State University, One Washington Square, San Jose, CA 95192-0058, USA; giselle.pignotti@sjsu.edu

[4] College of Nursing and Health Innovation, Arizona State University, 500 North 3rd Street, Phoenix, AZ 85004, USA; mike.todd@asu.edu

* Correspondence: sonia.vega.lopez@asu.edu; Tel.: +1-602-827-2268; Fax: +1-602-827-2253

Received: 7 August 2015; Accepted: 22 September 2015; Published: 2 October 2015

Abstract: Despite their low cost and high nutrient density, the contribution of eggs to nutrient intake and dietary quality among Mexican-American postpartum women has not been evaluated. Nutrient intake and dietary quality, as assessed by the Healthy Eating Index 2010 (HEI-2010), were measured in habitually sedentary overweight/obese (body mass index (BMI) = 29.7 $\pm$ 3.5 kg/m^2) Mexican-American postpartum women (28 $\pm$ 6 years) and compared between egg consumers (n = 82; any egg intake reported in at least one of three 24-h dietary recalls) and non-consumers (n = 57). Egg consumers had greater intake of energy (+808 kJ (193 kcal) or 14%; p = 0.033), protein (+9 g or 17%; p = 0.031), total fat (+9 g or 19%; p = 0.039), monounsaturated fat (+4 g or 24%; p = 0.020), and several micronutrients than non-consumers. Regarding HEI-2010 scores, egg consumers had a greater total protein foods score than non-consumers (4.7 $\pm$ 0.7 *vs.* 4.3 $\pm$ 1.0; p = 0.004), and trends for greater total fruit (2.4 $\pm$ 1.8 *vs.* 1.9 $\pm$ 1.7; p = 0.070) and the total composite HEI-2010 score (56.4 $\pm$ 12.6 *vs.* 52.3 $\pm$ 14.4; p = 0.082). Findings suggest that egg intake could contribute to greater nutrient intake and improved dietary quality among postpartum Mexican-American women. Because of greater energy intake among egg consumers, recommendations for overweight/obese individuals should include avoiding excessive energy intake and incorporating eggs to a nutrient-dense, fiber-rich dietary pattern.

Keywords: diet; eggs; healthy eating index; Hispanic women; nutrient intake

1. Introduction

Hispanics, the largest minority group in the United States (U.S.) [1], have a higher prevalence of obesity and cardiometabolic disease risk factors relative to other ethnic groups, disproportionately increasing their risk for chronic conditions such as cardiovascular disease and diabetes [2,3]. Among women of reproductive age, excess weight gain during pregnancy and failure to lose weight postpartum have been associated with long-term obesity and further risk for chronic diseases [4]. This is of particular concern for postpartum Hispanic women due to higher pre-pregnancy obesity rates [5] and the presence of many contributors to excessive weight retention after childbirth [6].

Several dietary factors are essential for the prevention and management of chronic diseases. Studies have shown that a higher dietary quality is inversely related to chronic disease risk factors such as waist circumference, low density lipoprotein (LDL)-cholesterol, insulin and C-reactive protein (CRP) [7,8]. Despite the known benefits of consuming adequate diets, available surveillance data on dietary composition suggest that, as for other ethnic groups, the diet of Mexican-American adults is in need for improvement, as indicated by reports of high intake of solid fats, added sugars, and sugar-sweetened beverages, and low intake of vitamins D and E, calcium and potassium, whole grains, dairy products, dark greens, and highly colored vegetables [9–13].

Due to their cholesterol content, the contribution of eggs to a healthful dietary pattern continues to be controversial [14–17]. Whereas some studies have identified eggs as part of a "healthful" or "prudent" dietary pattern with greater Healthy Eating Index (HEI) scores [18,19], others have identified eggs as components of dietary patterns associated with greater risk for adverse outcomes including overweight and obesity, metabolic syndrome, and insulin resistance [20,21]. However, data from prospective cohort studies suggest that egg intake is not associated with increased risk of coronary heart disease, stroke, and mortality, although it may be associated with increased risk of type 2 diabetes [22,23]. Eggs are an inexpensive food with high quality protein and a rich source of nutrients including choline, folate, selenium, and vitamins A, B, D, E, and K, and, if fortified, ω-3 fatty acids [24]. The nutritional value of eggs can be an important contributor to the health of women of reproductive age and to positive pregnancy outcomes particularly in disadvantaged populations with limited access to more costly healthy foods [24,25]. Folate, choline and docosahexaenoic acid (DHA), all of which can be supplied by eggs, are important nutrients during reproductive age for their role in the prevention of adverse pregnancy outcomes related to fetal central nervous system development [25–27].

The World Agricultural Supply and Demand Estimates Report [28] shows that the U.S. had an annual per capita consumption of 263 eggs in 2014, while Mexico is reported to have the highest consumption in the Americas with 335 eggs per person/year. Data from the 2001–2002 National Health and Nutritional Examination Survey (NHANES) suggested that eggs accounted for 7% of the servings from meat and beans group among the general U.S. population [29]. Estimates using NHANES III data suggested that 18.7% of U.S. adults were egg consumers (*i.e.*, individuals who reported intake of at least one egg-group product in a 24-h recall) [30]. Compared to non-consumers, egg consumers were less likely to have inadequate intakes of vitamins B12, A, E, and C. Furthermore, relative to other ethnic groups, a greater proportion of Mexican Americans (31.8%) were egg consumers [30].

Despite the known nutritional content of eggs and their potential benefit towards the health of reproductive-age women, information regarding their contribution to a healthful diet among Hispanic women of reproductive age is limited to a report with a diverse sample of pregnant women, most of them of Caribbean descent [31]. Thus, the objective of the present study was to compare nutrient intake and dietary quality, as assessed by the Healthy Eating Index 2010 (HEI-2010) [32], an algorithm that measures conformance to the 2010 Dietary Guidelines for Americans [33], between egg-consumers and non-consumers among Mexican-American postpartum women.

2. Study Design

2.1. Participants

Participants were 139 habitually sedentary overweight or obese (BMI between 25 and 35 kg/m^2) Mexican-American postpartum women (18–40 years old, at least six weeks but less than six months after childbirth) enrolled into *Madres para la Salud* (Mothers for Health; *Madres*), a social support community-based intervention promoting physical activity [34]. Exclusion criteria included currently engaged in regular, strenuous physical activity; currently pregnant or planning on becoming pregnant within the next 12 months; using antidepressants or anti-inflammatory medications; and having a BMI less than 25 or greater than 35 kg/m^2. Only baseline data were used for the current analysis. The study was approved by Arizona State University's Institutional Review Board, and all participants provided written consent to participate. The study was registered at ClinicalTrials.gov (Identifier: NCT01908959).

2.2. Measures

Trained bilingual research staff collected and processed all baseline sociodemographic, anthropometric and diet data prior to the randomization allocation. Standard procedures were used to measure in triplicate height, weight, and waist circumference.

Three unannounced 24-h recalls using a five-step, multiple-pass method were collected to assess baseline dietary intake data [35]. The dietary recalls were randomly collected during all seven days of the week, including two week days and one weekend day. The Nutrition Data System for Research (NDSR) software version 2009, developed by the Nutrition Coordinating Center (NCC), University of Minnesota, Minneapolis, MN, was used to analyze dietary data. Dietary variables of interest were estimates of total energy intake, amount and percentage of energy provided by macronutrients, and selected micronutrients. Egg intake was reported as servings per day, with one serving being equivalent to one large egg. Participants were classified as egg consumers if they reported any egg intake (including egg products) in at least one of the three 24-h dietary recalls (mean egg intake >0 servings/day).

Diet quality was assessed by calculating the HEI-2010, as described elsewhere [32]. Briefly, the HEI-2010 includes 12 components divided into adequacy components that should be included in the diet (total fruit, whole fruit, total vegetables, greens and beans, whole grains, dairy, total protein foods, seafood and plant proteins, and fatty acids) and moderation components that should be limited (refined grains, sodium, and empty calories). Individual components are scored from 0 to 5, 10, or 20 points; the total HEI-2010 score is calculated as the sum of all individual components, for a total of 100 possible points [36]. Maximum scores correspond to conformance to the dietary guidelines, reflecting higher consumption of adequacy components and lower consumption of moderation components. The scoring standards are assessed as food group and nutrients consumed per intake of 4184 kJ (1000 kcal), percentage of total energy intake, or a ratio, providing information on a density basis rather than absolute amounts [32]. The recommended approach to calculating HEI scores using NDSR was followed [37].

2.3. Statistical Analysis

All statistical analyses were conducted with software IBM SPSS Statistics for Windows, version 21.0 (IBM Corp., Armonk, NY, USA). Descriptive characteristics of participants and dietary data are presented in text and tables as mean ± standard deviation (SD). Nutrient intake for carbohydrates, protein, fat, and saturated fat was expressed as percentages of total energy. We used independent groups *t*-tests to compare egg consumers and non-consumers on each of the nutrient intake measures, each HEI-2010 component, and the HEI-2010 total score.

3. Results

3.1. Participant Characteristics

Participants were 139 women (28 ± 6 years old) self-identified as Mexican or Mexican-American (Table 1). Per study design, all participants were overweight or obese (mean BMI = 29.7 ± 3.5 kg/m^2) with mean waist and hip circumferences of 86 ± 9 cm and 106 ± 8 cm, respectively, and mean body fat of 38.6% ± 4.6%. Based on dietary intake data from three dietary recalls, 57 women (41% of participants) were classified as egg non-consumers, whereas 82 women (59% of participants) were classified as egg consumers. There were no significant differences in age, BMI, waist or hip circumferences, or body fat percent between egg consumers and non-consumers.

Table 1. Characteristics of study participants [a].

Characteristics	All (*n* = 139)	Egg Non-Consumers (*n* = 57)	Egg Consumers (*n* = 82)	*p* Value
Age (year)	28.3 ± 5.6	28.8 ± 5.4	27.9 ± 5.7	0.331
Body mass index (kg/m^2)	29.7 ± 3.5	29.3 ± 3.3	29.9 ± 3.7	0.321
Waist circumference (cm)	86.0 ± 9.0	86.1 ± 9.6	85.9 ± 8.7	0.895
Hip circumference (cm)	105.5 ± 7.6	105.4 ± 7.5	105.5 ± 7.8	0.934
Body fat (%)	38.6 ± 4.6	38.6 ± 4.7	38.5 ± 4.6	0.963

[a] Data shown as mean ± SD.

3.2. Nutrient Intake

Intake of total energy, macronutrient, and select micronutrient intake data for egg consumers and non-consumers are displayed in Table 2. Relative to non-consumers, egg consumers had 14% greater energy intake (*p* = 0.033), associated with consuming 17% more protein (*p* = 0.031) and 19% more fat (*p* = 0.039). There were no significant differences between egg non-consumers and consumers in the absolute amount of saturated and polyunsaturated fat, including ω-3 fatty acids, but monounsaturated fat intake was 24% greater for egg consumers than non-consumers (*p* = 0.020). There were no significant differences between egg non-consumers and consumers in the proportion of energy provided by macronutrients (data not shown), with the exception of monounsaturated fat (10.5% ± 2.4% of energy for non-consumers *vs.* 11.6% ± 3.1% of energy for consumers; *p* = 0.026). As expected, egg consumers had greater intake of dietary cholesterol (109%; *p* < 0.0001) than non-consumers. Whereas there were no significant differences between groups in total or added sugars intake, egg consumers had greater intake of total fiber (22%; *p* = 0.035) and soluble fiber (29%; *p* = 0.017) relative to non-consumers.

Regarding micronutrient intake (Table 2), there were no significant differences between groups in dietary vitamin A, vitamin C, vitamin E, vitamin K, thiamin, niacin, vitamin B6, folate, calcium, or iron. However, egg consumers had greater intakes of vitamin D (31%; *p* = 0.033), riboflavin (29%; *p* = 0.006), vitamin B12 (32%; *p* = 0.031), choline (59%; *p* < 0.0001), sodium (23%; *p* = 0.008), potassium (21%; *p* = 0.011), and phosphorus (19%; *p* = 0.012) than non-consumers. There were no significant differences in dietary lutein + zeaxanthin between groups.

Table 2. Comparison of total energy, macronutrient, and select micronutrient intake between egg consumers and egg non-consumers among postpartum Mexican American adult women [a].

Nutrient	DRI [b]	All (*n* = 139)	Egg Non-Consumers (*n* = 57)	Egg Consumers (*n* = 81)	*p* Value
Energy (kJ)		6137 ± 2208	5660 ± 1934	6468 ± 2334	0.033
Energy (kcal)		1466 ± 528	1353 ± 462	1546 ± 561	0.033
Total Carbohydrate (g)	160	195 ± 69	184 ± 61	203 ± 74	0.113
Total Protein (g)	0.66/kg	59 ± 24	53 ± 22	62 ± 25	0.031
Total Fat (g)		52 ± 25	47 ± 24	56 ± 26	0.039
Saturated Fat (g)		18 ± 9	16 ± 8	19 ± 9	0.131
Monounsaturated Fat (g)		19 ± 10	17 ± 9	21 ± 10	0.020
Polyunsaturated Fat (g)		11 ± 6	10 ± 7	12 ± 6	0.138
ω-3 Fatty Acids (g)		1.09 ± 0.77	0.99 ± 0.83	1.15 ± 0.71	0.205
Cholesterol (mg)		228 ± 148	139 ± 124	291 ± 131	0.0001
Total sugars (g)		93.7 ± 41.3	88.4 ± 37.2	97.3 ± 43.8	0.213
Added sugars (g)		62.9 ± 35.3	61.6 ± 33.4	63.8 ± 36.7	0.715
Total dietary fiber (g)	25	13.5 ± 7.0	12.0 ± 5.0	14.6 ± 8.0	0.035
Soluble fiber (g)		4.1 ± 2.6	3.5 ± 1.5	4.5 ± 3.1	0.017
Vitamin A (μg) [c]	500	625 ± 396	563 ± 401	668 ± 389	0.126
Vitamin C (mg)	60	62.3 ± 53.8	54.0 ± 44.2	68.2 ± 59.2	0.128

Table 2. *Cont.*

Nutrient	DRI [b]	All (*n* = 139)	Egg Non-Consumers (*n* = 57)	Egg Consumers (*n* = 81)	*p* Value
Vitamin D (µg)	10	4.95 ± 3.53	4.19 ± 3.39	5.48 ± 3.55	0.033
Vitamin E (mg)	12	4.92 ± 3.02	4.48 ± 3.21	5.22 ± 2.87	0.159
Vitamin K (µg)	90	42.5 ± 42.6	38.6 ± 34.8	45.2 ± 47.2	0.375
Thiamin (mg)	0.9	1.22 ± 0.57	1.16 ± 0.54	1.26 ± 0.58	0.268
Riboflavin (mg)	0.9	1.67 ± 0.86	1.43 ± 0.76	1.83 ± 0.90	0.006
Niacin (mg)	11	16.7 ± 7.9	15.9 ± 7.9	17.3 ± 8.0	0.328
Vitamin B6 (mg)	1.1	1.60 ± 1.09	1.44 ± 1.00	1.70 ± 1.14	0.165
Total folate (µg)	320	332 ± 210	295 ± 197	357 ± 217	0.090
Vitamin B12 (µg)	2.0	4.74 ± 3.48	3.98 ± 3.00	5.27 ± 3.70	0.031
Choline (mg)	425	237 ± 110	176 ± 79	279 ± 110	0.0001
Sodium (mg)	1500	2569 ± 1132	2266 ± 945	2780 ± 1206	0.008
Potassium (mg)	4700	1788 ± 781	1587 ± 629	1927 ± 848	0.011
Calcium (mg)	800	779 ± 358	735 ± 301	826 ± 390	0.142
Phosphorus (mg)	580	1018 ± 415	913 ± 349	1091 ± 443	0.012
Iron (mg)	8.1	12.6 ± 7.0	11.4 ± 6.4	13.4 ± 7.3	0.091
Lutein + Zeaxanthin (µg)		680 ± 979	547 ± 648	773 ± 1150	0.181

[a] Data shown as mean ± SD; [b] DRI = Dietary Reference Intake for women 31–50 years old; displayed as Adequate Intake for fiber, choline, vitamin K, sodium and potassium, and as Estimated Average Requirement for all other nutrients, when applicable; [c] Retinol Equivalents.

3.3. Healthy Eating Index 2010

Estimated mean HEI-2010 individual component and total scores for egg non-consumers and consumers are presented in Table 3. There were no significant differences in adequacy component scores between groups, with the exception of the total protein foods score, which was greater in egg consumers than in non-consumers (*p* = 0.004). There was a non-significant trend for egg consumers to have a greater total fruit score relative to non-consumers (*p* = 0.070). There were no significant differences between groups in moderation component scores, although relative to non-consumers, there were trends for egg consumers to have a lower score (greater intake) for sodium (score of 4.5 ± 3.5 *vs.* 3.5 ± 3.0 out of 10; *p* = 0.074) and a greater score (lower intake) for empty calories (score of 8.8 ± 5.7 *vs.* 10.6 ± 5.3 out of 20; *p* = 0.059). The total composite HEI-2010 score did not differ significantly between groups, although was slightly greater for egg consumers (52 ± 14 *vs.* 56 ± 13 out of 100 points for egg non-consumers and consumers, respectively; *p* = 0.082).

Table 3. Estimated mean total Healthy Eating Index (HEI)-2010 and component scores among between egg consumers and egg non-consumers among postpartum Mexican American adult women, expressed as absolute score and percentage of the maximum score [a].

Component (Score Range)	All (*n* = 139)	Egg Non-Consumers (*n* = 57)	Egg Consumers (*n* = 82)	*p* Value
Adequacy Components				
Total Fruit (0–5)	2.2 ± 1.7	1.9 ± 1.7	2.4 ± 1.8	0.070
Whole Fruit (0–5)	2.4 ± 1.9	2.1 ± 1.9	2.6 ± 1.9	0.168
Total Vegetables (0–5)	2.5 ± 1.2	2.6 ± 1.3	2.5 ± 1.1	0.710
Greens and Beans (0–5)	1.6 ± 1.6	1.8 ± 1.9	1.4 ± 1.4	0.227
Whole Grains (0–10)	7.6 ± 3.2	7.6 ± 3.4	7.6 ± 3.1	0.885
Dairy (0–10)	5.9 ± 3.3	5.8 ± 3.3	6.0 ± 3.3	0.729
Total Protein Foods (0–5)	4.5 ± 0.9	4.3 ± 1.0	4.7 ± 0.7	0.004
Seafood and Plant Proteins (0–5)	2.8 ± 2.1	2.2 ± 2.1	2.7 ± 2.1	0.173
Fatty Acids (0–0)	4.3 ± 2.9	3.9 ± 2.8	4.6 ± 3.0	0.116

[a] Data shown as mean ± SD.

Table 3. *Cont.*

Component (Score Range)	All (*n* = 139)	Egg Non-Consumers (*n* = 57)	Egg Consumers (*n* = 82)	*p* Value
Moderation Components				
Refined Grains (0–10)	7.5 ± 3.1	7.0 ± 3.2	7.8 ± 3.1	0.127
Sodium (0–10)	3.9 ± 3.3	4.5 ± 3.5	3.5 ± 3.0	0.074
Empty Calories (0–20)	9.8 ± 5.5	8.8 ± 5.7	10.6 ± 5.3	0.059
Total Score (0–100)	54.7 ± 13.5	52.3 ± 14.4	56.4 ± 12.6	0.082

[a] Data shown as mean ± SD.

4. Discussion

This study assessed the contribution of eggs to dietary quality among an understudied group of the population, Mexican-American postpartum women, by comparing nutrient intake and HEI-2010 scores between egg-consumers and non-consumers. This report is of importance because there is limited information regarding contributors to nutrient intake and dietary quality among Mexican-American women of reproductive age. Study findings indicated that egg consumers had greater intakes of energy, protein, fat, monounsaturated fat, cholesterol, total and soluble fiber, vitamin D, riboflavin, vitamin B12, choline, sodium, potassium, and phosphorus, and a modestly higher HEI-2010 score than non-consumers. Similarly, in the only study of its kind conducted in a diverse sample of pregnant Hispanic women, egg consumers had higher intakes of several nutrients including protein, fat, vitamins K and E, cholesterol, total polyunsaturated fatty acids, and DHA [31]. Comparable information among postpartum women is lacking.

In the current study, a greater proportion of participants (59% or *n* = 82) reported consuming eggs than what has been reported for U.S. adults (19%) or Mexican-American adults (32%) using NHANES III data [30]. A majority of study participants (78%) were immigrants of Mexican origin who had been in the U.S. for 12 ± 7 years [34,38,39]. Several reports indicate that multiple factors that are part of the immigration experience, such as acculturation, generational status, and time in the U.S., are associated with lifestyle modifications often associated with less healthful dietary patterns in part due to immigrants' lack of familiarity with available foods in their new environment [40–43]. However, eggs are a low-cost common protein source in the Mexican diet, as evidenced by the high per capita consumption of eggs in Mexico compared to other countries [28], which may have made eggs a nutritious and familiar dietary choice among the generally low-socioeconomic status study participants [34,38,39]. Nevertheless, the possibility cannot be ruled out that the methodology used in the current study (three 24-h recalls) may have better allowed to capture individual instances of egg intake than using only one 24-h recall for NHANES.

In the current study, energy intake was greater for egg consumers than non-consumers. Considering that participants were overweight or obese, this increased energy intake could be of concern because it could potentially translate into long-term weight gain, even when mean total energy intake was lower than what has been reported among U.S. adult women (7543 ± 59 kJ/day (1803 ± 14 kcal/day) according to NHANES 2009-2010 data [44]). The greater energy intake among egg consumers could have been in part attributed to greater fat intake. Differences in fatty acid intake were due to greater monounsaturated fatty acids in the diet of egg consumers *vs.* non-consumers, which explains the greater, albeit non-significant, HEI-2010 fatty acid ratio score ((polyunsaturated fatty acids + monounsaturated fatty acids)/saturated fatty acids) for egg consumers. Although these differences cannot be solely attributed to the fatty acid contribution from eggs, it is noteworthy that roughly 50% of fatty acids in eggs are monounsaturated [45]. Regarding polyunsaturated fatty acids, fortified eggs can be an important dietary contributor to ω-3 fatty acids. A study including Mexican pregnant women reported that 20% of total DHA intake was supplied by eggs [27]. In a diverse sample of pregnant Hispanic women, a greater proportion of egg consumers than non-consumers had DHA consumption in the highest tertile of intake [31]. In the current study, differences in ω-3 fatty acid intake between egg non-consumers and consumers were not statistically significant. Although as expected in the current study egg consumers had greater dietary cholesterol than non-consumers, intake levels did not exceed current recommendations for cholesterol intake (300 mg/day) [46].

Adequate protein intake is crucial for women of reproductive age to maintain maternal and fetal tissue accretion during pregnancy and milk production during lactation [47–49]. In fact, a recent report [50] suggested that protein needs for pregnancy may be even higher than current dietary reference intake recommendations of 1.1 g/kg of body weight/day [46]. In the current study, both absolute protein intake and the HEI-2010 score for total protein foods were greater for egg consumers than non-consumers, although as previously reported the total protein HEI-2010 score was indicative of appropriate consumption of protein-containing foods for all participants [38]. Intake of animal protein was also greater for egg consumers than for non-consumers, although non-significantly different (data not shown). However, the high-quality nature of egg protein [24] may provide an additional nutritional advantage to women who incorporate eggs as part of their diet in the postpartum period.

In the present study, egg-consumers had a greater intake of vitamin D compared to non-consumers. According to NHANES 2003–2006 data, eggs were ranked the third main source of vitamin D (after milk and fish/seafood), contributing with about 5% of vitamin D intake among adults in the United States [51]. This is important considering that it is estimated that between 40% and 80% of U.S. adults, depending on gender and age range, have inadequate vitamin D intake [52]. Furthermore, results from a meta-analysis study showed that low maternal vitamin D levels during pregnancy are associated with risk of preeclampsia, gestational diabetes, preterm birth and small-for-gestational age [53].

All participants in the current study had HEI-2010 scores suggesting intake of diets with low quality or in need for improvement (55 ± 14 relative to a maximum score of 100). A report using NHANES data suggested that at the population level HEI-2010 total score was 53 [54]. Furthermore, participants were not meeting intake recommendations for several nutrients, including fiber, Ca, vitamin E, vitamin C and folate. Egg consumers had a greater HEI-2010 score for total protein foods, and trends towards greater scores for total fruit and empty calories, and lower score for sodium. These differences resulted in a modestly greater total HEI-2010 score for egg consumers.

The main risk associated with egg consumption in the U.S. is salmonellosis, mainly due to consumption of raw or undercooked eggs [55]. The risk is particularly important during pregnancy since salmonellosis may be transmitted to the fetus, increasing the risk of preterm delivery and intrauterine death [55,56]. In a study about food safety, most pregnant women were aware about recommendations to avoid raw eggs; however, they still reported consumption of eggs with runny yolk (35%) and cookie dough containing raw eggs (40%), indicating the need to improve instructions given to this target group [57]. Nevertheless, the potential benefits associated with their high nutritional quality outweigh risks as long as eggs are properly cooked before consumption.

Prior reports from the current study have documented that participants included a large proportion of women living under disadvantaged socio-economic conditions in neighborhoods with limited food access [34,38,39]. In general, Hispanic households have been documented to have greater food insecurity rates than the general population [58]. Thus, an additional benefit of egg intake for the target population in the current study as well as other Hispanic subgroups is associated with their low cost. In general, the cost of foods is directly associated with protein but inversely associated with carbohydrate content [59]. In contrast, relative to other animal sources of protein, eggs are an inexpensive nutrient-dense, high-protein, low-carbohydrate food [24,59]. According to the Nutrient Rich Foods Index, developed as an effort to aid consumers select nutritious food choices under financial constraints, eggs are a low cost source of protein, vitamin A, vitamin B12, riboflavin, calcium and zinc, providing excellent nutritional value for the money [60].

An important limitation of the current report is that dietary assessment was conducted using three 24-h dietary recalls, a method subject to intake underreporting, particularly among women and Hispanic individuals [61,62], as indicated by the relatively low energy intake observed in the current

Nutrients **2015**, *7*, 8402–8412

study. Although this limitation was addressed by calculating the HEI-2010 scores on an energy-density basis when assessing dietary quality [32], differences observed in individual nutrient intakes between egg consumers and non-consumers, particularly macronutrients, are likely a result of absolute energy intake and not solely due to egg consumption. Moreover, data from 24-h dietary recalls may not be the best indicator of habitual food consumption, including eggs.

5. Conclusions

The current report suggests that Mexican-American women who consumed eggs had greater nutrient intake and higher dietary quality than non-consumers. Whereas these data do not indicate that egg intake directly improves dietary quality, it could potentially be an indicator of a healthier dietary pattern. Despite the greater energy intake observed among egg consumers, the low cost and high nutritional quality of eggs make them an ideal protein source that is likely to provide greater benefit than risk to the target population, especially if dietary recommendations focus on consuming eggs as part of a dietary pattern that also includes nutrient-dense and fiber-rich foods and maintaining a healthy body weight.

Acknowledgments: The data for this study were collected with support from the National Institutes of Health, National Institute of Nursing Research NIH/NINR 1 R01NR010356-01A2, *Madres para la Salud* (Mothers for Health) and 3R01NR010356-02S1. Research assistance for data analysis and manuscript development was supported by training funds from the National Institute on Minority Health and Health Disparities of the National Institutes of Health (NIMHD/NIH), award P20 MD002316.

Author Contributions: S.V.-L. and C.K. conceived and designed the study; G.A.P.P. collected the data; S.V.-L. and M.T. analyzed the data; and S.V.-L. and G.A.P.P. interpreted the data and wrote the manuscript.

Conflicts of Interest: The authors declare no conflict of interest.

References

1. Colby, S.L.; Ortman, J.M. *Projections of the Size and Composition of the U.S. Population: 2014 to 2060*; U.S. Census Bureau, Ed.; U.S. Census Bureau: Washington, DC, USA, 2014; pp. 25–1143.
2. Pan, L.; Galuska, D.A.; Sherry, B.; Hunter, A.S.; Rutledge, G.E.; Dietz, W.H.; Balluz, L.S. *Differences in Prevalence of Obesity among Black, White and Hispanic Adults—United States, 2006–2008*; Centers for Disease Control and Prevention (CDC): Atlanta, GA, USA, 2009; Volume 58, pp. 740–744.
3. Daviglus, M.L.; Talavera, G.A.; Avilés-Santa, M.L.; Allison, M.; Cai, J.; Cirqui, M.H.; Gellman, M.; Giachello, A.L.; Gouskova, N.; Kaplan, R.C.; *et al.* Prevalence of major cardiovascular risk factors and cardiovascular diseases among Hispanic/Latino individuals of diverse backgrounds in the United States. *JAMA* **2012**, *308*, 1775–1784. [PubMed]
4. Rooney, B.L.; Schauberger, C.W.; Mathiason, M.A. Impact of perinatal weight change on long-term obesity and obesity-related illnesses. *Obstet. Gynecol.* **2005**, *106*, 1349–1356. [PubMed]
5. Ogden, C.L.; Carroll, M.D.; Curtin, L.R.; McDowell, M.A.; Tabak, C.J.; Flegal, K.M. Prevalence of overweight and obesity in the United States, 1999–2004. *JAMA* **2006**, *295*, 1549–1555. [CrossRef] [PubMed]
6. Records, K.; Keller, C.; Ainsworth, B.; Permana, P.A. Overweight and obesity in postpartum Hispanic women. *Health Care Women Int.* **2008**, *29*, 649–667. [CrossRef] [PubMed]
7. Chiuve, S.E.; Fung, T.T.; Rimm, E.B.; Hu, F.B.; McCullough, M.L.; Wang, M.; Stampfer, M.J.; Willett, W.C. Alternative dietary indices both strongly predict risk of chronic disease. *J. Nutr.* **2012**, *142*, 1009–1018. [CrossRef] [PubMed]
8. Nicklas, T.A.; O'Neil, C.E.; Fulgoni, V.L., III. Diet quality is inversely related to cardiovascular risk factors in adults. *J. Nutr.* **2012**, *142*, 2112–2118. [CrossRef]
9. Carrera, P.M.; Gao, X.; Tucker, K.L. A study of dietary patterns in the Mexican-American population and their association with obesity. *J. Am. Diet. Assoc.* **2007**, *107*, 1735–1742. [CrossRef] [PubMed]
10. Ervin, R.B.; Ogden, C.L. *Consumption of Added Sugars among U.S. Adults, 2005–2010*; National Center for Health Statistics: Hyattsville, MD, USA, 2013.

11. Kirkpatrick, S.I.; Dodd, K.W.; Reedy, J.; Krebs-Smith, S.M. Income and race/ethnicity are associated with adherence to food-based dietary guidance among US adults and children. *J. Acad. Nutr. Diet.* **2012**, *112*, 624–626. [CrossRef] [PubMed]

12. Ogden, C.L.; Kit, B.K.; Carroll, M.D.; Park, S. *Consumption of Sugar Drinks in the United States, 2005–2008*; US Department of Health and Human Services, Centers for Disease Control and Prevention, National Center for Health Statistics: Hyattsville, MD, USA, 2011.

13. Hoerr, S.L.; Tsuei, E.; Liu, Y.; Franklin, F.A.; Nicklas, T.A. Diet quality varies by race/ethnicity of Head Start mothers. *J. Am. Diet. Assoc.* **2008**, *108*, 651–659. [CrossRef] [PubMed]

14. Lichtenstein, A.H.; Appel, L.J.; Brands, M.; Carnethon, M.; Daniels, S.; Franch, H.A.; Franklin, B.; Kris-Etherton, P.; Harris, W.S.; Howard, B.; *et al.* Diet and lifestyle recommendations revision 2006. A scientific statement from the American Heart Association Nutrition Committee. *Circulation* **2006**, *114*, 82–96. [CrossRef] [PubMed]

15. Spence, J.D.; Jenkins, D.J.A.; Davignon, J. Dietary cholesterol and egg yolks: Not for patients at risk of vascular disease. *Can. J. Cardiol.* **2010**, *26*, e336–e339. [CrossRef]

16. Fernandez, M.L. Rethinking dietary cholesterol. *Curr. Opin. Clin. Nutr. Metab. Care* **2012**, *15*, 117–121. [CrossRef] [PubMed]

17. Fernandez, M.L. Effects of eggs on plasma lipoproteins in healthy populations. *Food Funct.* **2010**, *1*, 156–160. [CrossRef] [PubMed]

18. Hsiao, P.Y.; Mitchell, D.C.; Coffman, D.L.; Allman, R.M.; Locher, J.L.; Sawyer, P.; Jensen, G.L.; Hartman, T.J. Dietary patterns and diet quality among diverse older adults: The University of Alabama at Birmingham study of aging. *J. Nutr. Health Aging* **2013**, *17*, 19–25. [PubMed]

19. Bouchard-Mercier, A.; Paradis, A.M.; Godin, G.; Lamarche, B.; Perusse, L.; Vohl, M.C. Associations between dietary patterns and LDL peak particle diameter: A cross-sectional study. *J. Am. Coll. Nutr.* **2010**, *29*, 630–637. [CrossRef] [PubMed]

20. Flores, M.; Macias, N.; Rivera, M.; Lozada, A.; Barquera, S.; Rivera-Dommarco, J.; Tucker, K.L. Dietary patterns in Mexican adults are associated with risk of being overweight or obese. *J. Nutr.* **2010**, *140*, 1869–1873. [CrossRef] [PubMed]

21. Amini, M.; Esmaillzadeh, A.; Shafaeizadeh, S.; Behrooz, J.; Zare, M. Relationship between major dietary patterns and metabolic syndrome among individuals with impaired glucose tolerance. *Nutrition* **2010**, *26*, 986–992. [CrossRef] [PubMed]

22. Rong, Y.; Chen, L.; Zhu, T.; Song, Y.; Yu, M.; Shan, Z.; Sands, A.; Hu, F.B.; Liu, L. Egg consumption and risk of coronary heart disease and stroke: Dose-response meta-analysis of prospective cohort studies. *BMJ* **2013**, *346*. [CrossRef] [PubMed]

23. Shin, J.Y.; Xun, P.; Nakamura, Y.; He, K. Egg consumption in relation to risk of cardiovascular disease and diabetes: A systematic review and meta-analysis. *Am. J. Clin. Nutr.* **2013**, *98*, 146–159. [CrossRef] [PubMed]

24. Applegate, E. Introduction: nutritional and functional roles of eggs in the diet. *J. Am. Coll. Nutr.* **2000**, *19*, 495S–498S. [CrossRef] [PubMed]

25. Iannotti, L.L.; Lutter, C.K.; Bunn, D.A.; Stewart, C.P. Eggs: The uncracked potential for improving maternal and young child nutrition among the world's poor. *Nutr. Rev.* **2014**, *72*, 355–368. [CrossRef] [PubMed]

26. Caudill, M.A. Pre- and postnatal health: Evidence of increased choline needs. *J. Am. Diet. Assoc.* **2010**, *110*, 1198–1206. [CrossRef] [PubMed]

27. Parra-Cabrera, S.; Stein, A.D.; Wang, M.; Martorell, R.; Rivera, J.; Ramakrishnan, U. Dietary intakes of polyunsaturated fatty acids among pregnant Mexican women. *Mater. Child Nutr.* **2011**, *7*, 140–147. [CrossRef] [PubMed]

28. U.S. Department of Agriculture. *World Agricultural Supply and Demand Estimates*; U.S. Department of Agriculture: Washington, DC, USA, 2015; p. 40.

29. Bachman, J.L.; Reedy, J.; Subar, A.F.; Krebs-Smith, S.M. Sources of food group intakes among the US population, 2001–2002. *J. Am. Diet. Assoc.* **2008**, *108*, 804–814. [CrossRef] [PubMed]

30. Song, W.O.; Kerver, J.M. Nutritional contribution of eggs to American diets. *J. Am. Coll. Nutr.* **2000**, *19*, 556S–562S. [CrossRef] [PubMed]

31. Bermudez-Millán, A.; Hromi-Fiedler, A.; Damio, G.; Segura-Perez, S.; Perez-Escamilla, R. Egg contribution towards the diet of pregnant Latinas. *Ecol. Food Nutr.* **2009**, *48*, 383–403. [CrossRef] [PubMed]

32. Guenther, P.M.; Casavale, K.O.; Reedy, J.; Kirkpatrick, S.I.; Hiza, H.A.; Kuczynski, K.J.; Kahle, L.L.; Krebs-Smith, S.M. Update of the Healthy Eating Index: HEI-2010. *J. Acad. Nutr. Diet.* **2013**, *113*, 569–580. [CrossRef] [PubMed]

33. U.S. Department of Agriculture; U.S. Department of Health and Human Services. *Dietary Guidelines for Americans, 2010*, 7th ed.U.S. Government Printing Office: Washington, DC, USA, 2010.

34. Keller, C.S.; Records, K.; Ainsworth, B.E.; Belyea, M.; Permana, P.A.; Coonrod, D.V.; Vega-López, S.; Nagle-Williams, A. Madres para la Salud: Design of a theory-based intervention for postpartum Latinas. *Contemp. Clin. Trials* **2011**, *32*, 418–427. [CrossRef] [PubMed]

35. Conway, J.M.; Ingwersen, L.A.; Moshfegh, A.J. Accuracy of dietary recall using the USDA five-step multiple-pass method in men: An observational validation study. *J. Am. Diet. Assoc.* **2004**, *104*, 595–603. [CrossRef] [PubMed]

36. Freedman, L.S.; Guenther, P.M.; Krebs-Smith, S.M.; Kott, P.S. A population's mean Healthy Eating Index-2005 scores are best estimated by the score of the population ratio when one 24-hour recall is available. *J. Nutr.* **2008**, *138*, 1725–1729. [PubMed]

37. Miller, P.E.; Mitchell, D.C.; Harala, P.L.; Pettit, J.M.; Smiciklas-Wright, H.; Hartman, T.J. Development and evaluation of a method for calculating the Healthy Eating Index-2005 using the Nutrition Data System for Research. *Public Health Nutr.* **2011**, *14*, 306–313. [CrossRef] [PubMed]

38. Pignotti, G.A.; Vega-López, S.; Keller, C.; Belyea, M.; Ainsworth, B.; Nagle Williams, A.; Records, K.; Coonrod, D.; Permana, P. Comparison and evaluation of dietary quality between older and younger Mexican-American women. *Public Health Nutr.* **2015**, *18*, 2615–2624. [CrossRef] [PubMed]

39. Keller, C.; Todd, M.; Ainsworth, B.; Records, K.; Vega-Lopez, S.; Permana, P.; Coonrod, D.; Nagle Williams, A. Overweight, obesity, and neighborhood characteristics among postpartum Latinas. *J. Obes.* **2013**, *2013*. [CrossRef] [PubMed]

40. Ayala, G.X.; Baquero, B.; Klinger, S. A systematic review of the relationship between acculturation and diet among Latinos in the United States: Implications for future research. *J. Am. Diet. Assoc.* **2008**, *108*, 1330–1344. [CrossRef] [PubMed]

41. Himmelgreen, D.; Romero Daza, N.; Cooper, E.; Martinez, D. "I don't make the soups anymore": Pre- to post-migration dietary and lifestyle chanes among Latinos living in West-Central Florida. *Ecol. Food Nutr.* **2007**, *46*, 427–444. [CrossRef]

42. Guendelman, S.; Abrams, B. Dietary intake among Mexican-American women: Generational differences and a comparison with white non-Hispanic women. *Am. J. Public Health* **1995**, *85*, 20–25. [CrossRef] [PubMed]

43. Perez-Escamilla, R. Acculturation, nutrition, and health disparities in Latinos. *Am. J. Clin. Nutr.* **2011**, *93*, 1163S–1167S. [CrossRef] [PubMed]

44. Ford, E.S.; Dietz, W.H. Trends in energy intake among adults in the United States: Findings from NHANES. *Am. J. Clin. Nutr.* **2013**, *97*, 848–853. [CrossRef] [PubMed]

45. Samman, S.; Kung, F.P.; Carter, L.M.; Foster, M.J.; Ahmad, Z.I.; Phuyal, J.L.; Petocz, P. Fatty acid composition of certified organic, conventional and omega-3 eggs. *Food Chem.* **2009**, *116*, 911–914. [CrossRef]

46. Institute of Medicine. *Dietary Reference Intakes for Energy, Carbohydrate, Fiber, Fat, Fatty Acids, Cholesterol, Protein, and Amino Acids (Macronutrients)*; The National Academies Press: Washington, DC, USA, 2005.

47. King, J.C. Physiology of pregnancy and nutrient metabolism. *Am. J. Clin. Nutr.* **2000**, *71*, 1218s–1225s. [PubMed]

48. Kalhan, S.C. Protein metabolism in pregnancy. *Am. J. Clin. Nutr.* **2000**, *71*, 1249s–1255s. [PubMed]

49. Manjarin, R.; Bequette, B.J.; Wu, G.; Trottier, N.L. Linking our understanding of mammary gland metabolism to amino acid nutrition. *Amino Acids* **2014**, *46*, 2447–2462. [CrossRef] [PubMed]

50. Stephens, T.V.; Payne, M.; Ball, R.O.; Pencharz, P.B.; Elango, R. Protein requirements of healthy pregnant women during early and late gestation are higher than current recommendations. *J. Nutr.* **2015**, *145*, 73–78. [CrossRef] [PubMed]

51. O'Neil, C.E.; Keast, D.R.; Fulgoni, V.L.; Nicklas, T.A. Food sources of energy and nutrients among adults in the US: NHANES 2003–2006. *Nutrients* **2012**, *4*, 2097–2120. [CrossRef] [PubMed]

52. Bailey, R.L.; Dodd, K.W.; Goldman, J.A.; Gahche, J.J.; Dwyer, J.T.; Moshfegh, A.J.; Sempos, C.T.; Picciano, M.F. Estimation of total usual calcium and vitamin D intakes in the United States. *J. Nutr.* **2010**, *140*, 817–822. [CrossRef] [PubMed]

53. Wei, S.Q.; Qi, H.P.; Luo, Z.C.; Fraser, W.D. Maternal vitamin D status and adverse pregnancy outcomes: A systematic review and meta-analysis. *J. Mater.Fetal Neonatal Med.* **2013**, *26*, 889–899. [CrossRef] [PubMed]

54. Guenther, P.M.; Casavale, K.O.; Kirkpatrick, S.I.; Reedy, J.; Hiza, H.A.B.; Kuczynski, K.J.; Kahle, L.L.; Krebs-Smith, S.M. *Diet Quality of Americans in 2001–02 and 2007–08 as Measured by the Healthy Eating Index-2010*; U.S. Department of Agriculture, Center For Nutrition Policu and Promotion: Washington, DC, USA, 2013; Volume 51.

55. Voetsch, A.C.; van Gilder, T.J.; Angulo, F.J.; Farley, M.M.; Shallow, S.; Marcus, R.; Cieslak, P.R.; Deneen, V.C.; Tauxe, R.V.; Emerging infections program FoodNet working group. FoodNet estimate of the burden of illness caused by nontyphoidal Salmonella infections in the United States. *Clin. Infect. Dis.* **2004**, *38*, S127–S134. [PubMed]

56. Kaiser, L.; Allen, L.H. Position of the American Dietetic Association: Nutrition and lifestyle for a healthy pregnancy outcome. *J. Am. Diet. Assoc.* **2008**, *108*, 553–561. [CrossRef]

57. Athearn, P.N.; Kendall, P.A.; Hillers, V.V.; Schroeder, M.; Bergmann, V.; Chen, G.; Medeiros, L.C. Awareness and acceptance of current food safety recommendations during pregnancy. *Matern. Child Health J.* **2004**, *8*, 149–162. [CrossRef] [PubMed]

58. Coleman-Jensen, A.; Gregory, C.; Singh, A. *Household Food Security in the United States in 2013*; U.S. Department of Agriculture Economic Research Service (ERS): Washington, D.C., USA, 2014.

59. Brooks, R.C.; Simpson, S.J.; Raubenheimer, D. The price of protein: Combining evolutionary and economic analysis to understand excessive energy consumption. *Obes. Rev.* **2010**, *11*, 887–894. [CrossRef] [PubMed]

60. Drewnowski, A. The Nutrient Rich Foods Index helps to identify healthy, affordable foods. *Am. J. Clin. Nutr.* **2010**, *91*, 1095S–1101S. [CrossRef] [PubMed]

61. Neuhouser, M.L.; Tinker, L.; Shaw, P.A.; Schoeller, D.; Bingham, S.A.; Horn, L.V.; Beresford, S.A.; Caan, B.; Thomson, C.; Satterfield, S.; *et al.* Use of recovery biomarkers to calibrate nutrient consumption self-reports in the Women's Health Initiative. *Am. J. Epidemiol.* **2008**, *167*, 1247–1259. [CrossRef] [PubMed]

62. Bothwell, E.K.G.; Ayala, G.X.; Conway, T.L.; Rock, C.L.; Gallo, L.C.; Elder, J.P. Underreporting of food intake among Mexican/Mexican-American women: Rates and correlates. *J. Am. Diet. Assoc.* **2009**, *109*, 624–632. [CrossRef] [PubMed]

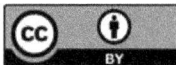

nutrients

MDPI

Review

The Fifty Year Rehabilitation of the Egg

Donald J. McNamara

Eggs for Health Consulting, 5905 Cozumel Pl., Las Vegas, NV 89131, USA; djmmcnamara@gmail.com;
Tel.: +1-202-550-7973

Received: 29 July 2015; Accepted: 15 October 2015; Published: 21 October 2015

Abstract: The 1968 American Heart Association announced a dietary recommendation that all individuals consume less than 300 mg of dietary cholesterol per day and no more than three whole eggs per week. This recommendation has not only significantly impacted the dietary patterns of the population, but also resulted in the public limiting a highly nutritious and affordable source of high quality nutrients, including choline which was limited in the diets of most individuals. The egg industry addressed the egg issue with research documenting the minimal effect of egg intake on plasma lipoprotein levels, as well as research verifying the importance of egg nutrients in a variety of issues related to health promotion. In 2015 dietary cholesterol and egg restrictions have been dropped by most health promotion agencies worldwide and recommended to be dropped from the 2015 Dietary Guidelines for Americans.

Keywords: eggs; dietary cholesterol; plasma cholesterol; lipoproteins; choline; xanthophylls

1. Introduction

Of the vast variety of foods that humans consume, only one has ever been specifically singled out for restriction in an effort to reduce cardiovascular disease (CVD) risk in the population—the egg. The most widely known dietary recommendation in the world is the 1968 admonition from the American Heart Association (AHA) to consume no more than three egg yolks per week [1]. For consumers this provided a recommendation they could easily incorporate into their lifestyles (in 1968 who knew what 10% of calories from saturated fat or 300 mg cholesterol actually meant); for health professionals it was easy to explain dietary equivalency (high dietary cholesterol equals high blood cholesterol equals high CVD risk) without getting into detailed explanations of fat, calories, *etc.*; and for the media it was an ideal icon for the hazards of our modern dietary patterns which lead to high CVD incidence. The only negative effect was on the egg industry which saw a substantial drop in per capita egg consumption over the subsequent years. The question many scientists raised was whether or not this recommendation would actually have any impact on CVD rates. But like the mistaken views in nutritional sciences, it was thought that it couldn't hurt. In the long run it turned out that not only was the recommendation based on misunderstood data and effectively useless, it actually did damage to the general public in terms of their nutritional needs.

2. The Egg Industry Responds

The egg industry was faced with a difficult situation in 1968: fight back and be accused of putting profits ahead of public health or simply give in to the dietary cholesterol phobia being promoted by the AHA and later on by the US government. The other challenge, should the industry decide to finance research in an attempt to prove the egg innocent of the charges, was the fact that in science the accusation that the findings of any study from "industry funded research" are often a quick nullification of the credibility of the results and the investigators involved. But the attacks from health promotion organizations and the media on how harmful meat, dairy and eggs were because of their fat and cholesterol content necessitated that the animal food commodity groups respond, and overall their responses were based on the use of science. The decline in egg consumption in the US after the AHA recommendations were publicized, and further still after the 26 March 1984 Time magazine cover (which referred to a drug study), prompted the US egg industry to establish the Egg Nutrition Center (ENC) to promote research and initiate health education efforts to address issues raised by the AHA in 1968, the Select Committee on Nutrition in 1977 (predecessor of the Dietary Guidelines Advisory Committee), and eventually the National Cholesterol Education Program (NCEP) of the Heart, Lung and Blood Institute of the National Institutes of Health (NIH). In addition, a number of non-government organizations (NGOs) had gotten on the bad egg, bad cholesterol bandwagon as an effective way to raise funds and there was a virtual avalanche of new food products touting "low-cholesterol" and "cholesterol-free" (cholesterol-free peanut butter?) in print, radio and TV advertising. And for most people the concept of "low cholesterol" was a confusion between dietary cholesterol and blood cholesterol. The evils of cholesterol, and eggs, were constantly presented to the consumer.

The egg industry's goal in forming ENC was to formulate a scientific basis for addressing the dietary cholesterol issue. ENC formed a scientific advisory panel in 1984 composed of clinical and university research scientists to help formulate a long range research plan, as well as to serve as consultants to the industry and spokespersons on behalf of the industry. Contrary to the "consensus" argument, not all nutritional scientists were convinced that the low-fat, low-cholesterol diet was the best answer to our CVD problems. I served on that original scientific advisory panel because I had carried out studies on the effects of egg intake on blood cholesterol levels and endogenous cholesterol metabolism [2] and had serious doubts regarding the contribution of dietary cholesterol to blood cholesterol levels and CVD risk [3].

The scientific bases for the original dietary cholesterol restriction was based on three lines of evidence: animal studies showing cholesterol in the diet increased plasma cholesterol levels and development of atherosclerosis; epidemiological evidence that high dietary cholesterol was associated with high CVD incidence; and clinical studies showing that high cholesterol intake resulted in increased serum cholesterol levels. While the evidence of harm seems strong, each line of evidence was open to debate. Animal studies often used herbivores which were hypersensitive to dietary cholesterol as compared to omnivores (rabbit *versus* dog). Studies in suitable animal models often required use of pharmacological levels of cholesterol in the diet in order to elicit a response. Epidemiological data in the 1960s and 1970s relied on simple correlation analyses to show associations and did not account for collinearity of nutrients (saturated fat and cholesterol found in animal products). Eventually multivariate analysis of dietary lipids and CVD incidence documented that dietary cholesterol was not an independent risk factor [4–6]. Clinical feeding studies had two limits: use of pharmacological levels of dietary cholesterol (for example, six eggs per day for six weeks) and in the early studies reliance on measurement of total plasma cholesterol as the marker of risk [6]. Use of physiological dietary cholesterol levels and analysis of lipoprotein cholesterol distribution, including LDL size, provide a very different perspective on risk assessment [6].

Over the years the egg industry funded a variety of animal and clinical studies investigating the effects of egg intake on plasma total and lipoprotein cholesterol levels and metabolism under various conditions. These studies indicated that eggs had little effect on CVD risk [6]. Retrospective analysis of existing clinical data also indicated that eggs and dietary cholesterol, when consumed at physiological, not pharmacological levels, did not significantly affect CVD risk profiles [6–8]. Retrospective review of epidemiological studies which involved analysis of egg intake showed that egg intake was not associated with CVD incidence [6]. The more modern epidemiological studies using multivariate analysis reported that dietary cholesterol was non-significant as an independent factor in CVD incidence [4–6]. Based on these facts, the egg industry considered that it was justified in its efforts to challenge the egg restriction recommendation. Of course, one could predict a backlash to such a challenge.

3. Speaking with One Voice

By 1995 there was a concerted effort to unify all the US national dietary recommendations (so as not to confuse the public) such that the AHA guidelines, the NCEP guidelines, the Dietary Guidelines for Americans, and the Nutrition Facts Panel from the Food and Drug Administration (FDA) all set the dietary cholesterol recommendation at less than 300 mg/day (For detailed reviews of the history of the rationale and implementation of dietary lipid guidelines and their subsequent demise, see Taubes [7] and Teicholz [8].) One question rarely raised by these various agencies or by the scientific community was why 300 mg/day, why not 250 or 400 mg/day or whatever. Determining how the 300 mg/day number was chosen back in 1968 remains a mystery without a satisfactory answer other than it was half of what the estimated cholesterol intake was at the time. Irrespective of the scientific rationale for the number, it became established dogma in the nutrition community. Since one large egg contained 213 mg of cholesterol, per capita egg consumption continued to be low. ENC continued to argue against egg recommendations and presented the science documenting no significant effect of eggs on CVD risk. The counter argument was that the evidence showed that egg intake did increase plasma cholesterol levels [9,10], although at a level which was miniscule and offset by comparable increases in both LDL and HDL cholesterol levels with no change in the LDL:HDL ratio (*i.e.*, no change in relative risk) [11,12]. (1995 was also the year that I accepted the position of Executive Director of ENC).

4. A New Approach

In 1995 the egg industry initiated a two pronged approach to dealing with the dietary cholesterol issue: detailed studies of the effects of egg intake on CVD risk factors and studies of the contribution of eggs to a healthy diet across the lifespan. It was clear to the egg industry that simply funding more egg feeding studies was not going to significantly impact the perception of eggs as potentially harmful. Attempts to fund research analyzing data from large epidemiological studies were met with great resistance due to the curse of "industry funded research" negation and the hesitation of some researchers to be seen as not going along with the "consensus" that dietary cholesterol was harmful. And it was clear that no matter how many feeding studies were presented that the various agencies involved were not going to simply change the recommendations because they were wrong. In view of these factors the egg industry decided that it needed to give the policy makers a reason to change; *i.e.*, implement the "do no harm" imperative.

ENC initiated research projects on a wide variety of themes to document why eggs should be included in the diet. The eventual outcomes of these studies were a surprise to both the egg industry and health agencies. Many of these findings are reported in the associated papers in this issue of the journal.

1. Nutritional Value of Eggs: It is widely recognized that eggs are a highly nutritious food based on their high quality protein and compliment of vitamins and minerals [13]. Eggs are one of the most widely available economical sources of animal protein. In addition, many of the nutrients in eggs can be increased by altering the hen's diet (Se, vitamin E, vitamin D, omega-3 fatty acids, xanthophylls and folate to name just a few). Due to the recommendation to eat no more than three whole eggs per week, and in some parts of Central and South America no more than two eggs per week, those in the lower socioeconomic classes have been scared away from an affordable source of high quality nutrition. It made little sense to restrict a highly nutritious food from the diets of those with sub-optimal nutrient intake whose main health issue was not the over consumption prevalent in the US. This became more obvious when considering the nutritional needs of growing children, pregnant women, and the elderly.

2. Egg Protein and Satiety: Egg protein, especially egg yolk protein, has a significantly greater satiety effect than other protein sources [14,15]. Studies have shown reduced caloric intake after an egg breakfast compared to a bagel breakfast [16], greater weight loss over 8 weeks with an egg as compared to a bagel breakfast as part of a hypocaloric diet [17], and larger changes in

satiety hormones with an egg breakfast [18]. The five decade long shift from eggs for breakfast to carbohydrate rich cereals might not have been the best approach to weight maintenance and probably contributed to our national obesity problem.

3.   Egg Protein and Sarcopenia: There are a number of factors which can impact the dietary availability of high quality animal protein for seniors: availability, affordability, preparation limits, and ease of chewing and digesting. Affordable sources of high-quality animal protein in the diet, especially eggs that are widely available and easy to cook, chew and digest, are of significant importance for growth and development in children as well as for reducing the rate of sarcopenia and maintaining lean muscle tissue mass in the elderly [19]. After 40 plus years of hearing about the dangers of egg cholesterol, many seniors studiously avoid eggs, probably to their detriment [20].

4.   Egg Xanthophylls: Lutein and Zeaxanthin: Eggs provide highly bioavailable forms of the xanthophylls lutein and zeaxanthin which are related to lower risks for age-related macular degeneration and cataracts [21–24] as well as some types of cancer [22,25] and carotid artery atherosclerosis [26]. Studies showed that egg lutein had high bioavailability [21] and that adding eggs to the diet could result in significant increases in macular pigment optical density [23,24]. What continues to make this line of investigation so intriguing is that the levels of lutein and zeaxanthin in an egg can easily be increased up to ten-fold by adding marigold extract to the hens' feed. In fact, today lutein enriched eggs are available in many parts of the world.

5.   Egg Choline: Eggs are an excellent source of choline [27], an essential nutrient which has been shown to be inadequate in the diets of 9 out of 10 adults in the U.S. Choline plays an important role in fetal and neonatal brain development [28] and inadequate choline intake during pregnancy increases the risk for neural tube defects such as spina bifida [29]. Choline intake is also associated with decreased plasma levels of homocysteine and inflammatory factors, which are related to increased cardiovascular disease risk [30]. Recent studies have also shown that high intake of choline is associated with reduced breast cancer incidence and mortality [31,32]. Unfortunately, studies also show that a majority of the population, including a majority of pregnant and lactating women, do not have adequate choline intakes and that adding an egg a day to the diet could alleviate this inadequacy [33]. The importance of choline in fetal and neonatal brain development has been shown in numerous studies and inadequate choline intakes during these critical periods can have very negative effects [34–36].

6.   The egg industry also supported a series of studies looking at the chronic and acute effects of egg intake on endothelial function in a variety of patients and found no evidence of adverse effects with daily egg ingestion on any cardiac risk factors in normolipidemic and hyperlipidemic adults or in adults with CVD [37–39].

5. An Outdated Hypothesis Slowly Put to Rest

In 1999 Hu *et al.* [40] published one of the first large, long term population studies on egg intake and CVD incidence. The results from over 117,000 men and women documented no differences in CVD risk between those consuming one egg a week *versus* one egg a day. Other large epidemiological studies have reported similar findings reporting that egg intake is not associated with CVD risk [41,42]. Meta-analyses have come to the same conclusion [43–45].

In 2002 the AHA dropped its specific egg restriction of 3–4 per week while keeping the less than 300 mg/day of dietary cholesterol guideline. While the US continued to recommend limits on dietary cholesterol, a large number of countries removed dietary cholesterol restrictions from their national dietary guidelines (Australia, Great Britain, Ireland to name a few). It took another twelve years for AHA to pronounce that "There is insufficient evidence to determine whether lowering dietary cholesterol reduces LDL-C." [46]. In an equally surprising turn of events, the 2015 Dietary Guidelines Advisory Committee (DGAC) stated in its report that "Previously, the Dietary Guidelines for Americans recommended that cholesterol intake be limited to no more than 300 mg/day. The 2015

Nutrients **2015**, *7*, 8716–8722

DGAC will not bring forward this recommendation because available evidence shows no appreciable relationship between consumption of dietary cholesterol and serum cholesterol, consistent with the conclusions of the AHA/ACC report." [47]. A recommendation known worldwide that lasted for 47 years has simply been discarded and we can all go back to including eggs in our diets. The United States, which had first promoted the "no more than 300 mg/day cholesterol" recommendation, was now one of the last countries to do away with it. It is interesting to note that it required a much greater amount of research to prove that egg intake was unrelated to CVD risk than it did to initially condemn it as a significant contributor to CVD incidence. This nutritional saga shows that dietary recommendations need to be based more on science than belief and that industry funded research can be a valid approach to address specific issues and when applying proper scientific methods, can be of benefit to both the industry and the public.

6. Conclusions

For almost 50 years eggs and dietary cholesterol have been thought to contribute to high plasma cholesterol levels and increased CVD risk. Based on this belief dietary recommendations in the US and most countries have included dietary cholesterol and egg restrictions. Half a century of research have shown that egg and/or dietary cholesterol intake is not associated with increased CVD risk. In addition, research studies have shown that egg intake addresses a number of nutrient inadequacies and can make important contributions to overall health across the life span. Dietary cholesterol and egg restrictions have now been removed from most national dietary recommendations.

Acknowledgments: The author thanks Eggs for Health Consulting for its support of this review.

Author Contributions: Donald J. McNamara is solely responsible for the concepts and opinions expressed in this article.

Conflicts of Interest: The author was Executive Director of the Egg Nutrition Center (1995–2008), a health education and research facility funded by the U.S. egg industry; and Founder of Eggs for Health Consulting (2009–2015), providing consulting services on egg nutrition to international egg promotion programs.

References

1. Committee on Nutrition; American Heart Association. *Diet and Heart Disease*; American Heart Association: Dallas, TX, USA, 1968.
2. McNamara, D.J.; Kolb, R.; Parker, T.S.; Batwin, H.; Samuel, P.; Brown, C.D.; Ahrens, E.H. Heterogeneity of cholesterol homeostasis in man. Response to changes in dietary fat quality and cholesterol quantity. *J. Clin. Invest.* **1987**, *79*, 1729–1739. [PubMed]
3. McNamara, D.J. Effects of fat-modified diets on cholesterol and lipoprotein metabolism. *Annu. Rev. Nutr.* **1987**, *7*, 273–290. [CrossRef] [PubMed]
4. Hegsted, D.M.; Ausman, L.M. Diet, alcohol and coronary heart disease in men. *J. Nutr.* **1988**, *118*, 1184–1189. [PubMed]
5. Kromhout, D.; Menotti, A.; Bloemberg, B.; Aravanis, C.; Blackburn, H.; Buzina, R.; Dontas, A.S.; Fidanza, F.; Giaipaoli, S.; Jansen, A.; *et al.* Dietary saturated and trans fatty acids and cholesterol and 25-year mortality from coronary heart disease: The seven countries study. *Prev. Med.* **1995**, *24*, 308–315. [CrossRef] [PubMed]
6. McNamara, D.J. Dietary cholesterol and atherosclerosis. *Biochim. Biophys. Acta* **2000**, *1529*, 310–320. [CrossRef]
7. Taubes, G. *Good Calories, Bad Calories*; Knopf: New York, NY, USA, 2007.
8. Teicholz, N. *The Big Fat Surprise: Why Butter, Meat and Cheese Belong in a Healthy Diet*; Simon & Schuster: New York, NY, USA, 2014.
9. Howell, W.H.; McNamara, D.J.; Tosca, M.A.; Smith, B.T.; Gaines, J.A. Plasma lipid and lipoprotein responses to dietary fat and cholesterol: A meta-analysis. *Am. J. Clin. Nutr.* **1997**, *65*, 1747–1764. [PubMed]
10. Clarke, R.; Frost, C.; Collins, R.; Appleby, P.; Peto, R. Dietary lipids and blood cholesterol: Quantitative meta-analysis of metabolic ward studies. *BMJ* **1997**, *314*, 112–117. [CrossRef] [PubMed]

11. Greene, C.M.; Zern, T.L.; Wood, R.; Shrestha, S.; Aggarwal, D.; Sharman, M.; Volek, J.S.; Fernandez, M.L. Dietary cholesterol provided by eggs does not result in an increased risk for coronary heart disease in an elderly population. *J. Nutr.* **2005**, *135*, 2793–2798. [PubMed]

12. Mutungi, G.; Waters, D.; Ratliff, J.; Puglisi, M.J.; Clark, R.M.; Volek, J.S.; Fernandez, M.L. Eggs distinctly modulate plasma carotenoid and lipoprotein subclasses in adult men following a carbohydrate restricted diet. *J. Nutr. Biochem.* **2010**, *21*, 261–267. [CrossRef] [PubMed]

13. Song, W.O.; Kerver, J.M. Nutritional contribution of eggs to American diets. *J. Am. Coll. Nutr.* **2000**, *19*, 556S–562S. [CrossRef] [PubMed]

14. Villaume, C.; Beck, B.; Rohr, R.; Pointel, J.P.; Debry, G. Effect of exchange of ham for boiled egg on plasma glucose and insulin responses to breakfast in normal subjects. *Diabetes Care* **1986**, *9*, 46–49. [CrossRef] [PubMed]

15. Pelletier, X.; Thouvenot, P.; Belbraouet, S.; Chayvialle, J.A.; Hanesse, B.; Mayeux, D.; Debry, G. Effect of egg consumption in healthy volunteers: Influence of yolk, white or whole-egg on gastric emptying and on glycemic and hormonal responses. *Ann. Nutr. Metab.* **1996**, *40*, 109–115. [CrossRef] [PubMed]

16. Vander Wal, J.S.; Marth, J.M.; Khosla, P.; Jen, K.L.; Dhurandhar, N.V. Short-term effect of eggs on satiety in overweight and obese subjects. *J. Am. Coll. Nutr.* **2005**, *24*, 510–515. [CrossRef] [PubMed]

17. Vander Wal, J.S.; Gupta, A.; Khosla, P.; Dhurandhar, N.V. Egg breakfast enhances weight loss. *Int. J. Obes. (Lond.)* **2008**, 1545–1551.

18. Ratliff, J.; Leite, J.O.; de Ogburn, R.; Puglisi, M.J.; VanHeest, J.; Fernandez, M.L. Consuming eggs for breakfast influences plasma glucose and ghrelin, while reducing energy intake during the next 24 h in adult men. *Nutr. Res.* **2010**, *30*, 96–103. [CrossRef] [PubMed]

19. Houston, D.K.; Nicklas, B.J.; Ding, J.; Harris, T.B.; Tylavsky, F.A.; Newman, A.B.; Lee, J.S.; Sahyoun, N.R.; Visser, M.; Kritchevsky, S.B.; *et al.* Dietary protein intake is associated with lean mass change in older, community-dwelling adults: The health, aging, and body composition (Health ABC) study. *Am. J. Clin. Nutr.* **2008**, *87*, 150–155. [PubMed]

20. Paddon-Jones, D.; Campbell, W.W.; Jacques, P.F.; Kritchevsky, S.B.; Moore, L.L.; Rodriguez, N.R.; van Loon, L.J. Protein and healthy aging. *Am. J. Clin. Nutr.* **2015**, *101*, 1339S–1345S. [CrossRef] [PubMed]

21. Chung, H.Y.; Rasmussen, H.M.; Johnson, E.J. Lutein bioavailability is higher from lutein-enriched eggs than from supplements and spinach in men. *J. Nutr.* **2004**, *134*, 1887–1893. [PubMed]

22. Ribaya-Mercado, J.D.; Blumberg, J.B. Lutein and zeaxanthin and their potential roles in disease prevention. *J. Am. Coll. Nutr.* **2004**, *23*, 567S–587S. [CrossRef] [PubMed]

23. Goodrow, E.F.; Wilson, T.A.; Houde, S.C.; Vishwanathan, R.; Scollin, P.A.; Handelman, G.; Nicolosi, R.J. Consumption of one egg per day increases serum lutein and zeaxanthin concentrations in older adults without altering serum lipid and lipoprotein cholesterol concentrations. *J. Nutr.* **2006**, *136*, 2519–2524. [PubMed]

24. Wenzel, A.J.; Gerweck, C.; Barbato, D.; Nicolosi, R.J.; Handelman, G.J.; Curran-Celentano, J. A 12-wk egg intervention increaes serum zeaxanthin and macular pigment optical density in women. *J. Nutr.* **2006**, *136*, 2568–2573. [PubMed]

25. Mignone, L.I.; Giovannucci, E.; Newcomb, P.A.; Titus-Ernstoff, L.; Trentham-Dietz, A.; Hampton, J.M.; Willett, W.C.; Egan, K.M. Dietary carotenoids and the risk of invasive breast cancer. *Int. J. Cancer* **2009**, *124*, 2929–2937. [CrossRef] [PubMed]

26. Dwyer, J.H.; Navab, M.; Dwyer, K.M.; Hassan, K.; Sun, P.; Shircore, A.; Hama-Levy, S.; Hough, G.; Wang, X.; Drake, T.; *et al.* Oxygenated carotenoid lutein and progression of early atherosclerosis: The Los Angeles Atherosclerosis Study. *Circulation* **2001**, *103*, 2922–2927. [CrossRef] [PubMed]

27. Zeisel, S.H. Choline: Critical role during fetal development and dietary requirements in adults. *Annu. Rev. Nutr.* **2006**, *26*, 229–250. [CrossRef] [PubMed]

28. Zeisel, S.H.; Niculescu, M.D. Perinatal choline influences brain structure and function. *Nutr. Rev.* **2006**, *64*, 197–203. [CrossRef] [PubMed]

29. Shaw, G.M.; Carmichael, S.L.; Yang, W.; Selvin, S.; Schaffer, D.M. Periconceptional dietary intake of choline and betaine and neural tube defects in offspring. *Am. J. Epidemiol.* **2004**, *160*, 102–109. [CrossRef] [PubMed]

30. Detopoulou, P.; Panagiotakos, D.B.; Antonopoulou, S.; Pitsavos, C.; Stefanadis, C. Dietary choline and betaine intakes in relation to concentrations of inflammatory markers in healthy adults: The Attica Study. *Am. J. Clin. Nutr.* **2008**, *87*, 424–430. [PubMed]

31. Xu, X.; Gammon, M.D.; Zeisel, S.H.; Lee, Y.L.; Wetmur, J.G.; Teitelbaum, S.L.; Bradshaw, P.T.; Neugut, A.I.; Santella, R.M.; Chen, J. Choline metabolism and risk of breast cancer in a population-based study. *FASEB J.* **2008**, *22*, 2045–2052. [CrossRef] [PubMed]

32. Xu, X.; Gammon, M.D.; Zeisel, S.H.; Bradshaw, P.T.; Wetmur, J.G.; Teitelbaum, S.L.; Neugut, A.I.; Santella, R.M.; Chen, J. High intakes of choline and betaine reduce breast cancer mortality in a population-based study. *FASEB J.* **2009**, *23*, 4022–4028. [CrossRef] [PubMed]

33. Yonemori, K.M.; Lim, U.; Koga, K.R.; Wilkens, L.R.; Au, D.; Boushey, C.J.; le marchand, L.; Kolonel, L.N.; Murphy, S.P. Dietary choline and betaine intakes vary in an adult multiethnic population. *J. Nutr.* **2013**, *143*, 894–899. [CrossRef] [PubMed]

34. Leermakers, E.T.; Moreira, E.M.; Kiefte-de Jong, J.C.; Darweesh, S.K.; Visser, T.; Voortman, T.; Bautista, P.K.; Chowdhury, R.; Gorman, D.; Bramer, W.M.; *et al.* Effects of choline on health across the life course: A systematic review. *Nutr. Rev.* **2015**, *73*, 500–522. [CrossRef] [PubMed]

35. Ruxton, C. Value of eggs during pregnancy and early childhood. *Nurs. Stand.* **2013**, *27*, 41–50. [CrossRef] [PubMed]

36. Shapira, N. Modified egg as a nutritional supplement during peak brain development: A new target for fortification. *Nutr. Health* **2009**, *20*, 107–118. [CrossRef] [PubMed]

37. Katz, D.L.; Gnanaraj, J.; Treu, J.A.; Ma, Y.; Kavak, Y.; Njike, V.Y. Effects of egg ingestion on endothelial function in adults with coronary artery disease: A randomized, controlled, crossover trial. *Am. Heart J.* **2015**, *169*, 162–169. [CrossRef] [PubMed]

38. Njike, V.; Faridi, Z.; Dutta, S.; Gonzalez-Simon, A.L.; Katz, D.L. Daily egg consumption in hyperlipidemic adults—Effects on endothelial function and cardiovascular risk. *Nutr. J.* **2010**, *9*, 28. [CrossRef] [PubMed]

39. Katz, D.L.; Evans, M.A.; Nawaz, H.; Njike, V.Y.; Chan, W.; Comerford, B.P.; Hoxley, M.L. Egg consumption and endothelial function: A randomized controlled crossover trial. *Int. J. Cardiol.* **2005**, *99*, 65–70. [CrossRef] [PubMed]

40. Hu, F.B.; Stampfer, M.J.; Rimm, E.B.; Manson, J.E.; Ascherio, A.; Colditz, G.A.; Rosner, B.A.; Spiegelman, D.; Speizer, F.E.; Sacks, F.M.; *et al.* A prospective study of egg consumption and risk of cardiovascular disease in men and women. *JAMA* **1999**, *281*, 1387–1394. [CrossRef] [PubMed]

41. Qureshi, A.I.; Suri, M.F.K.; Ajmed, S.; Nasar, A.; Divani, A.A.; Kirmani, J.F. Regular egg consumption does not increase the risk of stroke and cardiovascular diseases. *Med. Sci. Monit.* **2007**, *131*, CR1–CR8.

42. Nakamura, Y.; Iso, H.; Kita, Y.; Ueshima, H.; Okada, K.; Konishi, M.; Inoue, M.; Tsugane, S. Egg consumption, serum total cholesterol concentrations and coronary heart disease incidence: Japan public health center-based prospective study. *Br. J. Nutr.* **2006**, *96*, 921–928. [CrossRef] [PubMed]

43. Shin, J.Y.; Xun, P.; Nakamura, Y.; He, K. Egg consumption in relation to risk of cardiovascular disease and diabetes: A systematic review and meta-analysis. *Am. J. Clin. Nutr.* **2013**, *98*, 146–159. [CrossRef] [PubMed]

44. Rong, Y.; Chen, L.; Zhu, T.; Song, Y.; Yu, M.; Shan, Z.; Sands, A.; Hu, F.B.; Liu, L. Egg consumption and risk of coronary heart disease and stroke: Dose-response meta-analysis of prospective cohort studies. *BMJ* **2013**, *346*, e8539. [CrossRef] [PubMed]

45. Tran, N.L.; Barraj, L.M.; Heilman, J.M.; Scrafford, C.G. Egg consumption and cardiovascular disease among diabetic individuals: A systematic review of the literature. *Diabetes Metab. Syndr. Obes.* **2014**, *7*, 121–137. [CrossRef] [PubMed]

46. Eckel, R.H.; Jakicic, J.M.; Ard, J.D.; de Jesus, J.M.; Houston Miller, N.; Hubbard, V.S.; Lee, I.M.; Lichtenstein, A.H.; Loria, C.M.; Millen, B.E.; *et al.* 2013 AHA/ACC guideline on lifestyle management to reduce cardiovascular risk. *J. Am. Coll. Cardiol.* **2014**, *63*, 2960–2984. [CrossRef] [PubMed]

47. Advisory Report to the Secretary of Health and Human Services and the Secretary of Agriculture. Available online: http://www.health.gov/dietaryguidelines/2015-scientific-report (accessed on 5 October 2015).

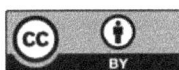

nutrients

MDPI

Review

Immune-Relevant and Antioxidant Activities of Vitellogenin and Yolk Proteins in Fish

Chen Sun and Shicui Zhang *

Laboratory for Evolution & Development, Institute of Evolution & Marine Biodiversity and Department of
Marine Biology, Ocean University of China, Qingdao 266003, China; sunchen@ouc.edu.cn
* Correspondence: sczhang@ouc.edu.cn; Tel./Fax: +86-532-82032787

Received: 15 July 2015; Accepted: 25 August 2015; Published: 22 October 2015

Abstract: Vitellogenin (Vtg), the major egg yolk precursor protein, is traditionally thought to provide
protein- and lipid-rich nutrients for developing embryos and larvae. However, the roles of Vtg as well
as its derived yolk proteins lipovitellin (Lv) and phosvitin (Pv) extend beyond nutritional functions.
Accumulating data have demonstrated that Vtg, Lv and Pv participate in host innate immune defense
with multifaceted functions. They can all act as multivalent pattern recognition receptors capable
of identifying invading microbes. Vtg and Pv can also act as immune effectors capable of killing
bacteria and virus. Moreover, Vtg and Lv are shown to possess phagocytosis-promoting activity as
opsonins. In addition to these immune-relevant functions, Vtg and Pv are found to have antioxidant
activity, which is able to protect the host from oxidant stress. These non-nutritional functions clearly
deepen our understanding of the physiological roles of the molecules, and at the same time, provide
a sound basis for potential application of the molecules in human health.

Keywords: vitellogenin; lipovitellin; phosvitin; immunity; antioxidant activity

1. Introduction

Most fishes are oviparous, with their eggs being fertilized externally [1]. Eggs or haploid
reproductive cells, which develop into viable embryos after fertilization, are the final product of oocyte
growth and differentiation [2]. Generally, several steps are involved in oocyte development: formation
of primordial germ-cells (PGCs), and transformation of PGCs into oogonia and then to oocytes.
Subsequently, massive maternal information and molecules needed for early embryo development
are deposited in growing oocytes during vitellogenesis, including RNAs, proteins, lipids, vitamins,
and hormones [2,3]. One of the most important proteins deposited in oocytes is vitellogenin (Vtg),
a member of the large lipid transfer protein (LLTP) superfamily [3–5]. Vtg is a high molecular mass
glycolipophosphoprotein, usually circulating in the blood (vertebrates)/hemolymph (invertebrates) as
a homodimer [4,6–8]. There are usually several isoforms of Vtg in a given species, which are encoded
by a multigene family [9,10]. For instance, three *vtg* genes have been identified in chicken *Gallus
gallus* [11,12], four in Africa frog *Xenopus laevis* [13,14], and six in nematode *Caenorhabditis elegans* [15].
Multiple *vtg* genes are also common in teleosts. It has been documented that there are seven *vtg* genes
in zebrafish *Danio rerio* [16,17], two *vtg* genes in carp *Cyprinus carpio* [18], four *vtg* genes in medaka
Oryzias latipes [10], three *vtg* genes in striped bass *Morone saxatilis* [19], and three *vtg* genes in white
perch *Morone americana* [20]. All vitellogenins (Vtgs) encoded by multiple genes display a similar
structure in vertebrates, such as fish, and invertebrates, particularly insects [21,22]. In most cases, Vtg
contains three conserved domains, the LPD_N (also known as vitellogenin_N or LLT domain), which
is identified at the N-terminus, the domain of unknown function (DUF) 1943, and the von Willebrand
factor type D domain (vWD), which is located at the C-terminus and distributed over a wide range
of proteins [21]. Occasionally, a domain of unknown function called DUF1944 is found to be present

in between DUF1943 and vWD in some Vtg proteins from vertebrates such as chicken and fish [22]. Beginning at the N-terminus, a complete fish Vtg consists of a signal peptide, a lipovitellin heavy chain (LvH), a phosphorylated serine-rich phosvitin (Pv), a lipovitellin light chain (LvL), and a β-component (β-C) plus a C-terminal coding region (CT) comprising the vWD (Figure 1) [4,19,20,23]. Notably, some teleostean Vtgs lack Pv and much of the carboxyl-terminus (β-component and C-terminal peptide), consisting of only LvH and LvL [23]. Pv are also absent in most invertebrate Vtg [8,16].

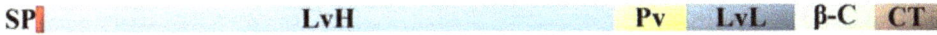

Figure 1. Schematic summary of structure of a complete teleost vitellogenin (Vtg). A short signal peptide (SP) is shown at the N-terminus, flowing by a lipovitellin heave chain (LvH), a phosphorylated serine-rich phosvitin (Pv), a lipovitellin light chain (LvL), and a β-component (β-C) plus a C-terminal coding region (CT).

Vtgs, the precursors of egg yolk proteins, are present in the females of nearly all oviparous species including fish, amphibians, reptiles, birds, most invertebrates and the platypus. Vtgs are usually synthesized in an extra-ovarian tissue (in the liver of vertebrates, the hepatopancreas of crustaceans and the fat body of insects) and transported by the circulation system to the ovary, where it is internalized into growing oocytes via receptor-mediated endocytosis during vitellogenesis with diverse proportional composition [2,7,19,24–31]. Interestingly, the rates of different Vtgs internalized by growing oocytes are not always equal to the rates of circulating Vtgs in the blood, which may be due to the regulation of the system of multiple ovarian receptors engaged in endocytosis of different Vtgs [32–35]. Once internalized into the oocytes, Vtgs are proteolytically cleaved by the aspartic protease cathepsin D to generate yolk proteins, such as Lv subunits, Pv and β-C [36–43]. Lv subunits and Pv are stored in yolk globules or platelets, while β-C remains in cytoplasm as a soluble fraction [44–46]. Lv, the largest yolk protein derived from the proteolytic processing of Vtgs, is an apoprotein delivering mainly phospholipids into developing oocytes [36,47]. Pv, the smallest yolk protein, largely consists of phosphorylated serine residues thought to stabilize nascent Vtg structure during lipid loading and to enhance solubility of Vtg in the blood [4,47]. β-C and CT, the small cleavage products of vWD that contains a highly conserved motif of repeated cysteine residues, are postulated to stabilize the Vtg dimer for cellular recognition and receptor binding, and to protect Vtg or its product yolk proteins from premature or inappropriate proteolysis [4,19,20]. All these yolk proteins are later used as the nutrients by developing embryos to nourish their cells [48,49].

Vtgs were once regarded as a female-specific protein [50,51]; however, synthesis, albeit in smaller quantities, has been shown to occur in male and even sexually immature animals [52–54], suggesting that Vtgs presumably fulfill a more general role independent of gender. Recently, both Vtgs and yolk proteins have been shown to be connected with the immune defense and antioxidant activity in fish, challenging the traditional view that Vtgs and yolk proteins were simple source of nutrients for the developing embryos. Below we will discuss the immune-relevant and antioxidant activities of Vtgs and yolk proteins in fish.

2. Immune-Relevant Activities of Vtgs and Yolk Proteins

2.1. Immune Roles of Vtgs

Accumulating data demonstrated several non-nutritional roles for Vtg. For instance, Vtgs were shown to be associated with the social organization, temporal division of labor and foraging specialization, regulation of hormonal dynamics and change in gustatory responsiveness in the honeybee *Apis mellifera*, an advanced eusocial insect (Figure 2) [55–58]. Recent studies show that Vtgs also play immune-relevant roles (Figure 2). The first solid evidence showing that Vtg preforms an immune-relevant role was the observation by Zhang *et al.*, that Vtg purified from the ovaries of the protochordate amphioxus (*Branchiostoma japonicum*) exhibited hemagglutinating activity against chick, toad and grass carp erythrocytes as well as antibacterial activity against the Gram-negative bacterium *E. coli* [59]. Soon after that, Vtg purified from the rosy barb *Puntius conchonius* was found to be capable of inhibiting the growth of the Gram-negative bacteria *E. coli*, *E. aerogenes* and *Pseudomonas putida* as well as the Gram-positive bacteria *Staphylococcus aureus*, *Bacillus subtilis* and *Streptococcus pyogenes* [60], and Vtg from the carp capable of suppressing the growth of *E. coli* and *S. aureus* in a dose dependent-manner [61]. Interestingly, Vtgs from protostomes also appear to have antibacterial activity. Vtg from the scallop (*Patinopecten yessoensis*) was recently shown to have antibacterial activity against Gram-positive and Gram-negative bacteria [62]. In addition, Vtg in the nematode *C. elegans* seems also involved in its antibacterial defense. A reduced survival was observed in the *vtg*-knockdown *C. elegans* after pathogen infection [63]. Another evidence for a role of invertebrate Vtg associated with resistance against bacteria was provided by the enhancement of resistance of nematode against the pathogen *Photorhabdus luminescens*, when the production of Vtg was stimulated by estrogen 17β-estradiol and phytoestrogen daidzein. However, reduction of Vtg caused by soy isoflavone genistein diminished the host resistance to *P. luminescens* [64]. Taken together, it appears that the antibacterial activity is a universal property of Vtgs from both vertebrates and invertebrates.

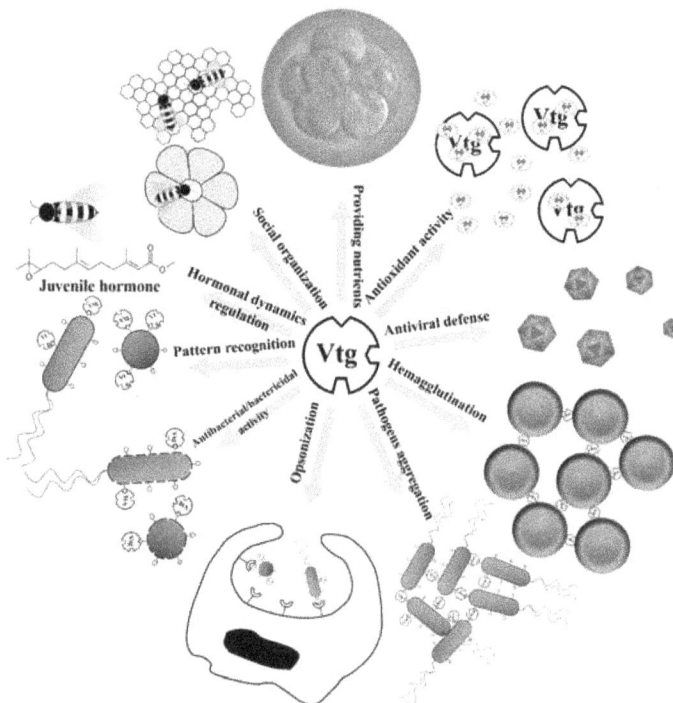

Figure 2. Multiple roles of vitellogenin (Vtg). Vtg is traditionally thought to provide protein- and lipid-rich nutrients for developing embryos and larvae. However, accumulating data demonstrate that its roles extend beyond the nutritional function. In the advanced eusocial insect honeybee, Vtgs were shown to be associated with the social organization, temporal division of labor and foraging specialization, regulation of hormonal dynamics and change in gustatory responsiveness. Recent studies show that Vtgs also play immune-relevant roles. Vtg is able to recognize the invading microbes as a multivalent pattern recognition receptor, kill bacteria or neutralize virus as an effector molecule as well as enhance phagocytosis as an opsonin. Besides, Vtg also exhibits activities to hemagglutinate erythrocytes and aggregate pathogens. In addition to immune roles, Vtg plays another novel role as an antioxidant.

Shi *et al.* showed that intraperitoneal injection of *E. coli* was able to enhance the level of serum Vtg in male *P. conchonius* [60]. This has recently been confirmed by Lu *et al.*, who showed that expression of *vtg* genes in the skin of zebrafish was induced following the challenge with Gram-negative bacterium *Citrobacter freundii* [65,66]. Moreover, an increased expression of *vtg* was also detectable in the insect *Bactericera cockerelli* after infected by "*Candidatus* Liberibacter solanacearum" via transcriptome analyses [67]. These data together suggest that Vtg may play an active role in the anti-infection of the host *in vivo*. Actually, Tong *et al.* showed that Vtg produced in male zebrafish as a consequence of induction by lipopolysaccharide (LPS) and lipoteichoic acid (LTA) is an acute phase reactant, with antibacterial activity against *E. coli* and *S. aureus* [68].

Vtg appears to play a multifaceted immune-relevant functions. Li *et al.* demonstrated that Vtg of the marine fish *Hexagrammos otakii* was able to bind to Gram-negative bacterium *E. coli* and Gram-positive bacterium *S. aureus* as well as fungus *Pichia pastoris* [69]. The binding to *E. coli* and *S. aureus* was also detected for carp and zebrafish Vtgs [61,68]. The binding of Vtgs to bacteria provides them ability to aggregate pathogens as well as to recognize the invading microbes [61]. Further examination via ELISA assay showed that Vtgs exhibited specific affinities to the components conserved within a class of microbes, called pathogen-associated molecular patterns (PAMPs), including LPS of Gram-negative bacteria, LTA of Gram-positive bacteria, peptidoglycan (PGN) of Gram-negative and positive bacteria, and glucan of fungi [61,69]. These observations indicate that Vtg first functions as a multivalent pattern recognition receptor capable of identifying invading Gram-negative and Gram-positive bacteria as well as fungi, and is involved in host immune defense as a detector. In a recent study attempting to search PGN recognition proteins in giant tiger shrimp (*Penaeus monodon*), an 83 kDa protein was isolated by *in vitro* PGN pull-down binding assay and identified as a Vtg-like protein via mass spectrometry as well as Western blots with monoclonal antibodies specific of Vtgs reported from *P. monodon* [70], implicating that invertebrate Vtg may also play a pattern recognition receptor role. Scanning electron microscopy as well as bacterial cell and protoplast lysis assays showed that *H. otakii* Vtg was able to kill pathogenic bacteria by lysing the whole cells (with cell walls) instead of protoplast (without cell walls) via interaction with LPS and LTA [71]. These show that Vtg functions as an effector molecule, capable of directly killing bacteria. Interestingly, Vtg was also shown to be able to enhance the phagocytosis of microbes by macrophages. Li *et al.* first reported that *H. otakii* Vtg could facilitate engulfing of the microbes *E. coli*, *S. aureus* and *P. pastoris* by head-kidney-derived macrophages *in vitro* [69]. Later, Vtg of carp was shown to possess similar phagocytosis-promoting activity [61]. In an *in-situ* study of impacts of urban wastewater on freshwater mussel *Elliptio complanata*, it was observed that the production of Vtg-like proteins was strongly associated with phagocytosis [72], suggesting a relation between Vtg and phagocytosis in invertebrates. Besides, *H. otakii* Vtg was found to be capable of binding to the cell surface of macrophages but not that of red blood cells [61,69]. Collectively, these observations indicate that Vtg is an opsonin functioning as a bridging molecule between host macrophages and invading pathogens, thereby leading to enhanced phagocytosis. Notably, Liu *et al.*, established that the *H. otakii* Vtg was able to opsonize the fungus *P. pastoris* for phagocytosis by macrophages isolated from sea bass *Lateolabrax japonicas*, implying that the opsonization of Vtg was not species-specific [73]. Further study revealed that Vtg-opsonized phagocytosis showed properties typical of type I phagocytosis, including pseudopod extension, tyrosine kinase dependence, and up-regulation of pro-inflammatory cytokine genes *tnf-α* and *il-1β* [73]. Therefore, Vtg is a pattern recognition receptor capable of identifying pathogens, a bactericidal molecule capable of damaging bacterial cell walls, and an opsonin capable of enhancing phagocytosis of pathogens by macrophages. The multifaceted immune-relevant activities of Vtg are in part endowed with its different domains. It was reported by Sun *et al.* that both DUF1943 and DUF1944 as well as vWD contribute to the function of Vtg as a pattern recognition receptor, and DUF1943 and DUF1944 (but not vWD) also contribute to the function of Vtg as an opsonin [21].

Recently, Garcia *et al.* showed that Atlantic salmon Vtg possessed neutralizing ability for infectious pancreatic necrosis virus [74], suggesting that Vtg is also involved in host antiviral immunity. This seems further supported by the observation that the mosquito (*Anopheles gambiae*) Vtg was able to interfere with anti-*plasmodium* response [75]. These denote that in addition to antibacterial activity, Vtg also has antiviral activity, which demands detailed study in the future.

2.2. Immune Roles of Yolk Proteins

Lv and Pv are the principal yolk proteins generated by the proteolytic cleavage of Vtg. As Vtg is an immune-competent molecule, it is thus reasonable to hypothesize that Lv and Pv also have similar immune activities. This hypothesis was first tested by Zhang and Zhang [76]. They demonstrated that the native Lv purified from ovulated eggs of the rosy barb *P. conchonius* was able to interact with LPS, LTA and PGN, as well as *E. coli* and *S. aureus*, but not with self-molecules such as the egg extracts prepared, indicating that Lv is a molecule capable of recognizing non-self components. Moreover, the bacterial binding activity of Lv enabled it to enhance the phagocytosis of bacteria by macrophages, suggesting that Lv is also an opsonin functional in developing embryos/larvae [76]. Similarly, Pv was also shown to play a critical role in the immunity of zebrafish embryos via acting as a pattern recognition receptor and an antimicrobial effector molecule [77]. In line with this, hen egg yolk Pv was also shown to be able to inhibit the growth of the Gram-negative bacterium *E. coli* and the Gram-positive bacterium *S. aureus* under thermal stress [78,79]. Of note, the affinity of Pv to LPS enabled the protein a capacity to neutralize endotoxin, promoting the survival rate of endotoxemia mice [79]. It was recently shown that a truncated Pv (Pt5) consisting of the C-terminal 55 residues of zebrafish Pv also displayed similar immune activities with Pv, including antimicrobial activity against *E. coli*, *Aeromonas hydrophila* and *S. aureus*, and specific affinity to LPS, LTA, and PGN [77]. Intraperitoneal injection of this Pv-derived peptide was able to increase the survival rate of zebrafish challenged with pathogenic *A. hydrophila* and to markedly decrease the number of the pathogen in multiple tissues, suggesting that Pt5 could inhibit multiplication/dissemination of pathogen in host as an antimicrobial agent. In addition to direct antimicrobial activity, Pt5 was also shown to be able to regulate the host immune responses via suppressing the expression of pro-inflammatory cytokine genes (*il-1β*, *il-6*, *tnf-α* and *ifn-γ*) and simultaneously enhancing the expression of anti-inflammatory cytokine genes (*il-10* and *il-4*), suggesting a dual role of Pt5 as both immune effector and modulator [80]. Recently, a mutant peptide of Pt5 (designated as Pt5e), generated by site-directed mutagenesis, was shown to have stronger bactericidal activity and LPS-neutralizing activity [81]. Besides, Sun *et al.* demonstrated that recombinant zebrafish Pv was capable of inhibiting the formation of the cytopathic effect in lymphocystis disease virus (LCDV)-infected cells and reducing the virus quantities in the infected cells as well as in the infected zebrafish, suggesting that Pv possesses an antiviral activity and participates in immune defense of host against the infection by viruses like LCDV [82]. Taken together, these data show that like Vtg, Lv and Pv are both immune-competent molecules involved in immune response of the host against invading pathogenic microbes.

3. Antioxidant Activities of Vtgs and Yolk Proteins

In addition to immune roles, another novel role of Vtg is antioxidant activity (Figure 2). It was first shown by Ando and Yanagida that Vtg from the eel *Anguilla japonica* was able to resist the copper-induced oxidation, and could protect the very low density lipoprotein (VLDL) against copper-induced oxidation [83]. This was the first observation reporting that Vtg has antioxidant activity, and serves to suppress the free-radical reactions in fish oocytes. Similar antioxidant activity was also suggested for the nematode (*C. elegans*) Vtg [84]. In the honeybee, Vtg was demonstrated to be able to reduce oxidative stress by scavenging free radicals, thereby increasing the lifespan in the facultatively sterile worker castes and reproductive queen castes [85,86]. The honeybee Vtg was also demonstrated in a recent study to be capable of recognizing cell damage through its binding to membrane and shielding living cells from damage by reactive oxygen species (ROS) [87]. It is clear that Vtg protects cells from ROS damage in both invertebrates and vertebrates.

It is well known that hen egg yolk Pv, as Vtg-derived major protein, show strong antioxidant activity owing to its high serine and phosphorus content, which makes this protein one of the strongest iron-chelating agents [88–90]. Very recently, we showed that zebrafish recombinant phosvitin (rPv) was an antioxidant agent capable of inhibiting the oxidation of the linoleic acid, and scavenging the 2,2-diphenyl-1-picrylhydrazyl (DPPH) radical. We also showed that zebrafish rPv is a cellular antioxidant capable of protecting radical-mediated oxidation of cellular biomolecules. Importantly, zebrafish rPv is non-cytotoxic to murine macrophages RAW264.7 [91]. These results show that Pv in fish is also a strong antioxidant agent. If Lv, another major Vtg-derived protein, has any antioxidant activity remains open, which is worthwhile exploring.

4. Potential Applications in Human Health

Antibiotics are globally utilized to control microbial infections in clinical practice up to date, however cases of resistance to the majority of antibiotic classes have been reported, which has become a serious threat to human health in many parts of the world [92,93]. It is thus essential to develop new antibiotic agents to combat these resistant pathogens. Antimicrobial proteins/peptides (AMPs) are potential candidates to solve this problem. As a protein/peptide with antimicrobial activity widely present in plants, animals and microbes, AMP commonly is a cationic and amphipathic molecule with a net positive charge and a high percentage of hydrophobic residues [94]. These structure characteristics provide AMP the ability to interact with the anionic cell wall and phospholipid membranes of microorganisms, which makes it more difficult for pathogens to evolve resistance [95]. Vtg and its derived protein Pv from oviparous species, especially teleost fishes, both display antibacterial activities with a broad antibacterial spectrum [59–62,68,71,77–79], and hence can be used as pro-drug to develop novel antibiotic agents. For example, based on the residual sequence of Pt5, the C-terminal peptide of zebrafish Pv, a total of six mutant peptides were generated by a single or double mutagenesis; among them, a mutant called Pt5e showed stronger antibacterial activities against *E. coli* and *S. aureus* [81], and was able to kill five strains of multiple drug resistance bacteria isolated from clinical cases via disturbing their cell membrane integrity (Data not shown).

Sepsis is a serious disease characterized by a systemic inflammatory response syndrome caused by infection. Severe sepsis is complicated by tissue damage and organ dysfunction, which can lead to sequential multi-organ failure followed by death [96]. The primary trigger of sepsis is thought to be LPS, or endotoxin, a major component of the cell wall of Gram-negative bacteria, which is released when bacteria grow or are abolished by antibiotics or host immunity. LPS, as a conserved molecular signature of Gram-negative bacteria, can specifically interact with Vtg, Lv, Pv and their derived peptides [21,61,62,69,71,76,77,79,81], making it possible to utilize these proteins/peptides to develop LPS-neutralizing agents for sepsis treatment. In line with this, both Pv and Pt5e exhibiting LPS-neutralizing ability had been shown to be able to promote the survival rate of endotoxemia mice. Moreover, both Pv and Pt5e displayed neither cytotoxicity to murine RAW264.7 macrophages nor hemolytic activity towards human red blood cells [79,81], suggesting that they can be a safe potential candidate for therapeutics of sepsis.

Antioxidant agents have attracted a great deal of attention in recent years because of their roles in prevention of chronic diseases and utilization as preservatives in food and cosmetics [97–99]. Vtg and its derived Pv both have antioxidant activities against ROS. As these proteins are components of our food source, they are thus natural antioxidant agents. These suggest that they can be can be an important antioxidant with a potential in preservation of food and cosmetics as well as in mediation of chronic disease states.

5. Conclusions

Vtg, the precursor of major egg yolk proteins, is traditionally thought to provide protein- and lipid-rich nutrients for developing embryos and larvae. However, accumulating data indicate that Vtg as well as its derived yolk proteins Lv and Pv also play non-nutritional functions: they are not only involved in immune defense but also antioxidant reaction. These non-nutritional functions clearly better and deepen our understanding of the physiological roles of the molecules, and at the same time, provide a sound basis for potential application of the molecules in human health.

Acknowledgments: This work was supported by Natural Science Foundation of China (No. 31402030; 31372505), Fundamental Research Funds for the Central Universities (201462004), China Postdoctoral Science Foundation (2015T80745; 2014M560580) and Qingdao Municipal Science and Technology Commission (No. 13-1-4-206-jch).

Author Contributions: C. Sun wrote the manuscript. S. C. Zhang read and revised the manuscript.

Conflicts of Interest: The authors declare no conflict of interest.

References

1. Jalabert, B. Particularities of reproduction and oogenesis in teleost fish compared to mammals. *Reprod. Nutr. Dev.* **2005**, *45*, 261–279. [CrossRef] [PubMed]
2. Lubzens, E.; Young, G.; Bobe, J.; Cerda, J. Oogenesis in teleosts: How eggs are formed. *Gen. Comp. Endocrinol.* **2010**, *165*, 367–389. [CrossRef]
3. Patiño, R.; Sullivan, C. Ovarian follicle growth, maturation, and ovulation in teleost fish. *Fish Physiol. Biochem.* **2002**, *26*, 57–70. [CrossRef]
4. Finn, R.N. Vertebrate yolk complexes and the functional implications of phosvitins and other subdomains in vitellogenins. *Biol. Reprod.* **2007**, *76*, 926–935. [CrossRef] [PubMed]
5. Smolenaars, M.M.; Madsen, O.; Rodenburg, K.W.; van der Horst, D.J. Molecular diversity and evolution of the large lipid transfer protein superfamily. *J. Lipid Res.* **2007**, *48*, 489–502. [CrossRef] [PubMed]
6. Avarre, J.C.; Lubzens, E.; Babin, P.J. Apolipocrustacein, formerly vitellogenin, is the major egg yolk precursor protein in decapod crustaceans and is homologous to insect apolipophorin II/I and vertebrate apolipoprotein B. *BMC Evol. Biol.* **2007**, *7*. [CrossRef] [PubMed]
7. Tufail, M.; Takeda, M. Molecular characteristics of insect vitellogenins. *J. Insect Physiol.* **2008**, *54*, 1447–1458. [PubMed]
8. Matozzo, V.; Gagne, F.; Marin, M.G.; Ricciardi, F.; Blaise, C. Vitellogenin as a biomarker of exposure to estrogenic compounds in aquatic invertebrates: A review. *Environ. Int.* **2008**, *34*, 531–545. [PubMed]
9. Wu, L.T.; Hui, J.H.; Chu, K.H. Origin and evolution of yolk proteins: Expansion and functional diversification of large lipid transfer protein superfamily. *Biol. Reprod.* **2013**, *88*. [CrossRef] [PubMed]
10. Finn, R.N.; Kolarevic, J.; Kongshaug, H.; Nilsen, F. Evolution and differential expression of a vertebrate vitellogenin gene cluster. *BMC Evol. Biol.* **2009**, *9*. [CrossRef] [PubMed]
11. Silva, R.; Fischer, A.H.; Burch, J.B. The major and minor chicken vitellogenin genes are each adjacent to partially deleted pseudogene copies of the other. *Mol. Cell. Biol.* **1989**, *9*, 3557–3562. [CrossRef] [PubMed]
12. Van het Schip, F.D.; Samallo, J.; Broos, J.; Ophuis, J.; Mojet, M.; Gruber, M.; Ab, G. Nucleotide sequence of a chicken vitellogenin gene and derived amino acid sequence of the encoded yolk precursor protein. *J. Mol. Biol.* **1987**, *196*, 245–260. [CrossRef]
13. Germond, J.E.; Walker, P.; ten Heggeler, B.; Brown-Luedi, M.; de Bony, E.; Wahli, W. Evolution of vitellogenin genes: Comparative analysis of the nucleotide sequences downstream of the transcription initiation site of four *Xenopus laevis* and one chicken gene. *Nucleic Acids Res.* **1984**, *12*, 8595–8609. [CrossRef] [PubMed]
14. Wahli, W.; Dawid, I.B.; Wyler, T.; Jaggi, R.B.; Weber, R.; Ryffel, G.U. Vitellogenin in *Xenopus laevis* is encoded in a small family of genes. *Cell* **1979**, *16*, 535–549. [CrossRef]
15. Blumenthal, T.; Squire, M.; Kirtland, S.; Cane, J.; Donegan, M.; Spieth, J.; Sharrock, W. Cloning of a yolk protein gene family from *Caenorhabditis elegans*. *J. Mol. Biol.* **1984**, *174*, 1–18. [CrossRef]
16. Wang, H.; Yan, T.; Tan, J.T.; Gong, Z. A zebrafish vitellogenin gene (*vg3*) encodes a novel vitellogenin without a phosvitin domain and may represent a primitive vertebrate vitellogenin gene. *Gene* **2000**, *256*, 303–310. [CrossRef]
17. Wang, H.; Tan, J.T.; Emelyanov, A.; Korzh, V.; Gong, Z. Hepatic and extrahepatic expression of vitellogenin genes in the zebrafish, *Danio rerio*. *Gene* **2005**, *356*, 91–100. [PubMed]
18. Kang, B.J.; Jung, J.H.; Lee, J.M.; Lim, S.G.; Saito, H.; Kim, M.H.; Kim, Y.J.; Saigusa, M.; Han, C.H. Structural and expression analyses of two *vitellogenin* genes in the carp, *Cyprinus carpio*. *Comp. Biochem. Physiol. Part B Biochem. Mol. Biol.* **2007**, *148*, 445–453. [CrossRef] [PubMed]

19. Williams, V.N.; Reading, B.J.; Hiramatsu, N.; Amano, H.; Glassbrook, N.; Hara, A.; Sullivan, C.V. Multiple vitellogenins and product yolk proteins in striped bass, *Morone saxatilis*: Molecular characterization and processing during oocyte growth and maturation. *Fish Physiol. Biochem.* **2014**, *40*, 395–415. [CrossRef] [PubMed]

20. Reading, B.J.; Hiramatsu, N.; Sawaguchi, S.; Matsubara, T.; Hara, A.; Lively, M.O.; Sullivan, C.V. Conserved and variant molecular and functional features of multiple egg yolk precursor proteins (vitellogenins) in white perch (*Morone americana*) and other teleosts. *Mar. Biotechnol.* **2009**, *11*, 169–187. [CrossRef] [PubMed]

21. Sun, C.; Hu, L.; Liu, S.; Gao, Z.; Zhang, S. Functional analysis of domain of unknown function (DUF) 1943, DUF1944 and von Willebrand factor type D domain (VWD) in vitellogenin 2 in zebrafish. *Dev. Comp. Immunol.* **2013**, *41*, 469–476. [CrossRef] [PubMed]

22. Hayward, A.; Takahashi, T.; Bendena, W.G.; Tobe, S.S.; Hui, J.H. Comparative genomic and phylogenetic analysis of vitellogenin and other large lipid transfer proteins in metazoans. *FEBS Lett.* **2010**, *584*, 1273–1278. [CrossRef] [PubMed]

23. Finn, R.N.; Kristoffersen, B.A. Vertebrate vitellogenin gene duplication in relation to the "3R hypothesis": Correlation to the pelagic egg and the oceanic radiation of teleosts. *PLoS ONE* **2007**, *2*, e169. [CrossRef] [PubMed]

24. Meusy, J.J. Vitellogenin, the extraovarian precursor of the protein yolk in Crustacea: A review. *Reprod. Nutr. Dev.* **1980**, *20*, 1–21. [CrossRef] [PubMed]

25. Girish, B.P.; Swetha, C.; Reddy, P.S. Hepatopancreas but not ovary is the site of vitellogenin synthesis in female fresh water crab, *Oziothelphusa senex senex*. *Biochem. Biophys. Res. Commun.* **2014**, *447*, 323–327. [CrossRef] [PubMed]

26. Mak, A.S.; Choi, C.L.; Tiu, S.H.; Hui, J.H.; He, J.G.; Tobe, S.S.; Chan, S.M. Vitellogenesis in the red crab *Charybdis feriatus*: Hepatopancreas-specific expression and farnesoic acid stimulation of vitellogenin gene expression. *Mol. Reprod. Dev.* **2005**, *70*, 288–300. [CrossRef] [PubMed]

27. Kolarevic, J.; Nerland, A.; Nilsen, F.; Finn, R.N. Goldsinny wrasse (*Ctenolabrus rupestris*) is an extreme *vtgAa*-type pelagophil teleost. *Mol. Reprod. Dev.* **2008**, *75*, 1011–1020. [CrossRef] [PubMed]

28. Sawaguchi, S.; Ohkubo, N.; Koya, Y.; Matsubara, T. Incorporation and utilization of multiple forms of vitellogenin and their derivative yolk proteins during vitellogenesis and embryonic development in the mosquitofish, *Gambusia affinis*. *Zool. Sci.* **2005**, *22*, 701–710. [CrossRef] [PubMed]

29. Amano, H.; Fujita, T.; Hiramatsu, N.; Kagawa, H.; Matsubara, T.; Sullivan, C.V.; Hara, A. Multiple vitellogenin-derived yolk proteins in gray mullet (*Mugil cephalus*): Disparate proteolytic patterns associated with ovarian follicle maturation. *Mol. Reprod. Deve.* **2008**, *75*, 1307–1317. [CrossRef] [PubMed]

30. Wallace, R.A.; Selman, K. Ultrastructural aspects of oogenesis and oocyte growth in fish and amphibians. *J. Electron Microsc. Tech.* **1990**, *16*, 175–201. [PubMed]

31. Conner, S.D.; Schmid, S.L. Regulated portals of entry into the cell. *Nature* **2003**, *422*, 37–44. [CrossRef] [PubMed]

32. Hiramatsu, N.; Todo, T.; Sullivan, C.V.; Schilling, J.; Reading, B.J.; Matsubara, T.; Ryu, Y.W.; Mizuta, H.; Luo, W.; Nishimiya, O.; *et al.* Ovarian yolk formation in fishes: Molecular mechanisms underlying formation of lipid droplets and vitellogenin-derived yolk proteins. *Gen. Comp. Endocrinol.* **2015**. [CrossRef] [PubMed]

33. Reading, B.J.; Hiramatsu, N.; Schilling, J.; Molloy, K.T.; Glassbrook, N.; Mizuta, H.; Luo, W.; Baltzegar, D.A.; Williams, V.N.; Todo, T.; *et al.* Lrp13 is a novel vertebrate lipoprotein receptor that binds vitellogenins in teleost fishes. *J. Lipid Res.* **2014**, *55*, 2287–2295. [CrossRef] [PubMed]

34. Reading, B.J.; Hiramatsu, N.; Sullivan, C.V. Disparate binding of three types of vitellogenin to multiple forms of vitellogenin receptor in white perch. *Biol. Reprod.* **2011**, *84*, 392–399. [CrossRef] [PubMed]

35. Williams, V.N.; Reading, B.J.; Amano, H.; Hiramatsu, N.; Schilling, J.; Salger, S.A.; Williams, T.I.; Gross, K.; Sullivan, C.V. Proportional accumulation of yolk proteins derived from multiple vitellogenins is precisely regulated during vitellogenesis in striped bass (*Morone saxatilis*). *J. Exp. Zool. A Ecol. Genet. Physiol.* **2014**, *321*, 301–315. [CrossRef] [PubMed]

36. Romano, M.; Rosanova, P.; Anteo, C.; Limatola, E. Vertebrate yolk proteins: A review. *Mol. Reprod. Dev.* **2004**, *69*, 109–116. [CrossRef] [PubMed]

37. Carnevali, O.; Carletta, R.; Cambi, A.; Vita, A.; Bromage, N. Yolk formation and degradation during oocyte maturation in seabream *Sparus aurata*: Involvement of two lysosomal proteinases. *Biol. Reprod.* **1999**, *60*, 140–146. [CrossRef] [PubMed]

38. Carnevali, O.; Cionna, C.; Tosti, L.; Lubzens, E.; Maradonna, F. Role of cathepsins in ovarian follicle growth and maturation. *Gen. Comp. Endocrinol.* **2006**, *146*, 195–203. [CrossRef] [PubMed]

39. Hiramatsu, N.; Ichikawa, N.; Fukada, H.; Fujita, T.; Sullivan, C.V.; Hara, A. Identification and characterization of proteases involved in specific proteolysis of vitellogenin and yolk proteins in salmonids. *J. Exp. Zool.* **2002**, *292*, 11–25. [CrossRef] [PubMed]

40. Fabra, M.; Cerda, J. Ovarian cysteine proteinases in the teleost *Fundulus heteroclitus*: Molecular cloning and gene expression during vitellogenesis and oocyte maturation. *Mol. Reprod. Dev.* **2004**, *67*, 282–294. [CrossRef] [PubMed]

41. Opresko, L.K.; Karpf, R.A. Specific proteolysis regulates fusion between endocytic compartments in Xenopus oocytes. *Cell* **1987**, *51*, 557–568. [CrossRef]

42. Sire, M.F.; Babin, P.J.; Vernier, J.M. Involvement of the lysosomal system in yolk protein deposit and degradation during vitellogenesis and embryonic development in trout. *J. Exp. Zool.* **1994**, *269*, 69–83. [CrossRef]

43. Retzek, H.; Steyrer, E.; Sanders, E.J.; Nimpf, J.; Schneider, W.J. Molecular cloning and functional characterization of chicken cathepsin D, a key enzyme for yolk formation. *DNA Cell Biol.* **1992**, *11*, 661–672. [CrossRef] [PubMed]

44. Babin, P.J. Apolipoproteins and the association of egg yolk proteins with plasma high density lipoproteins after ovulation and follicular atresia in the rainbow trout (*Salmo gairdneri*). *J. Biol. Chem.* **1987**, *262*, 4290–4296. [PubMed]

45. Matsubara, T.; Ohkubo, N.; Andoh, T.; Sullivan, C.V.; Hara, A. Two forms of vitellogenin, yielding two distinct lipovitellins, play different roles during oocyte maturation and early development of barfin flounder, *Verasper moseri*, a marine teleost that spawns pelagic eggs. *Dev. Biol.* **1999**, *213*, 18–32. [CrossRef] [PubMed]

46. Tyler, C.R.; Sumpter, J.P.; Bromage, N.R. *In vivo* ovarian uptake and processing of vitellogenin in the rainbow trout, *Salmo gairdneri*. *J. Exp. Zool.* **1988**, *246*, 171–179. [CrossRef]

47. Yilmaz, O.; Prat, F.; Ibanez, A.J.; Amano, H.; Koksoy, S.; Sullivan, C.V. Estrogen-induced yolk precursors in European sea bass, *Dicentrarchus labrax*: Status and perspectives on multiplicity and functioning of vitellogenins. *Gen. Comp. Endocrinol.* **2015**. [CrossRef] [PubMed]

48. Finn, R.N.; Fyhn, H.J. Requirement for amino acids in ontogeny of fish. *Aquac. Res.* **2010**, *41*, 684–716. [CrossRef]

49. Arukwe, A.; Goksoyr, A. Eggshell and egg yolk proteins in fish: Hepatic proteins for the next generation: Oogenetic, population, and evolutionary implications of endocrine disruption. *Comp. Hepatol.* **2003**, *2*. [CrossRef]

50. Pan, M.L.; Bell, W.J.; Telfer, W.H. Vitellogenic blood protein synthesis by insect fat body. *Science* **1969**, *165*, 393–394. [CrossRef] [PubMed]

51. Nath, P.; Sundararaj, B.I. Isolation and identification of female-specific serum lipophosphoprotein (vitellogenin) in the catfish, *Heteropneustes fossilis* (Bloch). *Gen. Comp. Endocrinol.* **1981**, *43*, 184–190. [CrossRef]

52. Shyu, A.B.; Raff, R.A.; Blumenthal, T. Expression of the vitellogenin gene in female and male sea urchin. *Proc. Natl. Acad. Sci. USA* **1986**, *83*, 3865–3869. [CrossRef] [PubMed]

53. Piulachs, M.D.; Guidugli, K.R.; Barchuk, A.R.; Cruz, J.; Simoes, Z.L.; Belles, X. The vitellogenin of the honey bee, *Apis mellifera*: Structural analysis of the cdna and expression studies. *Insect Biochem. Mol. Biol.* **2003**, *33*, 459–465. [CrossRef]

54. Scharf, M.E.; Wu-Scharf, D.; Zhou, X.; Pittendrigh, B.R.; Bennett, G.W. Gene expression profiles among immature and adult reproductive castes of the termite *Reticulitermes flavipes*. *Insect Mol. Biol.* **2005**, *14*, 31–44. [CrossRef] [PubMed]

55. Amdam, G.V.; Norberg, K.; Hagen, A.; Omholt, S.W. Social exploitation of vitellogenin. *Proc. Natl. Acad. Sci. USA* **2003**, *100*, 1799–1802. [CrossRef] [PubMed]

56. Amdam, G.V.; Norberg, K.; Page, R.E., Jr.; Erber, J.; Scheiner, R. Downregulation of *vitellogenin* gene activity increases the gustatory responsiveness of honey bee workers (*Apis mellifera*). *Behav. Brain Res.* **2006**, *169*, 201–205. [CrossRef] [PubMed]

57. Guidugli, K.R.; Nascimento, A.M.; Amdam, G.V.; Barchuk, A.R.; Omholt, S.; Simoes, Z.L.; Hartfelder, K. Vitellogenin regulates hormonal dynamics in the worker caste of a eusocial insect. *FEBS Lett.* **2005**, *579*, 4961–4965. [CrossRef] [PubMed]

58. Nelson, C.M.; Ihle, K.E.; Fondrk, M.K.; Page, R.E.; Amdam, G.V. The gene *vitellogenin* has multiple coordinating effects on social organization. *PLoS Biol.* **2007**, *5*, e62. [CrossRef] [PubMed]
59. Zhang, S.; Sun, Y.; Pang, Q.; Shi, X. Hemagglutinating and antibacterial activities of vitellogenin. *Fish Shellfish Immunol.* **2005**, *19*, 93–95. [CrossRef] [PubMed]
60. Shi, X.; Zhang, S.; Pang, Q. Vitellogenin is a novel player in defense reactions. *Fish Shellfish Immunol.* **2006**, *20*, 769–772. [CrossRef] [PubMed]
61. Liu, Q.H.; Zhang, S.C.; Li, Z.J.; Gao, C.R. Characterization of a pattern recognition molecule vitellogenin from carp (*Cyprinus carpio*). *Immunobiology* **2009**, *214*, 257–267. [CrossRef] [PubMed]
62. Wu, B.; Liu, Z.; Zhou, L.; Ji, G.; Yang, A. Molecular cloning, expression, purification and characterization of vitellogenin in scallop *Patinopecten yessoensis* with special emphasis on its antibacterial activity. *Deve. Comp. Immunol.* **2015**, *49*, 249–258. [CrossRef] [PubMed]
63. Fischer, M.; Regitz, C.; Kull, R.; Boll, M.; Wenzel, U. Vitellogenins increase stress resistance of *Caenorhabditis elegans* after *Photorhabdus luminescens* infection depending on the steroid-signaling pathway. *Microbes Infect.* **2013**, *15*, 569–578. [CrossRef] [PubMed]
64. Fischer, M.; Regitz, C.; Kahl, M.; Werthebach, M.; Boll, M.; Wenzel, U. Phytoestrogens genistein and daidzein affect immunity in the nematode *Caenorhabditis elegans* via alterations of vitellogenin expression. *Mol. Nutr. Food Res.* **2012**, *56*, 957–965. [CrossRef] [PubMed]
65. Lu, A.; Hu, X.; Wang, Y.; Shen, X.; Zhu, A.; Shen, L.; Ming, Q.; Feng, Z. Comparative analysis of the acute response of zebrafish *Danio rerio* skin to two different bacterial infections. *J. Aquat. Anim. Health* **2013**, *25*, 243–251. [CrossRef] [PubMed]
66. Lu, A.; Hu, X.; Xue, J.; Zhu, J.; Wang, Y.; Zhou, G. Gene expression profiling in the skin of zebrafish infected with Citrobacter freundii. *Fish Shellfish Immunol.* **2012**, *32*, 273–283. [CrossRef] [PubMed]
67. Nachappa, P.; Levy, J.; Tamborindeguy, C. Transcriptome analyses of *Bactericera cockerelli* adults in response to "*Candidatus* Liberibacter solanacearum" infection. *Mol. Genet. Genom.* **2012**, *287*, 803–817. [CrossRef] [PubMed]
68. Tong, Z.; Li, L.; Pawar, R.; Zhang, S. Vitellogenin is an acute phase protein with bacterial-binding and inhibiting activities. *Immunobiology* **2010**, *215*, 898–902. [CrossRef] [PubMed]
69. Li, Z.; Zhang, S.; Liu, Q. Vitellogenin functions as a multivalent pattern recognition receptor with an opsonic activity. *PLoS ONE* **2008**, *3*, e1940. [CrossRef] [PubMed]
70. Udompetcharaporn, A.; Junkunlo, K.; Senapin, S.; Roytrakul, S.; Flegel, T.W.; Sritunyalucksana, K. Identification and characterization of a QM protein as a possible peptidoglycan recognition protein (PGRP) from the giant tiger shrimp *Penaeus monodon*. *Dev. Comp. Immunol.* **2014**, *46*, 146–154. [CrossRef] [PubMed]
71. Li, Z.; Zhang, S.; Zhang, J.; Liu, M.; Liu, Z. Vitellogenin is a cidal factor capable of killing bacteria via interaction with lipopolysaccharide and lipoteichoic acid. *Mol. Immunol.* **2009**, *46*, 3232–3239. [CrossRef] [PubMed]
72. Bouchard, B.; Gagne, F.; Fortier, M.; Fournier, M. An *in-situ* study of the impacts of urban wastewater on the immune and reproductive systems of the freshwater mussel *Elliptio complanata*. *Comp. Biochem. Physiol. C Toxicol. Pharm.* **2009**, *150*, 132–140. [CrossRef] [PubMed]
73. Liu, M.; Pan, J.; Ji, H.; Zhao, B.; Zhang, S. Vitellogenin mediates phagocytosis through interaction with FcγR. *Mol. Immunol.* **2011**, *49*, 211–218. [CrossRef] [PubMed]
74. Garcia, J.; Munro, E.S.; Monte, M.M.; Fourrier, M.C.; Whitelaw, J.; Smail, D.A.; Ellis, A.E. Atlantic salmon (*Salmo salar* L.) serum vitellogenin neutralises infectivity of infectious pancreatic necrosis virus (IPNV). *Fish Shellfish Immunol.* **2010**, *29*, 293–297. [CrossRef] [PubMed]
75. Rono, M.K.; Whitten, M.M.; Oulad-Abdelghani, M.; Levashina, E.A.; Marois, E. The major yolk protein vitellogenin interferes with the anti-*plasmodium* response in the malaria mosquito *Anopheles gambiae*. *PLoS Biol.* **2010**, *8*, e1000434. [CrossRef] [PubMed]
76. Zhang, J.; Zhang, S. Lipovitellin is a non-self recognition receptor with opsonic activity. *Mar. Biotechnol.* **2011**, *13*, 441–450. [CrossRef] [PubMed]
77. Wang, S.; Wang, Y.; Ma, J.; Ding, Y.; Zhang, S. Phosvitin plays a critical role in the immunity of zebrafish embryos via acting as a pattern recognition receptor and an antimicrobial effector. *J. Biol. Chem.* **2011**, *286*, 22653–22664. [CrossRef] [PubMed]

78. Sattar Khan, M.A.; Nakamura, S.; Ogawa, M.; Akita, E.; Azakami, H.; Kato, A. Bactericidal action of egg yolk phosvitin against *Escherichia coli* under thermal stress. *J. Agric. Food Chem.* **2000**, *48*, 1503–1506. [CrossRef] [PubMed]

79. Ma, J.; Wang, H.; Wang, Y.; Zhang, S. Endotoxin-neutralizing activity of hen egg phosvitin. *Mol. Immunol.* **2013**, *53*, 355–362. [CrossRef] [PubMed]

80. Ding, Y.; Liu, X.; Bu, L.; Li, H.; Zhang, S. Antimicrobial-immunomodulatory activities of zebrafish phosvitin-derived peptide Pt5. *Peptides* **2012**, *37*, 309–313. [CrossRef] [PubMed]

81. Hu, L.; Sun, C.; Wang, S.; Su, F.; Zhang, S. Lipopolysaccharide neutralization by a novel peptide derived from phosvitin. *Int. J. Biochem. Cell Biol.* **2013**, *45*, 2622–2631. [CrossRef] [PubMed]

82. Sun, C.; Hu, L.; Liu, S.; Hu, G.; Zhang, S. Antiviral activity of phosvitin from zebrafish *Danio rerio*. *Deve. Comp. Immunol.* **2013**, *40*, 28–34. [CrossRef] [PubMed]

83. Ando, S.; Yanagida, K. Susceptibility to oxidation of copper-induced plasma lipoproteins from Japanese eel: Protective effect of vitellogenin on the oxidation of very low density lipoprotein. *Comp. Biochem. Physiol. Part C Pharmacol. Toxicol. Endocrinol.* **1999**, *123*, 1–7. [CrossRef]

84. Nakamura, A.; Yasuda, K.; Adachi, H.; Sakurai, Y.; Ishii, N.; Goto, S. Vitellogenin-6 is a major carbonylated protein in aged nematode, Caenorhabditis elegans. *Biochem. Biophys. Res. Commun.* **1999**, *264*, 580–583. [CrossRef] [PubMed]

85. Seehuus, S.C.; Norberg, K.; Gimsa, U.; Krekling, T.; Amdam, G.V. Reproductive protein protects functionally sterile honey bee workers from oxidative stress. *Proc. Natl. Acad. Sci. USA* **2006**, *103*, 962–967. [CrossRef] [PubMed]

86. Corona, M.; Velarde, R.A.; Remolina, S.; Moran-Lauter, A.; Wang, Y.; Hughes, K.A.; Robinson, G.E. Vitellogenin, juvenile hormone, insulin signaling, and queen honey bee longevity. *Proc. Natl. Acad. Sci. USA* **2007**, *104*, 7128–7133. [CrossRef] [PubMed]

87. Havukainen, H.; Munch, D.; Baumann, A.; Zhong, S.; Halskau, O.; Krogsgaard, M.; Amdam, G.V. Vitellogenin recognizes cell damage through membrane binding and shields living cells from reactive oxygen species. *J. Biol. Chem.* **2013**, *288*, 28369–28381. [CrossRef] [PubMed]

88. Lu, C.L.; Baker, R.C. Characteristics of egg yolk phosvitin as an antioxidant for inhibiting metal-catalyzed phospholipid oxidations. *Poult. Sci.* **1986**, *65*, 2065–2070. [CrossRef] [PubMed]

89. Ishikawa, S.; Yano, Y.; Arihara, K.; Itoh, M. Egg yolk phosvitin inhibits hydroxyl radical formation from the fenton reaction. *Biosci. Biotechnol. Biochem.* **2004**, *68*, 1324–1331. [CrossRef] [PubMed]

90. Guérin-Dubiard, C.; Anton, M.; Dhene-Garcia, A.; Martinet, V.; Brulé, G. Hen egg and fish egg phosvitins: Composition and iron binding properties. *Eur. Food Res. Technol.* **2002**, *214*, 460–464. [CrossRef]

91. Hu, L.; Sun, C.; Luan, J.; Lu, L.; Zhang, S. Zebrafish phosvitin is an antioxidant with non-cytotoxic activity. *Acta Biochim. Biophys. Sin.* **2015**, *47*, 349–354. [CrossRef] [PubMed]

92. Maria-Neto, S.; de Almeida, K.C.; Macedo, M.L.; Franco, O.L. Understanding bacterial resistance to antimicrobial peptides: From the surface to deep inside. *Biochim. Biophys. Acta* **2015**. [CrossRef] [PubMed]

93. Grundmann, H.; Klugman, K.P.; Walsh, T.; Ramon-Pardo, P.; Sigauque, B.; Khan, W.; Laxminarayan, R.; Heddini, A.; Stelling, J. A framework for global surveillance of antibiotic resistance. *Drug Resist. Updates* **2011**, *14*, 79–87. [CrossRef] [PubMed]

94. Wiesner, J.; Vilcinskas, A. Antimicrobial peptides: The ancient arm of the human immune system. *Virulence* **2010**, *1*, 440–464. [CrossRef] [PubMed]

95. Brown, K.L.; Hancock, R.E. Cationic host defense (antimicrobial) peptides. *Curr. Opin. Immunol.* **2006**, *18*, 24–30. [CrossRef] [PubMed]

96. Uppu, D.S.; Ghosh, C.; Haldar, J. Surviving sepsis in the era of antibiotic resistance: Are there any alternative approaches to antibiotic therapy? *Microb. Pathog.* **2015**, *80*, 7–13. [CrossRef] [PubMed]

97. Knight, J.A. The biochemistry of aging. *Adv. Clin. Chem.* **2000**, *35*, 1–62. [PubMed]

98. Lupo, M.P. Antioxidants and vitamins in cosmetics. *Clin. Dermatol.* **2001**, *19*, 467–473. [CrossRef]

99. Bonilla, J.; Atares, L.; Chiralt, A.; Vargas, M. Recent patents on the use of antioxidant agents in food. *Recent Pat. Food Nutr. Agric.* **2011**, *3*, 123–132. [CrossRef] [PubMed]

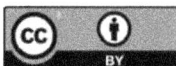

nutrients

MDPI

Review

The Nutraceutical Properties of Ovotransferrin and Its Potential Utilization as a Functional Food

Francesco Giansanti [1,2,*], Loris Leboffe [2,3], Francesco Angelucci [1] and Giovanni Antonini [2,3]

1   Department of Health, Life and Environmental Sciences, University of L'Aquila, L'Aquila I-67100, Italy; francesco.angelucci@univaq.it
2   Interuniversity Consortium INBB Biostructures and Biosystems National Institute, Rome I-00136, Italy; loris.leboffe@uniroma3.it (L.L.); giovanni.antonini@uniroma3.it (G.A.)
3   Department of Sciences, Roma Tre University, Rome I-00146, Italy
*   Correspondence: francesco.giansanti@cc.univaq.it; Tel.: +39-0862-433245; Fax: +39-0862-433273

Received: 29 September 2015; Accepted: 23 October 2015; Published: 4 November 2015

Abstract: Ovotransferrin or conalbumin belong to the transferrin protein family and is endowed with both iron-transfer and protective activities. In addition to its well-known antibacterial properties, ovotransferrin displays other protective roles similar to those already ascertained for the homologous mammalian lactoferrin. These additional functions, in many cases not directly related to iron binding, are also displayed by the peptides derived from partial hydrolysis of ovotransferrin, suggesting a direct relationship between egg consumption and human health.

Keywords: ovotransferrin; nutraceutical; functional food; antioxidant

1. Introduction

Ovotransferrin (Otrf) or conalbumin belongs to the family of transferrin iron-binding glycoproteins. In mammals, two different soluble iron-binding glycoproteins are present: (i) serum transferrin, involved in iron transport and delivery to cells and (ii) lactoferrin, involved in the so-called natural immunity. Differently, Otrf is the only soluble glycoprotein of the transferrin protein family present in avian. Otrf is present both in avian plasma and egg white and possesses both iron-transfer and protective properties [1]. Otrf represents about 12%–13% of total egg white proteins and contributes to promoting the growth and development of the chicken embryo mainly preventing the growth of micro-organisms together with other proteins such as lysozyme [2], cystatin [3,4], ovomacroglobulin [5] and avidin [6]. Galliformes (chicken, *Gallus gallus* and turkey, *Meleagris gallopavo*) appear to possess albumens with greater antimicrobial activity than those of the anseriformes (duck, *Anas platyrhynchos*), possibly due to higher concentrations of ovotransferrin and of the broad active c-type lysozyme [7]. However, recent evidence indicates that Otrf is endowed not only with the antibacterial activity related to iron withholding, but also with other roles related to the protection of the growing embryo, including: regulation of iron absorption; immune response; and anti-bacterial, anti-viral and anti-inflammatory properties. Some of these properties are shared by both the human protein homologues and peptides deriving from its partial enzymatic hydrolysis [8], being in this latter case also increased.

The state of the art hereby described suggests that Otrf and its peptides can be used as functional food ingredients and as important components for nutraceuticals, being characterized both by protective functions and by substantial nutritional benefits; for these reasons, the utilization of Otrf and its peptides in functional foods can present several additional advantages over other natural compounds.

2. Ovotransferrin Synthesis and Structure

Otrf is a monomeric glycoprotein containing 686 amino acids, with a molecular weight of 77.9 kDa and an isoelectric point of 6.0 [9,10].

The avian transferrin gene is transcripted in the liver and the oviduct. In the liver, the transferrin is secreted in the serum, where it is involved in iron transport and storage, while the oviduct transferrin (ovotransferrin) is secreted at high levels in the egg white. In particular, progesterone and oestrogen regulate the expression of Otrf in the oviduct: oestrogen can interact with chromatin through a nuclear receptor protein stimulating transcription and synthesis of the protein precursor [11]. Instead, the transcription of serum Otrf may depend on iron concentration [12]. Although the serum transferrin and Otrf have the same amino acidic sequence, they differ in the glycosylation sites. The glycan of Otrf is constituted by four residues of mannose and four residues of N-acetylglucosamine whereas serum transferrin is composed of two residues of mannose, two residues of galactose, three residues of N-acetylglucosamine, and one or two residues of sialic acid at its C-terminus [13–15].

Like the mammalian transferrins, the single chain of Otrf consists of two globular lobes (N- and C-lobes), interconnected by a α-helix of nine amino acidic residues (residues 333–341) that can be released by tryptic digestion. Each lobe contains an iron binding site and is divided in two domains, (domains N1 and N2 in the N-lobe and domains C1 and C2 in the C-lobe, respectively; Figure 1A) [16–18].

As shown in Figure 1, the domains are linked by anti-paralleled β-strands. The N- and C-lobes show about 38% sequence homology; indeed, it is has been hypothesized that all members of transferrin family resulted from gene fusion and duplication [19]. Fifteen disulfide bridges stabilize the structure. Six of them are conserved in both lobes, while three are present only in the C-lobe, conferring to the lobes a different metal affinity.

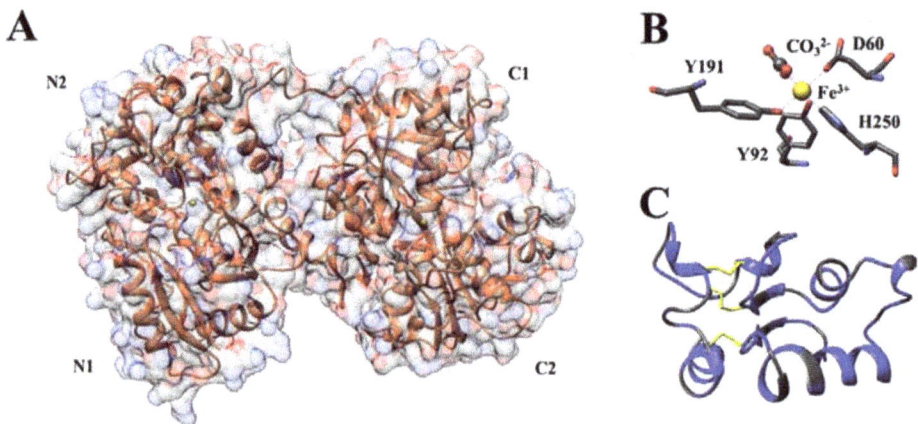

Figure 1. (**A**) Ribbon representation and the solvent-accessible surface (in transparency) of holo-Otrf (PDB ID:1OVT) [16]. N1, N2 and C1, C2 indicate the subdomains of each lobe. (**B**) The N-lobe iron binding site of hen's ovotransferrin (PDB ID:1OVT). The amino acids involved in iron binding are shown in sticks. H-bonds are displayed by purple broken lines. Both in (**A**) and (**B**), the iron is indicated as a yellow sphere. (**C**) Schematic ribbon representation of the OTAP-92 peptide. The three disulfide linkages are represented in yellow, while the hydrophobic residues are highlighted in blue. The peptide is shown with the same conformation displayed in the intact protein. Molecular graphic images were produced using the UCSF chimera package [20].

Each lobe has the capability to reversibly bind one Fe^{3+} ion along with one CO_3^{2-} anion. Although each lobe displays a high sequence homology, they show different iron-binding properties. In particular, the (approximate) iron binding affinity is 1.5×10^{18} M^{-1} for the C-lobe and 1.5×10^{14} M^{-1} for the N-lobe. As mentioned before, this difference is due to the presence, in the C-lobe, of an extra interdomain disulfide bond, Cys478-Cys671, which confers less flexibility and possibly less affinity towards Fe^{3+} ion [21].

From a stereochemical point of view, the iron binding pocket is conserved among all members of transferrins [16–18,22–24]. As shown in Figure 1B, in the N-lobe there are two phenolate oxygens of two tyrosine residues (Tyr92 and Tyr191), a carboxylate oxygen of the aspartic acid (Asp60), and the imidazole nitrogen of the histidine (His250), together with two oxygens of the synergistically bound $CO_3{}^{2-}$ anion. In C-lobe, the corresponding amino acids are Asp 395, Tyr524, Tyr431 and His592, respectively. In this latter, Arg460 keeps in place the carbonate moiety while in the N-lobe Arg121 plays the same role. Upon iron binding, each lobe of Otrf undergoes large conformational change; the observed movement is necessary to bury the metal inside the polypeptide chain given that, in its absence, the iron-coordinating amino acidic residues are solvent exposed.

3. Antibacterial Activity of Ovotransferrin and Its Peptides

Among the several protective functions of Otrf, the most important one is likely to be the antibacterial activity, which is directly related to the Otrf's ability to bind iron (Fe^{3+}), making it unavailable for bacterial growth [25,26]. This bacteriostatic activity is reversed by adding iron ions to the medium and it is blocked by iron saturation [27]; moreover, it can be enhanced by (i) adding carbonate ion [28] which is one of the iron ligands in the Otrf metal binding site [29]; (ii) increasing the pH from 6 to 8 [27]; (iii) and immobilizing Otrf by covalent linkage to Sepharose 4B [30]. An increase of the bacteriostatic activity towards *E. coli* O157:H7 as iron chelator was demonstrated using a combination of ovotransferrin, NaHCO$_3$, and EDTA [31]. The antibacterial activity was demonstrated also in an *in vivo* study using newborn guinea pigs orally infected with *E. coli* 0111 B4 [32]. On the contrary, citrate exerts an antagonistic effect in those bacteria that possess a receptor for iron-citrate complex [32]. The most sensitive species to the iron deprivation effect of Otrf are *Pseudomonas* spp., *Escherichia coli*, *Streptococcus mutans*, while the most resistant ones are *Proteus* spp., and *Klebsiella* spp. [32], according to the ability of these latter bacteria to produce molecules (*i.e.*, siderophores) able to compete with Otrf for iron binding. However, it is worth noting that some bacterial species that are also human pathogens, e.g., *Neisseria meningitidis*, *Neisseria gonorrhoeae* and *Moraxella catarrhalis*, have developed a mechanism for acquiring iron directly from transferrin-like proteins through surface receptors capable of specifically binding ovotransferrin [33].

Other studies suggested that part of the antibacterial activity of Otrf is not simply due to the removal of iron from the medium, but also involves more complex mechanisms related to a direct binding of Otrf to the bacterial surface. As a matter of fact, it has been initially demonstrated that the antibacterial activity of Otrf decreased when the protein is separated by dialysis from the bacteria, a condition in which it can exert only the iron-chelating property [34]. Accordingly, it was shown that Otrf is able to permeate the *E. coli* outer membrane and access the inner membrane, causing both ion leakage inside bacteria and the uncoupling of the respiration-dependent energy production [35]. The antibacterial effect of Otrf towards *Salmonella enterica* (*serovar Choleraesuis*) has been also demonstrated to be dependent on culture conditions that either favor or hinder binding Otrf to the bacterial surface [36]. These data suggest that this Otrf function, not related to iron binding, could be due to a cationic bactericidal domain which, as other transferrins, is located in the N-lobe [35].

The isolation of the bactericidal domain of Otrf, was carried out by Zhou and Smith in 1990 by a partial acid proteolysis. OTAP-92 is a peptide of 9.9 kDa, consisting of 92 aminoacidic residues (Leu109-Asp200) showing strong sequence similarity with defensins [37]. This peptide is characterized by three disulfide bridges (Cys115-Cys197, Cys160-174, and Cys171-Cys182) and several positively charged residues (Figure 1, panel C).

It has been suggested that the antibacterial action of OTAP-92 may be due to its relatively high alkalinity and to the cysteine array. Both these features are shared by native antibacterial peptides [38,39] and by insect defensins whose mechanism of action involves the blocking of the voltage-dependent K$^+$ channels [38–42].

As concerning the possible biotechnological applications of the Otrf antibacterial activity, Ko and coworkers [31] showed that a combination of Otrf, NaHCO$_3$, EDTA and/or Lysozyme have a potential growth inhibition effect against *E. coli* O157:H7 or *L. monocytogenes*, demonstrating also a potential application of Otrf as a natural preservative for food (*i.e.*, pork chops and commercial hams) [31,43,44].

4. Antiviral Activity of Ovotransferrin and Its Peptides

The antiviral activity of Otrf was firstly demonstrated towards the avian herpesvirus Marek's disease virus (MDV), and no correlation between antiviral efficacy and iron saturation was found [45]. It has been postulated that the ovotransferrin antiviral activity towards MDV is associated with two Otrf fragments: DQKDEYELL (hOtrf219-27) and KDLLFK (hOtrf269-301 and hOtrf633-638) capable of blocking Marek's disease virus infection in chicken embryo fibroblasts (CEF), even though the infection blocking efficiency of the isolated peptides is lower than that of the intact protein [46]. Interestingly, from an evolutionary point of view, these two Otrf peptides share sequence homology with two protein fragments, derived from human and bovine lactoferrin, known to be effective against *Herpes simplex* Virus (HSV-1) [47].

5. Antioxidant Activity of Ovotransferrin and Its Peptides

Ovotransferrin is a superoxide dismutase-mimicking protein exhibiting a superoxide radical (O$_2$$^{•-}$)-scavenging activity. Furthermore, self-cleaved Otrf exhibited O$_2$$^{•-}$ scavenging capacity greater than intact protein [48,49]. Accordingly, it has been shown that, after digestion by thermolysin and pepsin, the resulting Otrf hydrolysates possessed significantly higher oxygen radical absorption capacity (1.69 µmol Trolox equivalent mg^{-1}) than natural ovotransferrin [50].

Kim and coworkers [51] demonstrated that the antioxidant effects of hen's ovotransferrin and of its hydrolyzed peptides is approximately 3.2–13.5 times higher than superoxide anion scavenging activity than Otrf, with the maximum activity displayed by octapeptides. Similar results were obtained for oxygen radical absorbance capacity assay and against the oxidative stress-induced DNA damage in human leukocytes [51]. In addition, Otrf-derived peptides showed synergistic antioxidant effects with Vitamin C, epigallocatechin gallate (EGCG), and caffeic acid [52]. Otrf hydrolyzate (obtained using enzymes such as protamex, alkalase, trypsin, and α-chymotrypsin) showed protective effects against oxidative stress including DNA damage in human leukocytes [53].

The conjugation of ovotransferrin with catechin (a polyphenol antioxidant found in tea, wine, fruits, with high affinity to bind protein) improved the oxygen radical absorbance capacity of the protein. The ovotransferrin-catechin conjugates were prepared using a hydrogen peroxide–ascorbic acid pair as radical initiator system and alkaline method [54]. Moreover, it has been also shown that catechin, after the conjugation reaction and after UPLC (Ultra-Performance Liquid Chromatography), MALDI-TOF (Matrix Assisted Laser Desorption Ionization Time-of-Flight) and Liquid chromatography-tandem mass spectrometry (LC-MS-MS) analysis, was bound to lysine (residues 327) of the Otrf peptide DLLFKDSAIMLK (residues 316–327) and to glutamic acid (residues 186) of the Otrf peptide FFSASCVPGATIE (residues 174–186) present in ovotransferrin N-lobe [54].

Autocleaved Otrf was shown to (i) hinder effectively the discoloration of ß-carotene (used as radical target in a bleaching test); (ii) prevent the oxidation of linoleic acid during five days of storage at 4 °C; and (iii) show strong Cu^{2+}- and Ca^{2+}-binding capacities, suggesting that it could be a good source of natural antioxidants. Once again, its metal-chelating activity could be at least partly responsible for the observed antioxidant mechanisms [55].

In conclusion, the use of Otrf-derived conjugates as a novel proteinaceous antioxidants as ingredient in the nutraceutical and functional food is desirable.

6. Anti-Inflammatory Activities of Ovotransferrin and Its Peptides

During inflammation in avians, Otrf, as well as the positive acute phase protein (APP), is up-regulated both *in vivo* and *in vitro* [56–63]; its levels in blood remain elevated as long as the inflammation persists [64,65]. Indeed, the use of blood Otrf concentration as an infection and inflammation marker in chickens has been hypothesized [66]. Otrf may act directly as an immunomodulator [63], even though its role in inflammation preventing microbial growth [67] and acting as an antioxidant against Fenton reaction products [36] cannot be ruled out.

More recently, two tripeptides, IRW and IQW, both derived from Otrf hydrolysis, were found to attenuate TNF-α-induced inflammatory responses and oxidative stress in vascular endothelial cells [68]. Furthermore, other peptides derived from ovomucoid showed an immunomodulating activity against T-cells and macrophage-stimulating activities *in vitro* [69], indicating that they also can be good candidates for pharmaceutical use in humans [70].

7. Other Protective Activities of Ovotransferrin and Its Peptides

In the last years, it has been reported that Otrf underwent thiol-linked auto-cleavage after reduction, and produced partially hydrolyzed products with very strong anticancer effects against colon (HCT-116) and breast cancer (MCF-7) by inducting apoptosis [71].

An antihypertensive subsidiary function of the Otrf was detected in the hen Otrf's peptide KVREGT, showing an IC_{50} value of 9.1 µM towards angiotensin I-converting enzyme [72]. Moreover, the same peptide displayed both a strong ACE-inhibitory and a vasodilatory activities [73].

Ovotransferrin has also shown both *in vitro* and *in vivo* development promoting activity, which has been associated to its iron binding/transport capabilities. Ovotransferrin is transiently expressed and secreted in large amounts during the *in vitro* differentiation of hypertrophic chondrocytes into osteoblast-like cells. Cells expressing ovotransferrin also co-express ovotransferrin receptors, suggesting a self-regulatory mechanism in the control of chondrocyte differentiation to osteoblast-like cells [74–79].

Otrf shares with human and bovine lactoferrin a proteolytic activity catalyzing the hydrolysis of several synthetic substrates [80]. Serine protease inhibitors PMSF (phenylmethylsulfonyl fluoride), LPS (lipopolysaccharide) and Pefabloc impair this proteolytic activity suggesting that it is similar to that of serine proteases [81,82]. This function is conserved in several mammalian lactoferrins but not in serum transferrins, and thus it is plausible that it belongs to the protective functions of Otrf, although the physiological target has not been identified, yet.

Lastly, Ibrahim *et al.* [83] demonstrated the efficiency of Otrf to serve as a drug carrier to improve the solubility of three water-insoluble antibiotics and to facilitate their specific delivery into microbial or infected cells. For a complete overview of the Otrf properties, see Table 1.

Table 1. Physiological and pharmacological activities of Ovotransferrin (Otrf) and its peptides identified to-date.

PROTEIN OR PEPTIDE	ACTIVITY	MECHANISM/S	REFERENCES
	ANTIMICROBIAL		
Ovotransferrin (whole molecule)	BACTERIAL SENSITIVITY (BACTERIOSTATIC)	• Otrf iron Binding (Iron withholding)	[25,27,30,32]
	BACTERIAL SENSITIVITY (BACTERICIDAL)	• Membrane damage	[7,25,32]

Table 1. *Cont.*

PROTEIN OR PEPTIDE	ACTIVITY	MECHANISM/S	REFERENCES
	ANTIMICROBIAL		
Ovotransferrin (whole molecule)	BACTERIAL RESISTANCE	• Bacterial production of Iron chelators or Tbp1 and 2	[33]
	ANTIBACTERIAL (FOOD PRESERVATIVE)	• In combination with EDTA and/or Lysozyme prevents *E. coli* O157:H7 or *L. monocytogenes*, proliferation	[43]
	ANTIVIRAL	• Viral adsorption inhibition	[45]
	ANTIOXIDANT	• Iron Binding • SuperOxide Dismutase (SOD)-like activity • Fenton's reaction inhibition • Catechin conjugation	[49,50]
	FLOGOSIS MARKER	• Otrf Belongs to Acute Phase Proteins (APP). • Recognition and protection against invading pathogens, and restoration of the physiological homeostasis. • Otrf upregulation of interleukin-6, nitric oxide, and matrix metalloproteinase.	[61,63,64,66]
	IMMUNE/ANTI-INFLAMMATION	• Modulation of macrophages and heterophils functions. • SOD-Like Activity	[49,63,64]
	PROTEOLYTIC	• Hydrolysis of Haemophilus colonization factors and of several synthetic substrates	[80]

Table 1. *Cont.*

PROTEIN OR PEPTIDE	ACTIVITY	MECHANISM/S	REFERENCES
	ANTIMICROBIAL GROWTH FACTOR:		
Ovotransferrin (whole molecule)	CARTILAGE NEOVASCULARIZATION	• Chemotactic factor for endothelial cells. • Iron delivery	[59]
	CHONDROGENESIS AND OSTEOGNESIS REGULATION	• Iron delivery	[77,78]
	MYOTROPHIC	• Iron delivery	[74]
	NEUROTROPHYC	• Iron delivery	[79]
	CARRIER FOR DRUG DELIVERY	• Binding and delivery of water insoluble antibiotics (sulphantibiotics)	[83]
Otrf peptide OTAP-92	ANTIMICROBIAL	• Bacterial Membrane damage	[41]
Otrf peptides219–227; 269–301; 633–638	ANTIVIRAL	• Viral adsorption inhibition	[46]
Reduced autocleaved Otrf (rac-Otrf)	ANTICANCER/ANTIPROLIFERATION	• Apoptosis induction	[71]
	ANTIOXIDANT	• Autocleaved Otrf as preservative to prevent ß-carotene discoloration	[55]
Otrf Peptides (IRW or IQW)	ANTINFLAMMATORY	• Attenuate TNF-α-induced inflammatory responses	[68]
Otrf peptide (KVREGT)	ANTIHYPERTENSIVE	• Inhibition of Angiotensin I-Converting Enzyme.	[72,73]
Otrf Peptides (DLLFKDSAIMLK) (FFSASCVPGATIE)	ANTIOXIDANT	• Catechin conjugation	[54]
Otrf peptides (mix obtained using: protamex, or alkalase, or trypsin, or α-chymotrypsin)	ANTIOXIDANT	• Synergistic antioxidant effects with vitamin C, epigallocatechin gallate (EGCG), and caffeic acid.	[52,53]

8. Conclusions

Many of the Otrf's protective properties, described in this review and outlined in Table 1, contribute, in addition to the well-known iron transfer activity, to the proper development of the chicken embryo. Moreover, the demonstration that several defensive properties of Otrf are also possessed by its proteolytic fragments and that these properties may be of importance for human wellness strongly support the use of egg white (preferably raw or cooked at low temperature to preserve ovotransferrin properties) and its derivatives as dietary additives in normal and pathological human conditions.

Author Contributions: The authors warrant that all of the authors have contributed substantially to the manuscript and approved the final submission.

Conflicts of Interest: The authors warrant the absence of any real or perceived conflicts of interest.

References

1. Giansanti, F.; Leboffe, L.; Pitari, G.; Ippoliti, R.; Antonini, G. Physiological roles of ovotransferrin. *Biochim. Biophys. Acta* **2012**, *1820*, 218–225. [CrossRef] [PubMed]
2. Deeming, D.C. Behavior patterns during incubation. In *Avian Incubation: Behaviour, Environment, and Evolution*; Deeming, D.C., Ed.; Oxford University Press: Oxford, UK, 2002; pp. 63–87.
3. Saxena, I.; Tayyab, S. Protein proteinase inhibitors from avian egg whites. *Cell. Mol. Life Sci.* **1997**, *53*, 13–23. [CrossRef] [PubMed]
4. Wesierska, E.; Saleh, Y.; Trziska, T.; Kopec, W.; Sierwinski, M.; Korzekwa, K. Antimicrobial activity of chicken egg white cystatin. *World J. Microbiol. Biotechnol.* **2005**, *21*, 59–64. [CrossRef]
5. Miyagawa, S.; Matsumaoto, K.; Kamata, R.; Okamura, R.; Maeda, H. Spreading of *Serratia marcescens* in experimental keratitis and growth suppression by chicken egg white ovomacroglobulin. *Jpn. J. Ophthalmol.* **1991**, *35*, 402–410. [PubMed]
6. Board, P.A.; Fuller, R. Non-specific antimicrobial defences of the avian egg, embryo and neonate. *Biol. Rev. Camb. Philos. Soc.* **1974**, *49*, 15–49. [CrossRef] [PubMed]
7. Wellman-Labadie, O.; Picman, J.; Hinke, M.T. Comparative antibacterial activity of avian egg white protein extracts. *Br. Poult. Sci.* **2008**, *49*, 125–132. [CrossRef] [PubMed]
8. Walther, B.; Sieber, R. Bioactive proteins and peptides in foods. *Int. J. Vitam. Nutr. Res.* **2011**, *81*, 181–192. [CrossRef] [PubMed]
9. Jeltsch, J.M.; Chambon, P. The complete nucleotide sequence of the chicken ovotransferrin mRNA. *Eur. J. Biochem.* **1982**, *122*, 291–295. [CrossRef] [PubMed]
10. Williams, J.; Elleman, T.C.; Kingston, I.B.; Wilkins, A.G.; Kuhn, K.A. The primary structure of hen ovotransferrin. *Eur. J. Biochem.* **1982**, *122*, 297–303. [CrossRef] [PubMed]
11. Sutherland, R.L.; Geynet, C.; Binart, N.; Catelli, M.G.; Schmelck, P.H.; Mester, J.; Lebeau, M.C.; Baulieu, E.E. Steroid receptors and effects of oestradiol and progesterone on chick oviduct proteins. *Eur. J. Biochem.* **1980**, *107*, 155–164. [CrossRef] [PubMed]
12. Dierich, A.; Gaub, M.P.; LePennec, J.P.; Astinotti, D.; Chambon, P. Cell-specificity of the chicken ovalbumin and conalbumin promoters. *EMBO J.* **1987**, *6*, 2305–2312. [PubMed]
13. Williams, J. A comparison of glycopeptides from the ovotransferrin and serum transferrin of the hen. *Biochem. J.* **1968**, *108*, 57–67. [CrossRef] [PubMed]
14. Iwase, H.; Hotta, K. Ovotransferrin subfractionation dependent upon chain differences. *J. Biol. Chem.* **1977**, *252*, 5437–5443. [PubMed]
15. Jacquinot, P.M.; Leger, D.; Wieruszeski, J.M.; Coddeville, B.; Montreuil, J.; Spik, G. Change in glycosylation of chicken transferrin glycans biosynthesized during embryogenesis and primary culture of embryo hepatocytes. *Glycobiology* **1994**, *4*, 617–624. [CrossRef] [PubMed]
16. Kurokawa, H.; Mikami, B.; Hirose, M. Crystal structure of diferric hen ovotransferrin at 2.4 Å resolution. *J. Mol. Biol.* **1995**, *254*, 196–207. [CrossRef] [PubMed]

17. Kurokawa, H.; Dewan, J.C.; Mikami, B.; Sacchettini, J.C.; Hirose, M. Crystal structure of hen apo-ovotransferrin: Both lobes adopt an open conformation upon loss of iron. *J. Biol. Chem.* **1999**, *274*, 28445–28452. [CrossRef] [PubMed]

18. Thakurta, G.P.; Choudhury, D.; Dasgupta, R.; Dattagupta, J.K. Structure of diferric hen serum transferrin at 2.8 Å resolution. *Acta Crystallogr. Sect. D* **2003**, *59*, 1773–1781. [CrossRef]

19. Williams, J. The evolution of transferrins. *Trends Biochem. Sci.* **1982**, *7*, 394–397. [CrossRef]

20. Pettersen, E.F.; Goddard, T.D.; Huang, C.C.; Couch, G.S.; Greenblatt, D.M.; Meng, E.C.; Ferrin, T.E. UCSF Chimera—A visualization system for exploratory research and analysis. *J. Comput. Chem.* **2004**, *25*, 1605–1612. [CrossRef] [PubMed]

21. Williams, J.; Moreton, K.; Goodearl, A.D. Selective reduction of a disulphide bridge in hen ovotransferrin. *Biochem. J.* **1985**, *228*, 661–665. [CrossRef] [PubMed]

22. Mizutani, K.; Yamashita, H.; Kurokawa, H.; Mikami, B.; Mikami, B. Alternative structural state of transferrin. The crystallographic analysis of iron-loaded but domain-opened ovotransferrin N-lobe. *J. Biol. Chem.* **1999**, *274*, 10190–10194. [CrossRef] [PubMed]

23. Lindley, P.F.; Bajaj, M.; Evans, R.W.; Garatt, R.C.; Hasnain, S.S.; Jhoti, H.; Kuser, P.; Neu, M.; Patel, K.; Sarra, R.; *et al.* The mechanism of iron uptake by transferrins: The structure of an 18 kDa NII-domain fragment from duck ovotransferrin at 2.3 Å resolution. *Acta Crystallogr. Sect. D* **1993**, *49*, 292–304. [CrossRef] [PubMed]

24. Kuser, P.; Hall, D.R.; Haw, M.L.; Neu, M.; Evans, R.W.; Lindley, P.F. The mechanism of iron uptake by transferrins: The X-ray structures of the 18 kDa NII domain fragment of duck ovotransferrin and its nitrilotriacetate complex. *Acta Crystallogr. Sect. D* **2002**, *58*, 777–783. [CrossRef]

25. Alderton, G.; Ward, W.H.; Fevold, H.L. Identification of the bacteria-inhibiting iron-binding protein of egg white as conalbumin. *Arch. Biochem.* **1946**, *11*, 9–13. [PubMed]

26. Bullen, J.J.; Rogers, H.J.; Griffiths, E. Role of iron in bacterial infection. *Curr. Top. Microbiol. Immunol.* **1978**, *80*, 1–35. [PubMed]

27. Antonini, E.; Orsi, N.; Valenti, P. Effetto delle transferrine sulla patogenicità delle Enterobacteriaceae. *G. Mal. Infett. Parassit.* **1977**, *29*, 481–489.

28. Valenti, P.; de Stasio, A.; Mastromarino, P.; Seganti, L.; Sinibaldi, L.; Orsi, N. Influence of bicarbonate and citrate on the bacteriostatic action of ovotransferrin towards staphylococci. *FEMS Microbiol. Lett.* **1981**, *10*, 77–79. [CrossRef]

29. MacGillivray, R.T.; Moore, S.A.; Chen, J.; Anderson, B.F.; Baker, H.; Luo, Y.; Bewley, M.; Smith, C.A.; Murphy, M.E.; Wang, Y.; *et al.* Two high-resolution crystal structures of the recombinant N-lobe of human transferrin reveal a structural change implicated in iron release. *Biochemistry* **1998**, *37*, 7919–7928. [CrossRef] [PubMed]

30. Valenti, P.; Antonini, G.; Fanelli, M.R.; Orsi, N.; Antonini, E. Antibacterial activity of matrixbound ovotransferrin. *Antimicrob. Agents Chemother.* **1982**, *21*, 840–841. [CrossRef] [PubMed]

31. Ko, K.Y.; Mendonca, A.F.; Ahn, D.U. Effect of ethylenediaminetetraacetate and lysozyme on the antimicrobial activity of ovotransferrin against *Listeria monocytogenes*. *Poult. Sci.* **2008**, *87*, 1649–1658. [CrossRef] [PubMed]

32. Valenti, P.; Antonini, G.; von Hunolstein, C.; Visca, P.; Orsi, N.; Antonini, E. Studies of the antimicrobial activity of ovotransferrin. *Int. J. Tissue React.* **1983**, *5*, 97–105. [PubMed]

33. Alcantara, J.; Schryvers, A.B. Transferrin binding protein two interacts with both the N-lobe and C-lobe of ovotransferrin. *Microb. Pathog.* **1996**, *20*, 73–85. [CrossRef] [PubMed]

34. Valenti, P.; Visca, P.; Antonini, G.; Orsi, N. Antifungal activity of ovotransferrin toward genus Candida. *Mycopathologia* **1985**, *89*, 169–175. [CrossRef] [PubMed]

35. Aguilera, O.; Quiros, L.M.; Fierro, J.F. Transferrins selectively cause ion efflux through bacterial and artificial membranes. *FEBS Lett.* **2003**, *548*, 5–10. [CrossRef]

36. Superti, F.; Ammendolia, M.G.; Berlutti, F.; Valenti, P. Ovotransferrin. In *Bioactive Egg Compounds*; Huopalahti, R., Lopez-Fandino, R., Eds.; Springer-Verlag: Berlin, Germany, 2007; pp. 43–48.

37. Zhou, Z.R.; Smith, D.L. Assignment of disulfide bonds in proteins by partial acid hydrolysis and mass spectrometry. *J. Protein Chem.* **1990**, *9*, 523–532. [CrossRef] [PubMed]

38. Strahilevitz, J.; Mor, A.; Nicolas, P.; Shai, Y. Spectrum of antimicrobial activity and assembly of dermaseptin-β and its precursor form in phospholipid membranes. *Biochemistry* **1994**, *33*, 10951–10960. [CrossRef] [PubMed]

39. Ehret-Sabatier, L.; Loew, D.; Goyffon, M.; Fehlbaum, P.; Hoffmann, J.A.; Dorsselaer, A.V.; Bulet, P. Characterization of novel cysteine-rich antimicrobial peptides from scorpion blood. *J. Biol. Chem.* **1996**, *271*, 29537–29544. [CrossRef] [PubMed]

40. Ibrahim, H.R.; Iwamori, E.; Sugimoto, Y.; Aoki, T. Identification of a distinct antibacterial domain within the N-lobe of Ovotransferrin. *Biochim. Biophys. Acta* **1998**, *1401*, 289–303. [CrossRef]

41. Ibrahim, H.R.; Sugimoto, Y.; Aoki, T. Ovotransferrin antimicrobial peptide (OTAP-92) kill bacteria through a membrane damage mechanism. *Biochim. Biophys. Acta* **2000**, *1523*, 196–205. [CrossRef]

42. Galvez, A.; Gimenez-Gallego, G.; Reuben, J.P.; Roy-Contancin, L.; Feigenbaum, P.; Kaczorowski, G.J.; Garcia, M.L. Purification and characterization of a unique, potent, peptidyl probe for the high conductance calcium-activated potassium channel from venom of the scorpion *Buthus tamulus*. *J. Biol. Chem.* **1990**, *265*, 11083–11090. [PubMed]

43. Ko, K.Y.; Mendoncam, A.F.; Ismail, H.; Ahn, D.U. Ethylenediaminetetraacetate and lysozyme improves antimicrobial activities of ovotransferrin against *Escherichia coli* O157:H7. *Poult. Sci.* **2009**, *88*, 406–414. [CrossRef] [PubMed]

44. Seol, K.H.; Lim, D.G.; Jang, A.; Jo, C.; Lee, M. Antimicrobial effect of kappa carrageenan-based edible film containing ovotransferrin in fresh chicken breast stored at 5 °C. *Meat Sci.* **2009**, *83*, 479–483. [CrossRef] [PubMed]

45. Giansanti, F.; Rossi, P.; Massucci, M.T.; Botti, D.; Antonini, G.; Valenti, P.; Seganti, L. Antiviral activity of ovotransferrin discloses an evolutionary strategy for the defensive activities of lactoferrin. *Biochem. Cell Biol.* **2002**, *80*, 125–130. [CrossRef] [PubMed]

46. Giansanti, F.; Massucci, M.T.; Giardi, M.F.; Nozza, F.; Pulsinelli, E.; Nicolini, C.; Botti, D.; Antonini, G. Antiviral activity of ovotransferrin derived peptides. *Biochem. Biophys. Res. Commun.* **2005**, *331*, 69–73. [CrossRef] [PubMed]

47. Siciliano, R.; Rega, B.; Marchetti, M.; Seganti, L.; Antonini, G.; Valenti, P. Bovine lactoferrin peptidic fragments involved in inhibition of *Herpes simplex* virus type 1 infection. *Biochem. Biophys. Res. Commun.* **1999**, *264*, 19–23. [CrossRef] [PubMed]

48. Ibrahim, H.R.; Haraguchi, T.; Aoki, T. Ovotransferrin is a redox-dependent autoprocessing protein incorporating four consensus self-cleaving motifs flanking the two kringles. *Biochim. Biophys. Acta* **2006**, *1760*, 347–355. [CrossRef] [PubMed]

49. Ibrahim, H.R.; Hoq, M.I.; Aoki, T. Ovotransferrin possesses SOD-like superoxide anion scavenging activity that is promoted by copper and manganese binding. *Int. J. Biol. Macromol.* **2007**, *41*, 631–640. [CrossRef] [PubMed]

50. Huang, W.Y.; Majumder, K.; Wu, J. Oxygen radical absorbance capacity of peptides from egg white protein ovotransferrin and their interaction with phytochemicals. *Food Chem.* **2010**, *123*, 635–641. [CrossRef]

51. Kim, J.; Moon, S.H.; Ahn, D.U.; Paik, H.D.; Park, E. Antioxidant effects of ovotransferrin and its hydrolysates. *Poult. Sci.* **2012**, *91*, 2747–2754. [CrossRef] [PubMed]

52. Huang, W.; Shen, S.; Nimalaratne, C.; Li, S.; Majumder, K.; Wu, J. Effects of addition of egg ovotransferrin-derived peptides on the oxygen Radical absorbance capacity of different teas. *Food Chem.* **2012**, *135*, 1600–1607. [CrossRef] [PubMed]

53. Moon, S.H.; Lee, J.H.; Lee, Y.J.; Chang, K.H.; Paik, J.Y.; Ahn, D.U.; Paik, H.D. Screening for cytotoxic activity of ovotransferrin and its enzyme hydrolysates. *Poult. Sci.* **2013**, *92*, 424–434. [CrossRef] [PubMed]

54. You, J.; Luo, Y.; Wu, J. Conjugation of ovotransferrin with catechin shows improved antioxidant activity. *J. Agric. Food Chem.* **2014**, *62*, 2581–2587. [CrossRef] [PubMed]

55. Moon, S.H.; Lee, J.H.; Ahnb, D.U.; Paika, H.D. *In vitro* antioxidant and mineral-chelating properties of natural and autocleaved ovotransferrin. *J. Sci. Food Agric.* **2015**, *95*, 2065–2070. [CrossRef] [PubMed]

56. Morgan, R.W.; Sofer, L.; Anderson, A.S.; Berneberg, E.L.; Cui, J.; Burnside, J. Induction of host gene expression following infection of chicken embryo fibroblasts with oncogenic Marek's disease virus. *J. Virol.* **2001**, *75*, 533–539. [CrossRef] [PubMed]

57. Kushner, I.; Mackiewicz, A. The acute phase response: An overview. In *Acute Phase Proteins: Molecular Biology, Biochemistry, and Clinical Applications*; Kushner, I., Baumann, H., Mackiewicz, A., Eds.; CRC Press: Boca Raton, FL, USA, 1993; pp. 3–19.

58. Gabay, C.; Kushner, I. Acute phase proteins and other systemic response to inflammation. *N. Engl. J. Med.* **1999**, *340*, 448–454. [PubMed]

59. Carlevaro, M.F.; Albini, A.; Ribatti, D.; Gentili, C.; Benelli, R.; Cermelli, S.; Cancedda, R.; Cancedda, F.D. Transferrin promotes endothelial cell migration and invasion: Implication in cartilage neovascularisation. *J. Cell Biol.* **1997**, *136*, 1375–1384. [CrossRef] [PubMed]

60. Hallquist, N.A.; Klasing, K.C. Serotransferrin, ovotransferrin and metallothionein levels during an immune response in chickens. *Comp. Biochem. Physiol. B* **1994**, *108*, 375–384. [CrossRef]

61. Tohjo, H.; Miyoshi, F.; Uchida, E.; Niiyama, M. Polyacrylamide gel electrophoretic patterns of chicken serum in acute inflammation induced by intramuscular injection of turpentine. *Poult. Sci.* **1995**, *74*, 648–655. [CrossRef] [PubMed]

62. Chamanza, R.; Toussaint, M.J.M.; van Ederen, A.M.; van Veen, L.; Hulskamp-Koch, C. Serum amyloid A and transferrin in chicken. A preliminary investigation of using acute phase variables to assess diseases in chickens. *Vet. Q.* **1999**, *21*, 158–162. [CrossRef] [PubMed]

63. Xie, H.; Huff, G.R.; Huff, W.E.; Balog, J.M.; Rath, N.C. Effects of ovotransferrin on chicken macrophages and heterophil-granulocytes. *Dev. Comp. Immunol.* **2002**, *26*, 805–815. [CrossRef]

64. Xie, H.; Huff, G.R.; Huff, W.E.; Balog, J.M.; Holt, P.; Rath, N.C. Identification of ovotransferrin as an acute phase protein in chickens. *Poult. Sci.* **2002**, *81*, 112–120. [CrossRef] [PubMed]

65. Rath, N.C.; Xie, H.; Huff, W.E.; Huff, G.R. Avian acute phase protein ovotransferrin modulates phagocyte function. In *New Immunology Research Development*; Muller, G.V., Ed.; Nova Science Publishers: New York, NY, USA, 2008; pp. 95–108.

66. Rath, N.C.; Anthony, N.B.; Kannan, L.; Huff, W.E.; Huff, G.R.; Chapman, H.D.; Erf, G.F.; Wakenell, P. Serum ovotransferrin as a biomarker of inflammatory diseases in chickens. *Poult. Sci.* **2009**, *88*, 2069–2074. [CrossRef] [PubMed]

67. Giansanti, F.; Giardi, M.F.; Massucci, M.T.; Botti, D.; Antonini, G. Ovotransferrin expression and release by chicken cell lines infected with Marek's disease virus. *Biochem. Cell Biol.* **2007**, *85*, 150–155. [CrossRef] [PubMed]

68. Majumder, K.; Chakrabarti, S.; Davidge, S.T.; Wu, J. Structure and activity study of egg protein ovotransferrin derived peptides (IRW and IQW) on endothelial inflammatory response and oxidative stress. *J. Agric. Food Chem.* **2013**, *61*, 2120–2129. [CrossRef] [PubMed]

69. Kovacs-Nolan, J.; Phillips, M.; Mine, Y. Advances in the value of eggs and egg components for human health. *J. Agric. Food Chem.* **2005**, *53*, 8421–8431. [CrossRef] [PubMed]

70. Abeyrathne, E.D.N.S.; Lee, H.Y.; Ahn, D.U. Egg white proteins and their potential use in food processing or as nutraceutical and pharmaceutical agents—A review. *Poult. Sci.* **2013**, *92*, 3292–3299. [CrossRef] [PubMed]

71. Ibrahim, H.R.; Kiyono, T. Novel anticancer activity of the autocleaved ovotransferrin against human colon and breast cancer cells. *J. Agric. Food Chem.* **2009**, *57*, 11383–11390. [CrossRef] [PubMed]

72. Lee, N.Y.; Cheng, J.T.; Enomoto, T.; Nakano, Y. One peptide derived from hen ovotransferrin as pro-drug to inhibit angiotensin converting enzyme. *J. Food Drug Anal.* **2006**, *14*, 31–35. [CrossRef]

73. Wu, J.; Acero-Lopez, A. Ovotransferrin: Structure, bioactivities and preparation. *Food Res. Int.* **2012**, *46*, 480–487. [CrossRef]

74. Shimo-Oka, T.; Hagiwara, Y.; Ozawa, E. Class specificity of transferrin as a muscle trophic factor. *J. Cell. Physiol.* **1986**, *126*, 341–351. [CrossRef] [PubMed]

75. Leitner, D.F.; Connor, J.R. Functional roles of transferrin in the brain. *Biochim. Biophys. Acta* **2012**, *1820*, 393–402. [CrossRef] [PubMed]

76. Paek, S.H.; Shin, H.Y.; Kim, J.W.; Park, S.H.; Son, J.H.; Kim, D.G. Primary culture of central neurocytoma: A case report. *J. Korean Med. Sci.* **2010**, *25*, 798–803. [CrossRef] [PubMed]

77. Cancedda, R.; Castagnola, P.; Cancedda, F.D.; Dozin, B.; Quarto, R. Developmental control of chondrogenesis and osteogenesis. *Int. J. Dev. Biol.* **2000**, *44*, 707–714. [PubMed]

78. Gentili, C.; Doliana, R.; Bet, P.; Campanile, G.; Colombatti, A.; Cancedda, F.D.; Cancedda, R. Ovotransferrin and ovotransferrin receptor expression during chondrogenesis and endochondral bone formation in developing chick embryo. *J. Cell Biol.* **1994**, *124*, 579–588. [CrossRef] [PubMed]

79. Bruinink, A.; Sidler, C.; Birchler, F. Neurotrophic effects of transferrin on embryonic chick brain and neural retinal cell cultures, *Int. J. Dev. Neurosci.* **1996**, *14*, 785–795. [CrossRef]

80. Leboffe, L.; Giansanti, F.; Antonini, G. Antifungal and antiparasitic activities of lactoferrin. *Anti-Infect. Agents Med. Chem.* **2009**, *8*, 114–127. [CrossRef]

81. Massucci, M.T.; Giansanti, F.; di Nino, G.; Turacchio, M.; Giardi, M.F.; Botti, D.; Ippoliti, R.; de Giulio, B.; Siciliano, R.A.; Donnarumma, G.; *et al.* Proteolytic activity of bovine lactoferrin. *Biometals* **2004**, *17*, 249–255. [CrossRef] [PubMed]

82. Hendrixson, D.R.; Qiu, J.; Shewry, S.C.; Fink, D.L.; Petty, S.; Baker, E.N.; Plaut, A.G.; St Geme, J.W., 3rd. Human milk lactoferrin is a serine protease that cleaves Haemophilus surface proteins at arginine-rich sites. *Mol. Microbiol.* **2003**, *47*, 607–617. [CrossRef] [PubMed]

83. Ibrahim, H.R.; Tatsumoto, S.; Ono, H.; van Immerseel, F.; Raspoet, R.; Miyata, T. A novel antibiotic-delivery system by using ovotransferrin as targeting Molecule. *Eur. J. Pharm. Sci.* **2015**, *66*, 59–69. [CrossRef] [PubMed]

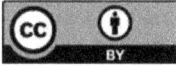

nutrients

MDPI

editorial
Eggs and Health Special Issue

Maria Luz Fernandez

Department of Nutritional Sciences, University of Connecticut, Storrs, CT 06269, USA;
maria-luz.fernandez@uconn.edu

Received: 23 November 2016; Accepted: 25 November 2016; Published: 2 December 2016

In 1968, the American Heart Association recommended the consumption of no more than 300 mg/day of dietary cholesterol and emphasized that no more than 3 eggs should be eaten per week, resulting in substantial reductions in egg consumption, not just by diseased populations but also by healthy individuals, and more importantly by poor communities in undeveloped counties who were advised against consuming a highly nutritious food. These recommendations did not take into account that eggs not only contain important nutrients for overall health but also components which exert protection against chronic disease. The newly-released 2015 dietary guidelines finally took into consideration the epidemiological information and the data from clinical interventions and eliminated an upper limit for dietary cholesterol. This special issue addresses the history of the recommendations for eggs [1], the components of eggs providing beneficial effects against disease [2–6], the relationship between egg intake and healthy eating index [7]; the protective effects of eggs against inflammation [8] and oxidative stress [9]. Finally, the controversies surrounding egg intake and risk for diabetes are presented in a review of epidemiological data [10] and in a clinical study [11].

The history of the recommendations of dietary cholesterol and the politics behind those recommendations as well as the perception of the public and the creation of the Egg Nutrition Center in the US are thoroughly discussed alongside the lines of evidence on which the original recommendations were based [1]. The number of studies supporting the lack of evidence of an association between dietary cholesterol and risk of heart diseases and the evidence-based research associated with the elimination of dietary cholesterol from the current dietary guidelines are presented in chronological order [1].

Eggs have been recognized as functional foods due to the presence of bioactive components, which may play a role in the prevention of chronic and infectious diseases [2]. The presence of antimicrobial, antioxidant, anti-cancer and hypotensive properties are discussed in this review [2]. Phospholipids are among the bioactive components of eggs [3]. Sphingomyelin and phosphatidyl choline have been postulated to regulate cholesterol absorption and inflammation and, interestingly, the incorporation of egg phospholipids into high density lipoprotein (HDL) appears to be a major factor in the cholesterol-accepting capacity of this lipoprotein [3]. Ovotransferrin, a protein present in egg, is well known for its antibacterial properties [4]. There is evidence that ovotransferrin and its peptides possess antiviral activity, as well as antioxidant and anti-inflammatory properties [4]. In addition, egg yolk proteins including vitellogenin, lipovitellin and phosvitin have also been shown to participate in the immune defense system, capable of killing bacteria and viruses as well as promoting phagocytosis activity [5]. A study conducted in rats demonstrated that egg white protein was very useful for the recovery of iron-deficiency anemia [6]. These roles of egg proteins in protecting against bacterial infection further document the association between egg consumption and health [4–6].

The role of eggs on the healthy eating index (HEI) was evaluated in 139 obese post-partum Mexican American women [7]. This article details the role of eggs as a component of the diet in some of these women and how egg-eaters achieved higher HEI scores, mainly by the higher consumption of high quality protein [7]. The anti-inflammatory properties of eggs have been demonstrated in numerous studies [8]. Among the egg components with anti-inflammatory properties are: phospholipids, the carotenoids, lutein and zeaxanthin and egg proteins. The mechanisms of action of these anti-inflammatory components is discussed in detail [8]. The components of eggs that have been shown to participate in the immune defense and act as anti-inflammatory agents, have also been shown to be anti-oxidants [9]. The role of eggs as an anti-oxidant food commodity due to the presence of specific egg proteins, carotenoids and phospholipids is thoroughly discussed in this review [9].

There is controversy regarding egg consumption and patients diagnosed with diabetes [10]. While it is clear that heart disease does not increase by egg intake, some of the epidemiological data appear to find a relationship between egg intake and diabetes [10]; thus, the authors emphasize the need for more clinical interventions in patients with diabetes. A clinical study compared the effects of two distinctive breakfasts in diabetic patients in a crossover design: one egg per day or 1 cup of oatmeal per day for 5 weeks each [11]. The authors report that there were no differences in the parameters related to cholesterol or glucose metabolism between dietary interventions. However, following egg consumption, there was a reduction of liver enzymes and inflammatory markers in these patients. [11]. Thus, this study demonstrates that, for this specific population, egg intake did not increase cardiovascular disease risk but was rather protective against inflammation. It is clear that more clinical interventions are needed so that more conclusive statements can be generated regarding egg intake and risk for people with diabetes.

Conflicts of Interest: The author declares no conflict of interest.

References

1. McNamara, D.J. The fifty year rehabilitation of the egg. *Nutrients* **2015**, *7*, 8716–8722. [CrossRef] [PubMed]
2. Miranda, J.M.; Anton, X.; Redonde-Valbuena, C.; Roca-Saavedra, P.; Rodriguez, J.A.; Lamas, A.; Franco, C.M.; Cepeda, A. Egg and egg-derived Foods: Effects on human Health and use as functional Foods. *Nutrients* **2015**, *7*, 706–729. [CrossRef] [PubMed]
3. Blesso, C.N. Egg phospholipids and cardiovascular health. *Nutrients* **2015**, *7*, 2731–2747. [CrossRef] [PubMed]
4. Giansanti, F.; Leboffe, L.; Angelucci, F.; Antonini, G. The nutraceutical properties of ovotransferrin and its potential utilization as a functional food. *Nutrients* **2015**, *7*, 9105–9115. [CrossRef] [PubMed]
5. Sun, C.; Zhang, S. Immune-relevant and antioxidant activities of vitellogenin and yolk proteins in fish. *Nutrients* **2015**, *7*, 8818–8829. [CrossRef] [PubMed]
6. Kobayashi, Y.; Wakasugy, E.; Yasui, R.; Kuwahata, M.; Kido, Y. Egg protein delays recovery while ovalbumin is useful in recovery from iron deficiency anemia. *Nutrients* **2015**, *7*, 4792–4803. [CrossRef] [PubMed]
7. Vega-Lopez, S.; Pignotti, G.A.P.; Tood, M.; Keller, C. Egg intake and dietary quality among overweight and obese Mexican-American postpartum women. *Nutrients* **2015**, *7*, 8402–8412. [CrossRef] [PubMed]
8. Andersen, C.J. Bioactive egg components and inflammation. *Nutrients* **2015**, *7*, 7789–7913. [CrossRef] [PubMed]
9. Nimalaratne, C.; Wu, J. Hen egg as an antioxidant food commodity, a review. *Nutrients* **2015**, *7*, 8274–8293. [CrossRef] [PubMed]
10. Fuller, N.R.; Sainsbury, A.; Caterson, I.D.; Markovik, T.P. Egg consumption and human cardio-metabolic health in people with and without diabetes. *Nutrients* **2015**, *7*, 7399–7420. [CrossRef] [PubMed]
11. Ballesteros, M.N.; Valenzuela, F.; Robles, A.E.; Artalejo, E.; Aguilar, D.; Andersen, C.J.; Valdez, H.; Fernandez, M.L. One egg per day improves inflammation when compared to an oatmeal-based breakfast without increasing other cardiometabolic risk factors in diabetic patients. *Nutrients* **2015**, *7*, 3449–3463. [CrossRef] [PubMed]

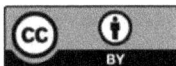

MDPI AG

St. Alban-Anlage 66

4052 Basel, Switzerland

Tel. +41 61 683 77 34

Fax +41 61 302 89 18

http://www.mdpi.com

Nutrients Editorial Office

E-mail: nutrients@mdpi.com

http://www.mdpi.com/journal/nutrients

www.ingramcontent.com/pod-product-compliance
Lightning Source LLC
Chambersburg PA
CBHW041217220326
41597CB00033BA/6000